NURSING KEY TOPICS REVIEW

Mental Health

ELSEVIER

ELSEVIER

3251 Riverport Lane
St. Louis, Missouri 63043

Senior Content Strategist: Jamie Blum
Senior Content Development Manager: Laurie Gower
Senior Content Development Specialist: Heather Bays
Publishing Services Manager: Julie Eddy
Project Manager: Mike Sheets
Design Direction: Margaret Reid

Printed in the United States of America

Last digit is the print number: 9 8 7 6 5 4 3 2 1

Reviewers

Melissa Bear, RN
Staff Nurse
DePaul Hospital
St. Louis, Missouri

Michelle Bonnheim
Nursing Student
California State University, Fresno
Fresno, California

Teresa S. Burckhalter, MSN, RN, BC
Adjunct Faculty
University of South Carolina Beaufort
Beaufort, South Carolina

Ms. Lorraine Chiappetta, MSN, RN, CNE
Professional Faculty
Nursing & Health Sciences
Washtenaw Community College
Ann Arbor, Michigan

Crystal Gallardo
CNA Nursing Assistant
Cypress College
Cypress, California

Carolyn M. Kruse, BS, DC
Educational Consultant/Owner
Kruisin Editorial
O'Fallon, Missouri

Katelynn Landers
Nursing Student
Brockton Hospital School of Nursing
Brockton, Massachusetts

Angela Lanzoni
Nursing Student
Brockton Hospital School of Nursing
Brockton, Massachusetts

Reagan Lizardi
Nursing Student
Polk State College
Lakeland, Florida

Michelle Luckett
Nursing Student
Polk State College
Winter Haven, Florida

Karla Psaros
Nursing Student
Brockton Hospital School of Nursing
Brockton, Massachusetts

Gina Rena
Nursing Student
Polk State College
Lakeland, Florida

Cianna Simpson
Nursing Student
Brockton Hospital School of Nursing
Brockton, Massachusetts

Lauren E. Snapp, NP
Nursing Student
East Tennessee State University
Johnson City, Tennessee

Briana Sundlie
Nursing Student
Cypress College
Cypress, California

Preface

The *Nursing Key Topics Review* book series was developed and designed with you, **the nursing student**, in mind. We know how difficult nursing school can be! How do you focus your study? How can you learn in the most time-efficient way possible? Where do you go when you need help?

We asked YOU, and this is what we learned:

- You think textbooks are useful, but they can be overwhelming (also . . . heavy)
- You want quick and easy access to manageable levels of nursing information
- You like questions and rationales to challenge you and make sure you know what you need to know

Nursing Key Topics Review is your solution, whether you're looking for a textbook supplement or a NCLEX examination study aid. Review questions interspersed throughout the text make it easy to test your knowledge. The bulleted outline format allows for quick comprehension. A mobile app with key points lets you take your review with you anywhere you go!

In short, *Nursing Key Topics Review* helps you narrow down what's important and tells you what to focus on. Be sure to look for all the titles in the series to make your studies more effective . . . and your journey a little bit lighter!

Contents

Psychiatric Mental Health Nursing

FUNDAMENTAL PRINCIPLES

Prevention

- Primary prevention helps reduce the incidence (occurrence) of mental disorders
    - Requires *proactive* involvement by care providers
    - *Primary* prevention means <u>preventing disorders</u> *before* they begin; for example, teaching the normal stages of child development and effective parenting skills to high-risk single women who are pregnant for the first time, or programs discouraging youngsters from ever starting to use drugs
- Secondary prevention efforts are aimed at the early detection of a crisis, thereby increasing opportunities for interventions to prevent the progression of symptoms and the worsening of the crisis.
    - Includes <u>early identification and treatment</u> to prevent increased disability
    - For example, providing comfort and arranging for the safety of a child who comes to school with multiple bruises and cigarette burns on his or her body or screening to identify alcohol use disorder
    - Tertiary prevention has two objectives:
        - (1) To <u>reduce the residual effects of a disorder</u> (such as in a support group) and thus improve quality of life
        - (2) To <u>promote rehabilitation</u> (such as teaching job skills to recovering clients) and improved ability to function

Promotion of Mental Health

- Goals:
    - Disseminating information to increase public knowledge and awareness of mental health and mental disorders
    - Ensuring access to health care
    - Encouraging and providing support for individuals, families, communities, and organizations that value principles and activities that promote mental health
    - Supporting organizations that assist others with meeting the many demands of daily living and that facilitate healthy socialization
    - Providing ongoing education and mentoring
    - Supporting clients with defining their personal life goals and in their efforts to achieve those goals
    - Reducing the stigma associated with mental disorders
- Nursing functions that meet these goals include:
    - Initial and ongoing assessments
    - Therapeutic communication
    - Facilitating family, group, and community seminars
    - Teaching and advocating
    - Role modeling and mentoring
    - Collaborating with clients and colleagues
    - Monitoring outcomes

- Sites for health promotion
  - Homes, schools, community agencies, and organizations are primary
  - Ambulatory care settings
  - Positive and supportive early life experiences, especially in the home, are invaluable
  - Nurses engage and interact with family members to strengthen homes and families; ideally, a home ensures that its members receive:
    - Physical sustenance, with adequate food, clothing, and shelter
    - Physical and psychological safety and security
    - Nurturing, love, and affection
    - Consideration, attention, support, and encouragement
    - Clear and unambiguous communication
    - Role modeling
    - Opportunities for socialization and actualization
    - Instructions for navigating through the world to meet one's own needs while considering the needs and rights of others
- Inhibitors of health promotion include environments in which any member is unable to fulfill their role; for example, dysfunctional families ineffectively coping with a member diagnosed with an addiction

Treatment

- Client-centered health care model establishes that the course of treatment is based on the client's preferences, needs, and values regarding care
- Clients are encouraged to make decisions and to actively engage in their own treatment plans to meet their needs
  - Steps of the nursing process help determine the best practice treatment for each client
  - Client-centered treatment objectives are based on the information gathered and used during the nursing process. It is important to assess the following:
    - The client's psychiatric diagnosis or diagnoses (ie, the type and severity of the disorder)
    - Current observable and reported symptoms and other responses
    - The client's potential highest level of functioning
    - Client motivation, readiness and willingness to participate in treatment and in maintaining wellness
    - Availability and access to treatment resources and options, including the cost of treatment
  - Specific treatment is tailored to and outlined for each individual
- Acute episodes and severe, persistent disorders are managed and treated differently
  - Acute: Hospitalization may be required for the alleviation and management of symptoms, the prescribing and monitoring of medications, the stabilization of the immediate condition, and the support or modification of current living situations
  - Severe, persistent (aka chronic): Treatment requires ongoing monitoring of the person's symptoms, medications, living conditions, and circumstances; collaboration with families and agencies; and advocating in the community
- Treatment plan
  - Clients' participation in their own care is a primary objective of all treatment plans
  - Nurses work collaboratively with the treatment team to involve clients, families, and others who will provide ongoing care
  - A family member's realistic expectations often increases in direct proportion to the perception of the client's condition and situation, level of knowledge, attitudes about the client's disorder, and personal experiences with mental disorders

- Time and the willing involvement of the client and family members often result in successful outcomes; support and guidance from skilled nurses and other health care professionals is often necessary as well
- Clients' rights in treatment
  - See Chapter 4 for information about a client's legal rights
  - A client's health and safety may become jeopardized by his or her severely impaired judgment and result in the loss of a client's right to make choices about treatment; examples:
    - when a person is unable to cognitively process information or make sound decisions about his or her own welfare because of mental incompetence or severe psychosis
    - when a person is so severely depressed that he or she is intent on committing suicide
  - If threats of violence toward the self or others become a factor, then the client's rights are suspended to protect the family or the public and also to protect the client from his or her own poor judgment and acting out of dangerous behaviors
- Evidence-based practice
  - The standard of practice for all health care institutions and health care providers is evidence-based practice (EBP)
  - EBP is not based on intuition or the repetition of interventions because they were always done that way before or because techniques were agreed upon and approved by experts or colleagues
  - The transition to EBP in nursing is steadily growing; as evidence-based research is completed and specific interventions are identified, the resulting practice outcomes will be reflected in client care and published in the literature
- Integrated care: The mind and the body
  - Two meanings relating to treatment. The integration of mind-body focus of care because mental disorders and physical illnesses are closely linked
  - Integration of care for clients who are diagnosed with both mental disorders and **other** medical disorders (comorbidity) and who often are treated in settings other than the psychiatric setting
  - Use of complementary therapies

Rehabilitation

- Prevents multiple "revolving door" episodes and their negative consequences
- Reintegrates clients into the community
- Supports clients as they more actively participate in their own treatment
- Staff teaches strategies while supporting clients and families as they learn and use techniques to effectively manage and cope with their symptoms, their inevitable stressors, and the challenges of daily living
- Communicating with others, building social networks, and establishing a meaningful role and purpose in life are also important objectives for clients
- The goal is to engage again in purposeful activities and meaningful social relationships within a healthy environment
- Nurses and other caregivers providers continue to include individual clients and significant others in all aspects of their care, including taking responsibility for decision making, engaging in their own treatment plans and interventions, completing collaborative evaluations, and setting long-term goals under the guidance of the interdisciplinary team
- Client recovery is faster and more effective when the team includes the client

Standards of Psychiatric Nursing Care

- The standards of practice developed by the American Nurses Association, the American Psychiatric Nurses Association, and the International Society of Psychiatric-Mental Health Nurses describe the professional activities that the nurse performs during the steps of the nursing process; they are the basis for:
  - Certification criteria
  - Nursing's legal definition, which is noted in the Nurse Practice Act in many states
  - The National Council of State Boards of Nursing Licensure Examination (NCLEX-RN)
- These standards are used as guidelines to help them make clinical decisions that provide quality psychiatric mental health care
- The standards of practice relating to the nursing process are discussed further in Chapter 3
- The nursing process is a sequence of steps used to meet the client's needs; an overview includes:
  - Standard I. Assessment
    - The nurse assesses the client's mental status, psychosocial state, physical health, pain level, and nonverbal behaviors—as well as physical parameters—with the use of various methods of data collection
    - Assessment is always the first step in the nursing process
    - It usually also includes cultural or sociocultural and spiritual dimensions.
  - Standard II. Nursing diagnosis
    - The nurse diagnoses the client with the use of subjective and objective data that are analyzed during the assessment phase. Nursing diagnoses are statements that describe a person's health state and responses to actual or potential health problems; they are based on reliable clinical judgments made by the nurse after an extensive nursing assessment as described in the previous section
    - Nursing diagnoses include actual, potential (at-risk), and wellness diagnoses.
    - Nursing diagnoses are based on client responses and needs that the nurse is able to treat; they differ from medical diagnoses in that the medical diagnosis names the disease
  - Standard III. Outcome identification
    - The nurse identifies client behaviors (outcomes) on the basis of nursing diagnosis statements and on behaviors that are the result of nursing interventions
    - Outcomes are based on assessment and nursing diagnosis.
    - Outcome statements are specific, measurable indicators that nurses use to evaluate the results of their interventions
  - Standard IV. Planning
    - The nurse plans and prioritizes client care with the client, the physician, and the interdisciplinary team; the planning phase consists of the total planning of the client's treatment to achieve quality outcomes in a safe, effective, and timely manner
  - Standard V. Implementation
    - The nurse sets in motion the interventions prescribed during the planning phase and implements them as meaningful actions
    - Interventions are the most powerful pieces of the nursing process
  - Standard VI. Evaluation
    - The nurse evaluates the achievement of client's outcomes or improvement in client's health status, which reflect the effectiveness of nursing interventions
    - Evaluation of the client's progress and the nursing activities involved are critical because this lets nurses know if interventions need modification. Also, evaluation is important because nurses are accountable for the standards of care in each discipline
  - Documentation can be considered a seventh standard of care

- Nurse relationship with client: See Nurse-Client Relationship
- Recognition of cultural differences: See Cultural and Spiritual Concepts

NURSE-CLIENT RELATIONSHIP

Overview

- The therapeutic interpersonal relationship that develops between the nurse and the client is an important factor for effecting client change and growth
- The relationship is therapeutic rather than social (Table 1.1); it is guided by standards and objectives
- The focus is on the client's needs and problems rather than on the nurse or other issues; interactions are client centered
- The relationship is purposeful and goal directed
- The relationship is objective rather than subjective in quality
- The relationship is time limited rather than open-ended
- Therapeutic communication requires a basic understanding and use of interviewing techniques (see Chapter 2).
- Therapeutic communication is one of the tools used to facilitate the nurse-client relationship.

Therapeutic Alliance

- Definition and description
  - A major objective for nurses when interacting with patents in any clinical psychiatric setting is to establish a therapeutic alliance
  - A professional bond that exists between the nurse and the client; it is the heart of the nurse-client relationship and often plays a significant role in the client's well-being
  - Acts as the cornerstone of nursing interventions in any psychiatric setting
  - The nurse provides a safe environment for this relationship to occur and grow
- Purpose:
  - Facilitates the interpersonal process
  - Primarily focuses on client-centered needs, issues, and short-term and long-term goals
  - Serves as a vehicle for clients to accomplish:
    - Freely discussing their needs and problems in the absence of judgment and criticism
    - Gaining insight into their problems, expectations, abilities, and support systems

TABLE 1.1 Differences Between a Social and a Professional Relationship

Social	Professional
Unstructured time frame	Structured time
Not goal directed	Goal directed
Focus on mutual needs	Focus on client's needs
Nontheoretical	Theory-based interaction
Independent relationships	Part of a treatment team
Informal duties	Legal and ethical duties
No financial concerns	Financial issues
	Confidentiality
	Documentation

From Nugent, P. M., Green, J. S., Hellmer Saul, M. A., & Pelikan, P. K. (2012). *Mosby's comprehensive review of nursing for the NCLEX-RN examination* (20th ed.). St Louis, MO: Mosby.

- ■ Learning and practicing new skills
- ■ Effecting life changes
- ■ Healing mental and emotional wounds
- ■ Promoting growth
- Formation: The alliance begins when the nurse demonstrates:
  - Knowledge of principles that guide the formation and maintenance of the nurse–client relationship and its inherent responsibilities
  - Understanding of the relational aspects of all nursing interventions and interactions
  - Knowledge of, understanding of, and commitment to maintaining healthy boundaries
  - Willingness to engage and interact with clients and to guide them on their return to wellness
  - Commitment to practice nursing interventions and interactions within prescribed reliable guidelines and to integrate time-tested EBP interpersonal skills
  - Inclusion of the client in a therapeutic process that focuses on the client's health
  - Encouragement of the client's responsibility for his or her own health within the client's capacity

Nursing Interventions

- Nursing interventions are discussed in detail in Chapter 3
- General nursing care of clients with mental health/psychiatric problems
  - Provide for the client's safety
  - Help prevent mental health problems and assist clients to cope with mental health problems
  - Accept and respect people as individuals and strive to separate the person from behavior that may be dysfunctional
  - Reorient client to person, place, time, and situation
  - Limit or reject inappropriate behavior without rejecting the individual
  - Help individuals set appropriate limits for themselves or set limits for them when they are unable to do so
  - Recognize that all behavior has meaning and is meeting the needs of the person performing it, regardless of how distorted or meaningless it appears to others
  - Accept the dependency needs of individuals while supporting and encouraging moves toward independence; build on ego strengths
  - Create a nonjudgmental environment that encourages individuals to express their feelings without judgment, punishment, or rejection; be aware of your own personal biases so that you do not demonstrate them
    - ■ Sitting quietly with the client conveys the message that the nurse cares and accepts the client's feelings; this helps establish trust
    - ■ For clients with psychiatric problems, provide an opportunity for the client to try out different behaviors in an accepting atmosphere and ultimately to replace pathologic responses with more effective responses
  - Recognize that individuals need to use maladaptive defenses until other healthier defenses can be substituted
  - Recognize how feelings, behavior, and thoughts are interrelated and influence relationships
  - Recognize that individuals frequently respond to the behavioral expectations of others, including family, peers, and authority figures (eg, health team members)
  - Develop an awareness of yourself and your professional role in the relationship with clients
  - Recognize that all individuals have a potential for movement toward higher levels of emotional health

- Include family members in the health care team when they can be supportive and with client approval; recognize that in many cultures family bonds and support are important
- Base interventions on research (evidence-based practice)

Phases of Therapeutic Relationship

- Preinteraction: Begins before nurse's initial contact with client
  - Self-exploration involves acknowledging one's own feelings, fears, personal values, and attitudes, including identification of misconceptions and prejudices that are socially learned
  - Self-awareness is necessary before establishing a relationship with others; it is the most difficult initial task when developing a nurse-client relationship
  - Oneself and a desire to help are the most important tools in a nurse-client relationship
  - Tasks include gathering data about client and planning for first interaction with client
- Orientation or introductory: The nurse, who is initially a stranger, establishes a trusting relationship with the client by consistency in communication and actions; clients should never be pushed to discuss areas of concern that are upsetting to them
  - Introduction of nurse, explanation of nurse's role in multidisciplinary team, and purpose of interaction
  - Contract outlining mutually agreed-upon goals is set
  - Confidentiality issues are discussed, and client rights are upheld
  - Termination begins during orientation phase by establishing time parameters
- Working: Nurse and client discuss areas of concern, and client is helped plan, implement, and evaluate a course of action
  - Problems need to be discussed and resolved
  - Contract can be formal or informal, and it may be written or verbal
    - Nurses usually use verbal and informal contracts with clients in acute-care settings in which the client and nurse meet on a regular basis
    - It may be necessary for the nurse to write a more specific and formalized contract for clients who seek therapy outside of an acute-care setting and when there is an expectation that a client behavior will continue (eg, a "no self-harm" contract) after discharge
  - New adaptive behaviors can be learned
  - Anxiety levels may increase; acting-out behaviors can and do occur; resistance to change needs to be anticipated, identified, and addressed
  - Issues that interfere with a therapeutic relationship during the working phase of a therapeutic relationship
    - Transference: The client superimposes feelings from other relationships onto the nurse-client relationship (eg, client gets angry easily at nurse who resembles a former significant other with whom the client had a contentious relationship)
    - Countertransference: The nurse superimposes feelings from other relationships onto the nurse-client relationship (eg, older nurse treats a younger client like a son or daughter)
    - Resistance: Client fails to engage in or sabotages treatment (eg, forgets appointments, keeps changing subject)
    - Blurring of a professional versus a social relationship
- Termination: End of therapeutic relationship between nurse and client; spacing meetings further apart near end facilitates termination
  - Goals and objectives achieved are summarized
  - Positive adaptive behaviors are reinforced
  - Feelings and experiences for both client and nurse are shared

- Rejection, anger, regression, or other negative behaviors may be expressed as a means of coping with the impending termination of the relationship
- Issues of loss must be discussed to facilitate a successful termination.
- If indicated, facilitating referral to another professional may be appropriate.

Boundaries

- Healthy boundaries
  - Help define the nurse's role, especially in the therapeutic alliance
  - Healthy boundaries differ from acting cold or distant toward clients
  - Warmth and genuineness are important qualities in any nurse
  - Trying to be a client's friend blurs boundaries and confuses roles
  - The nurse helps clients increase their awareness and knowledge of the presence or absence of their own boundaries, as well as understanding the purposes that others have for maintaining boundaries
  - The nurse also helps clients practice boundary setting
  - Box 1.1 illustrates some examples that the nurse may use to assist clients with the recognition of boundary violations
  - Some social conversation usually occurs at the beginning of meetings and helps establish or maintain rapport

---

BOX 1.1 Signs of Unhealthy Boundaries

- Going against personal values or rights to please another
- Not noticing when someone displays inappropriate boundaries
- Not noticing when someone invades your boundaries
- Talking at an intimate level during the first meeting with someone
- Feeling in love with a new acquaintance
- Feeling in love with anyone who reaches out
- Being overwhelmed by or preoccupied with a person
- Acting on first sexual impulse
- Being sexual for your partner rather than for yourself
- Accepting food, gifts, touch, or sex that you do not want
- Touching a person without asking
- Taking as much as you can for the sake of getting
- Giving as much as you can for the sake of giving
- Allowing someone to take as much as they can from you
- Letting others direct your life
- Letting others describe your reality
- Letting others define you
- Believing others can anticipate your needs
- Expecting others to fill your needs automatically
- Refusing to act so someone will take care of you
- Self-abuse
- Sexual and physical abuse
- Food and drug abuse
- Loaning money you do not have
- Flirting or sending mixed sexual messages
- Telling all

From Fortinash, K. M., & Holoday, P. A. (2012). *Psychiatric mental health nursing* (5th ed.). St. Louis, MO: Mosby.

- Occasionally during meetings, superficial or social conversations briefly reappear
- The nurse then returns to the preferred topic and keeps the conversation focused and therapeutic
- Boundary violations
  - Occur when the nurse goes *beyond the established therapeutic relationship standards* and enters into a social *or personal relationship* with the client
  - Some clients also attempt to violate boundaries by asking personal information or touching the nurse inappropriately
  - Violations are more frequent if:
    - The nurse spends more time with the client
    - The nurse treats the client at odd hours or in a nontreatment setting
    - The nurse accepts compensation or gifts for treatment
    - The nurse's language or clothing is unprofessional
    - The nurse's self-disclosure or physical contact lacks therapeutic value
  - Violating professional boundaries can result in:
    - Legal and professional sanctions for the nurse
    - Loss of therapeutic objectivity in the relationship
    - Inability to achieve the desired outcomes for client growth and recovery
  - Clients who have mental illnesses are vulnerable; they may become too dependent on the nurse who they trust to guide them in their recovery
  - Professional nursing ethical standards must be maintained to preserve the therapeutic nature of the nurse-client relationship and to achieve positive client treatment outcomes

APPLICATION AND REVIEW

1. A nurse educator is presenting information about the nursing process to a class of nursing students. What definition of the nursing process should be included in the presentation?
   1. Procedures used to implement client care
   2. Sequence of steps used to meet the client's needs
   3. Activities employed to identify a client's problem
   4. Mechanisms applied to determine nursing goals for the client
2. A nurse on the medical-surgical unit tells other staff members, "That client can just wait for the lorazepam; I get so annoyed when people drink too much." What does this nurse's comment reflect?
   1. Demonstration of a personal bias
   2. Problem solving based on assessment
   3. Development of client acuity to set priorities
   4. Consideration of the complexity of client care
3. A teenager begins to cry when talking with the nurse about the problem of not being able to make friends. What is the **most** therapeutic nursing intervention?
   1. Sitting quietly with the client
   2. Telling the client that crying is not helpful
   3. Suggesting that the client play a board game
   4. Recommending how the client can change this situation
4. A client has been told to stop smoking by the health care provider. The nurse discovers a pack of cigarettes in the client's bathrobe. What is the nurse's **initial** action?
   1. Notify the health care provider
   2. Report this to the nurse manager

3. Tell the client that the cigarettes were found
4. Discard the cigarettes without commenting to the client

5. A client with internal bleeding is in the intensive care unit (ICU) for observation. At the change of shift an alarm sounds, indicating a decrease in blood pressure. What is the **initial** nursing action?
   1. Perform an assessment of the client before resuming the change-of-shift report
   2. Continue the change-of-shift report and include the decrease in blood pressure
   3. Lower the diastolic pressure limits on the monitor during the change-of-shift report
   4. Turn off the alarm temporarily and alert the oncoming nurse to the decrease in blood pressure

6. A client is admitted for surgery. Although not physically distressed, the client appears apprehensive and withdrawn. What is the nurse's **best** action?
   1. Explore the patient's nonverbal behavior, saying, "You look worried."
   2. Have a copy of hospital regulations available
   3. Explain that that there is no reason to be concerned
   4. Reassure the client that the staff is available to answer questions

7. A client has a right above-the-knee amputation after trauma sustained in a work-related accident. Upon awakening from surgery, the client states, "What happened to me? I don't remember a thing." What is the nurse's **initial** response?
   1. "Tell me what you think happened"
   2. "You will remember more as you get better"
   3. "You were in a work-related accident this morning"
   4. "It was necessary to amputate your leg after the accident"

8. After being medicated for anxiety, a client says to a nurse, "I guess you are too busy to stay with me." How should the nurse respond?
   1. "I'm so sorry, but I have to see other clients"
   2. "I have to go now, but I will come back in 10 minutes"
   3. "You'll be able to rest after the medicine starts working"
   4. "You'll feel better after I've made you more comfortable"

9. A client with hemiplegia is staring blankly at the wall and reports feeling "like half a person" and feeling inadeqate What is the **initial** nursing action?
   1. Use techniques to distract the client
   2. Include the client in decision making
   3. Offer to spend more time with the client
   4. Help the client problem-solve personal issues

10. A nurse in the ambulatory preoperative unit identifies that a client is more anxious than most clients. What is the nurse's **best** intervention?
    1. Attempt to identify the client's concerns
    2. Reassure the client that the surgery is routine
    3. Report the client's anxiety to the health care provider
    4. Provide privacy by pulling the curtain around the client

See Answers on pages 15-19.

CLINICAL CONCEPTS AND TECHNIQUES

Overview

- Useful clinical concepts
  - *Safety:* Always the first and foremost intervention; the primary objective of the entire staff

- *Helping:* A fundamental element of nursing; nurses must examine their own motives for helping
- *Altruism:* Having and showing compassion, generosity, goodwill, charity, kindness, and benevolence toward others
- *Power and control:* Nurses recognize the imbalance of power and control between the nurse and the client in some psychiatric settings
- Useful clinical techniques
  - *Make observations versus inferences;* an *inference* is an interpretation of a response or behavior
  - *Accept the client's feelings, but not all behaviors*
  - *Desire to protect others*
  - *Insight* into clients' disorders, problems, needs, and outcomes is beneficial to both clients and nurses, and it is essential for growth
  - *Identify and overcome fears*
  - *Stress management*
  - *Increase your own knowledge and skills*
  - *Set priorities*
  - *Explain to clients the rationale for not keeping* secrets
  - *Recognize variations of change*
  - *Identify and reinforce strengths*
  - *Offer alternatives versus resolutions*
  - *Use simple, concrete, and direct language with clients*
  - *Manage your own frustration*
  - *Encourage clients to take responsibility for their own actions, decisions, choices, and lives whenever they are capable*
- Patterns to avoid:
  - *Avoid evaluative responses (Ex:* "That was *so great* that you divorced him"). If the nurse can approve, it implies the nurse can disapprove also.
  - *Avoid giving advice*
  - *Avoid false reassurances, clichés, and global statements (Ex:* "Everything happens for a reason.")
  - *Avoid rescue fantasy and heroics;* you are <u>not</u> the only person who can help a client

Considerations Fundamental to a Therapeutic Relationship

- Client is unique and worthy of respect
- Client needs to feel accepted
  - Acceptance is an active process designed to convey respect for another through empathetic understanding
  - Acceptance of others implies and requires acceptance of self
  - Nurse's identification of own attitudes and feelings and their effect on perception is necessary before developing a nonjudgmental attitude
  - Acceptance requires that clients be permitted and even encouraged to express feelings and attitudes even though they may be divergent from a general viewpoint; setting limits might be required for inappropriate behavior in a manner that does not reject client
  - Acceptance requires a nonjudgmental environment
- The high stress/anxiety of most health settings is created in part by the health problem itself; by the treatments and procedures; by the nontherapeutic behavior of personnel; by the strange environment; by the inability to use usual coping skills (eg, exercise, talking with friends); and by the change in lifestyle, body image, and/or self-concept

- Previous patterns of behavior may become inadequate under stress: health problems may produce change in family or community
- Health problems may produce change in self-perception and role identity
- All behavior has meaning and usually results from an attempt to cope with stress or anxiety
- Value systems influence behavior
- Cultural differences exist among people; one's own culture is an integral part of an individual
- Personal meaning of experiences to clients is important
- Clients have potential for growth
  - Clients need to learn about their own behaviors
  - Exchanging experiences with others provides a new learning environment and reassurance that reactions are valid and feelings are shared
  - Participating in groups increases knowledge of interpersonal relationships and helps individuals to identify strengths and resources
  - Identifying client's strengths and resources emphasizes positive attributes that form a basis for future growth
- Behavioral changes are possible only when client has other defenses to maintain equilibrium
- Providing information may not alter client's behavior
- Use of defense mechanisms needs to be identified
- Maintaining confidentiality supports a trusting relationship
- Use of therapeutic interviewing techniques communicates acceptance and supports expression of feelings
- Nurses need to identify and cope with their own anxiety

Nursing Process

- The steps of the nursing process are themselves clinical concepts and techniques, as well as standards of psychiatric nursing care; they are reviewed in Chapter 3

CULTURAL AND SPIRITUAL CONCEPTS

Cultural Heritage

- Culture defines for its people what is important and what is true and real
- Age, ethnicity, gender, education, income, and belief system (eg, worldview, religion, or spirituality) make up the sociocultural profile of clients
- A group's culture influences its members' worldview, nonverbal communication patterns, etiquette norms, ways of viewing the person and the family, and the "right" way to think and behave in society
- When clients face increased stressors, suffering, or pain, belief systems play a greater role in their lives
- Ethnocentrism: A belief that one's beliefs and culture are better than those of others
- Assimilation: The process in which a person or group from a different ethnic background become absorbed into a new culture; integration of common values, beliefs, attitudes, and behaviors of dominant culture
- Common sociocultural stressors such as stereotyping, intolerance, stigma, prejudice, discrimination, and racism
- Language does not define a culture; for example, many different countries have Spanish as their native language, but each has its own distinct heritage, culture, and traditions
- Subcultures exist within cultures; subcultures are ethnic and religious groups with characteristics that differ from the dominant culture

- Individuals may choose to not actively practice their cultural heritage; thus assumptions about belief systems and behaviors based on a person's ethnicity or heritage are not useful
- Cultural heritage has a strong influence on communication patterns (see Chapter 2)

Culture and Health

- Clients' perceptions of health and illness, their help-seeking behavior, and adherence to treatment depend on beliefs, social norms, and cultural values
- Psychiatric mental health nursing is based on personality and developmental theories advanced by Europeans and Americans and grounded in Western cultural ideals and values, which is not always congruent with other cultures
- Complementary health therapies may be based on philosophies and techniques other than conventional Western medicine, often derived from those used by other cultures
- Immigrants (especially refugees) and minority groups who suffer from the effects of low socioeconomic status, including poverty and discrimination, are at particular risk for mental illness
- Culture-bound or culture-specific illnesses are those specific to one culture and do not conform to Western nomenclature
  - They have defined symptoms and treatments within that culture
  - There may be culturally specific language to describe mental illnesses
  - Assessment of culture-bound syndromes is part of the nursing process
- Different cultures may explain or exhibit symptoms differently for the same mental health problem
- Exploring specific cultural issues with the client gives the nurse the best understanding of how to care for a particular patient in a culturally competent way.

Cultural Differences

- Take into consideration how culture affects:
  - Health care practices and beliefs
  - Family roles, social organization, and social support
    - Consider legal and social aspects of consent by adults versus consent to treat minors
  - Client-provider communication, including nonverbal behavior
  - Perceptions of time
- Nurses are as influenced by their own professional and ethnic cultures as clients are by theirs
- Nurses must guard against ethnocentric tendencies when caring for clients, because cultural imposition does not promote client health and well-being
- Degree of compatibility between client's and nurse's belief systems often determines greater satisfaction with treatment, adherence to therapeutic regimens, and treatment outcomes
- Nurses need to experience ethnic diversity through multiple cultural encounters, which helps prevent them from stereotyping their clients

Culturally Competent Care

- Nurses must consider their own personal and cultural background and views about other cultures; education about other cultures is critical to providing culturally competent care
- Awareness of, acceptance of, and respect for beliefs, values, traditions, and practices that are different from one's own is cultural competency
- Transcultural nursing (Leininger): Sensitivity to beliefs and practices about health and illness various populations promotes culturally competent care
- Culturally competent nurses have an understanding of cultural diversity to provide care within a context that is appropriate for clients

- Nurses must have a holistic perspective to assess sociocultural context of clients from different cultures
- Nurses must appreciate that clients bring their own cultures, attitudes, and belief systems to a situation
- Nurses need to perform culturally sensitive assessment interviews
- Nurses must adapt health care to meet clients' cultural needs and preferences, especially so it shows respect and does not violate the culture or religion of the client
- Together, nurse and client should agree on the nature of a client's coping responses and set goals and behavioral outcomes within client's sociocultural context
- Achieving cultural competence is aided by knowledge, skills, and encounters with others of different cultures

Spiritual Concepts

- Spiritual concepts are important for mental health nursing, because spirituality can overlap with a client's emotional and mental distress to affect such concepts as the purpose and meaning in life, hope and faith, and peace and forgiveness
- A client's spirituality influences his view about health and illness, pain and suffering, and life and death

Spiritual Assessment and Diagnoses

- The use of a tool, such as the questions within the HOPE acronym (Anandarajah and Hight, 2001), can facilitate spiritual assessment
  - H: What helps you have **h**ope
  - O: The role of **o**rganized religion play for the client
  - P: **P**ersonal spirituality and **p**ractices
  - E: What are the **e**ffects on medical issues and **e**nd-of-life
- Based on the spiritual and cultural assessment, nurses can help clients reach out to religious, spiritual, or cultural healers to help resolve spiritual distress
- Shadowing a chaplain is an excellent way to understand how they can help clients

APPLICATION AND REVIEW

11. A physician is admitted to the psychiatric unit of a community hospital. The client, who was restless, loud, aggressive, and resistive during the admission procedure, states, "I will take my own blood pressure." What is the nurse's **most** therapeutic response?
    1. "Right now you are just another client"
    2. "If you would rather, I'm sure you will do it correctly"
    3. "I will get the attendants to assist me if you do not cooperate"
    4. "I am sorry, but I cannot allow that because I must take your blood pressure"
12. What is the **most** difficult initial task when developing a nurse-client relationship?
    1. Remaining therapeutic and professional
    2. Being able to understand and accept a client's behavior
    3. Developing an awareness of self and the professional role in the relationship
    4. Accepting responsibility for identifying and evaluating the real needs of a client
13. What is the **most** important tool a nurse brings to the therapeutic nurse-client relationship?
    1. Oneself and a desire to help
    2. Knowledge of psychopathology
    3. Advanced communication skills
    4. Years of experience in psychiatric nursing

14. When a nurse is working with a client with psychiatric problems, a primary goal is the establishment of a therapeutic nurse-client relationship. What is the **major** purpose of this relationship?
    1. Increase nonverbal communication
    2. Present an outlet for suppressed hostile feelings
    3. Assist the client in acquiring more effective behavior
    4. Provide the client with someone who can make decisions
15. A daughter of a Chinese-speaking client approaches a nurse and asks multiple questions while maintaining direct eye contact. What culturally related concept does the daughter's behavior reflect?
    1. Prejudice
    2. Stereotyping
    3. Assimilation
    4. Ethnocentrism
16. A nurse manager works on a unit in which the nursing staff members are uncomfortable taking care of clients from cultures that are different from their own. How should the nurse manager initially address this situation?
    1. Assign articles about various cultures so that they can become more knowledgeable
    2. Relocate the nurses to units in which they are not required to care for clients from a variety of cultures
    3. Rotate the nurses' assignments so they have an equal opportunity to care for clients from other cultures
    4. Plan a workshop that offers opportunities to learn about the cultures they might encounter when at work
17. A client is hospitalized for an elective surgical procedure. The client tells a nurse about the emotional stress of recently disclosing being a homosexual to family and friends. What is the nurse's **first** consideration when planning care?
    1. Exploring the client's emotional conflict
    2. Identifying personal feelings toward this client
    3. Planning to discuss this situation with the client's family
    4. Developing a rapport with the client's health care provider
18. Which statement best describes the practice of psychiatric nursing?
    1. Helps people with present or potential mental health problems
    2. Ensures clients' legal and ethical rights by being a client advocate
    3. Focuses interpersonal skills on people with physical or emotional problems
    4. Acts in a therapeutic way with people who are diagnosed as having a mental disorder
19. What is the **priority** when the nurse is establishing a therapeutic environment for a client?
    1. Providing for the client's safety
    2. Accepting the client's individuality
    3. Promoting the client's independence
    4. Explaining to the client what is being done

See Answers on pages 15-19.

ANSWER KEY: REVIEW QUESTIONS

1. **2** The nursing process is a step-by-step method that scientifically provides for a client's nursing needs **1** Identifying procedures used to implement care is only one step in the nursing process. **3** Sequencing steps to meet the client's needs is only one step in the nursing process. **4** Determination of nursing goals for the client is only one step in the nursing process
   Client Need: Management of Care; **Cognitive Level:** Comprehension; **Integrated Process:** Teaching/Learning; **Nursing Process:** Planning/Implementation

2. **1 When nurses make judgmental remarks and client needs are not placed first, the standards of care are violated and quality of care is compromised**

   2 Assessments should be objective, not subjective and biased. **3** There is no information about the client's acuity to come to the conclusion that the nurse is working on development of client acuity to set priorities. **4** The nurse's statement does not reflect information about complexity of care

   Client need: Psychosocial Integrity; **Cognitive Level:** Application; **Integrated Process:** Communication/Documentation; **Nursing Process:** Evaluation/Outcomes

3. **1 Sitting quietly with the client conveys the message that the nurse cares and accepts the client's feelings; this helps establish trust**

   2 Telling the client that crying is not helpful is negating feelings and the client's right to cry when upset. **3** Distraction closes the door on further communication of feelings. **4** After a trusting relationship has been established, the nurse can help the client explore the problem in more depth

   Client Need: Psychosocial Integrity; **Cognitive Level:** Application; **Integrated Process:** Caring; **Nursing Process:** Planning/Implementation

4. **3 An honest nurse-client relationship should be maintained so that trust can develop**

   1 Although other health care team members may need to be informed eventually, the initial action should involve only the nurse and client. **2** Although other health care team members may need to be informed eventually, the initial action should involve only the nurse and client. **4** Discarding the cigarettes without commenting to the client does not promote trust or communication between the client and nurse

   Client Need: Psychosocial Integrity; **Cognitive Level:** Application; **Integrated Process:** Communication/Documentation; **Nursing Process:** Planning/Implementation

---

Memory aid: Trust should be spelled "tHrust" so you could see that the H stands for Honesty. Honesty is necessary to establishing trust!

---

5. **1 The cause of the alarm should be investigated and appropriate intervention instituted; after the client's needs are met, then other tasks can be performed**

   2 An alarm should never be ignored; the client's status takes priority over the change-of-shift report. **3** The diastolic pressure limit has been ordered by the health care provider and should not be changed for the convenience of the nurse. **4** Alarms should always remain on; the alarm indicates that the client's blood pressure has decreased and immediate assessment is required

   Client Need: Management of Care; **Cognitive Level:** Application; **Nursing Process:** Planning/Implementation

6. **1 The technique of sharing your observation for the purpose of clarifying is the best response so you can assess the reason for the apprehension rather than guess the cause.**

   2 Having a copy of hospital regulations available is part of orienting the client to the unit. This alone is not enough when orienting a client to the hospital. **3** Because no one can guarantee that there is no reason to be concerned, that response may be false reassurance. **4** Saying that the staff is available to answer questions implies that staff members are available *only* if the client has specific questions

   Client Need: Psychosocial Integrity; **Cognitive Level:** Application; **Integrated Process:** Caring, Communication/Documentation; **Nursing Process:** Planning/Implementation

7. **3 Telling the client that he was in a work-related accident is truthful and provides basic information that may prompt recollection of what occurred; it is a starting point**

   1 Asking the client for his or her recollections ignores the client's question; avoidance may increase anxiety. **2** Telling clients they will remember more as they get better ignores the client's question; the frustration of trying to remember will increase anxiety. **4** Stating that an amputation was necessary is too blunt for the initial response to the client's question; the client may not be ready to hear this at this time

Client Need: Psychosocial Integrity; Cognitive Level: Application; Integrated Process: Caring, Communication/Documentation; Nursing Process: Planning/Implementation

8. **2 Telling the client that you will come back in 10 minutes demonstrates that the nurse cares about the client and will have time for the client's special emotional needs; this approach allays anxiety and reduces emotional stress**

1 Apologizing because you need to see other clients indicates that the nurse's other tasks are more important than the client's needs. 3 Saying that the client will be able to rest after the medicine starts working is false reassurance and not therapeutic. 4 Promising that the client will feel better after you make the client more comfortable does not respond to the client's need and cuts off communication

Client Need: Psychosocial Integrity; Cognitive Level: Application; Integrated Process: Caring, Communication/Documentation; Nursing Process: Planning/Implementation

9. **3 Because of the profound effect of paralysis on body image, the nurse should foster an environment that permits exploration of feelings without judgment, punishment, or rejection**

1 Attempts to distract the client may be interpreted as denial of the client's feelings and will not resolve the underlying problem. 2 Including the client in decision making is an important part of nursing care, but it is not related to the client's feelings. 4 Helping the client problem-solve personal issues is an important part of nursing care, but it is not related to the client's feelings

Client Need: Psychosocial Integrity; Cognitive Level: Application; Integrated Process: Caring; Nursing Process: Planning/Implementation

10. **1 The nurse should assess the situation before planning an intervention**

2 Reassuring the client that the surgery is routine minimizes concerns and cuts off communication. 3 Reporting the client's anxiety to the health care provider would be premature as more information is needed. 4 The nurse needs more information; pulling the curtain may make the client feel isolated, which may increase anxiety

Client Need: Psychosocial Integrity; Cognitive Level: Application; Integrated Process: Caring; Nursing Process: Assessment/Analysis

11. **4 Stating that you cannot allow the client to take his or her own blood pressure because you must take the blood pressure simply states facts without getting involved in role conflict**

1 Being a health care professional is a big part of this client's self-esteem, and by this remark the nurse is threatening that self-esteem. 2 Allowing the client to take his or her own blood pressure will confuse the client's role on the unit, and a client who is a health care professional cannot be responsible for checking vital signs. 3 Threats will make the situation worse and set the tone for future negative nurse-client interactions

Client Need: Psychosocial Integrity; Cognitive Level: Application; Integrated Process: Communication/Documentation; Nursing Process: Planning/Implementation

12. **3 The nurse's major tool in mental health nursing is the therapeutic use of self; mental health nurses must learn to identify their own feelings and understand how they affect the situation**

1 Although remaining therapeutic and professional may be difficult, an awareness of self is still the most difficult. 2 Although being able to understand and accept a client's behavior may be difficult, an awareness of self is still the most difficult. 4 Accepting responsibility for identifying and evaluating the real needs of a client implies that the nurse is working alone in caring for the client

Client Need: Management of Care; Cognitive Level: Comprehension; Nursing Process: Planning/Implementation

13. **1 The nurse brings to a therapeutic relationship the understanding of self and basic principles of therapeutic communication; this is the unique aspect of the helping relationship**

2 Knowledge of psychopathology supports the psychotherapeutic management model, but it is not the most important tool used by the nurse in a therapeutic relationship. 3 Advanced communication skills support the psychotherapeutic management model, but they are not the most important tool used by the nurse in a therapeutic relationship. 4 Years of experience in psychiatric nursing support the psychotherapeutic management model, but it is not the most important tool used by the nurse in a therapeutic relationship

Client Need: Psychosocial Integrity; **Cognitive Level:** Comprehension; **Integrated Process:** Caring; **Nursing Process:** Planning/Implementation

14. **3 The therapeutic nurse-client relationship provides an opportunity for the client to try out different behaviors in an accepting atmosphere and ultimately to replace pathologic responses with more effective responses**

    1 Verbal, not nonverbal, communication is the objective of the therapeutic relationship. **2** The nurse, although accepting of the client's hostile feelings, uses the therapeutic relationship to redirect hostile feelings into more acceptable behaviors. **4** The nurse provides the support and acceptance that encourage clients to make their own decisions

    Client Need: Psychosocial Integrity; **Cognitive Level:** Comprehension; **Integrated Process:** Caring; **Nursing Process:** Planning/Implementation

15. **3 Assimilation involves incorporating the behaviors of a dominant culture; maintaining eye contact is characteristic of the American culture and not of Asian cultures**

    1 Prejudice is a negative belief about another person or group and does not characterize this behavior. **2** Stereotyping is the perception that all members of a group are alike. **4** Ethnocentrism is the perception that one's beliefs are better than those of others

    Client Need: Psychosocial Integrity; **Cognitive Level:** Analysis; **Nursing Process:** Planning/Implementation

16. **4 A workshop provides an opportunity to discuss cultural diversity; it should include identification of one's own feelings; also, it provides an opportunity for participants to ask questions**

    1 Assigning articles about cultures will provide information, but it does not promote a discussion about the topic. **2** Relocating the nurses to units in which they will not have to care for clients from a variety of cultures is not feasible or desirable because clients from other cultures are found in all settings. **3** Rotating the nurses' assignments so they have opportunities to care for clients from other cultures probably will increase tension on the unit

    Client Need: Psychosocial Integrity; **Cognitive Level:** Application; **Nursing Process:** Planning/Implementation

17. **2 Nurses must identify their own feelings and prejudices because these may affect the ability to provide objective, nonjudgmental nursing care**

    1 Exploring a client's emotional well-being can be accomplished only after the nurse works through one's own feelings. **3** The focus should be on the client, not the family. **4** Health team members should work together for the benefit of all clients, not just this client

    Client Need: Psychosocial Integrity; **Cognitive Level:** Application; **Integrated Process:** Caring; **Nursing Process:** Assessment/Analysis

18. **1 An important aspect of the role of the psychiatric nurse is primary, secondary, and tertiary interventions to promote emotional equilibrium**

    2 Ensuring clients' legal and ethical rights by being a client advocate is only a small part of the role of the psychiatric nurse, a role usually shared with others on the health team. **3** Focusing interpersonal skills on people with physical or emotional problems is only a small part of the role of the psychiatric nurse, a role usually shared with others on the health team. **4** Acting in a therapeutic way with people who are diagnosed as having a mental disorder is only a part of the role of the psychiatric nurse, because psychiatry is concerned with people with varying degrees of mental and emotional disorders

    Client Need: Psychosocial Integrity; **Cognitive Level:** Comprehension; **Integrated Process:** Caring; **Nursing Process:** Planning/Implementation

19. **4 In the Latino culture, usually there is a strong family bond, and the support of the family is essential during problematic times**

    1 Socioeconomic status does not play more than the usual role in deciding on appropriate health care options. **2** Latino clients tend to be present, not future, time oriented. **3** Latino clients frequently believe in fate and that outcomes are influenced by external controls (eg, divine being, authority figures)

    Client Need: Psychosocial Integrity; **Cognitive Level:** Application; **Integrated Process:** Caring; **Nursing Process:** Planning/Implementation

20. **1 Safety is the priority before any other intervention is provided**

2 Accepting the client's individuality is important but less of a priority. **3** Promoting the client's independence is a later nursing action. **4** Although explaining to the client what is being done is important, it is not the priority

Client Need: Management of Care; **Cognitive Level:** Comprehension; **Integrated Process:** Caring; **Nursing Process:** Planning/Implementation

2 Therapeutic Communication

COMMUNICATION PROCESS

- A dynamic process in which two or more people share types of information

Overview

- Need to communicate is universal
- Through communication, humans maintain contact with reality, validate findings with others to interpret reality, and develop a concept of self in relation to others
- Validation is enhanced when communication conveys an understanding of feelings
- Requires sender, message, medium, receiver, and response or feedback
  - Usually there is a stimulus or a reason for the communication to occur
  - The individual who initiates the transmission of information is the sender
  - Each transmission is both verbal and nonverbal
    - Nonverbal communication is generally thought to be more powerful than verbal communication
  - The information that is being sent and received, such as feelings or ideas, is the message
  - The method by which the message is sent is the medium; the medium can be seen (visual), heard (verbal), felt (tactile), or smelled (scent)
  - The receiver both receives and interprets the message; in an ideal situation, the receiver will interpret the message exactly as the sender intends it, thus resulting in accurate communication
  - The feedback that the receiver provides to the sender is a means of measuring the accuracy of the message
  - Feedback is a continual process because it is a response to the message and because it provides a new stimulus to the sender, thus causing the original sender to become the receiver; in any interaction, the sender and the receiver continually reverse roles
- Variables in communication include the culture and experience of both the client and the nurse; the client's coping ability and psychopathology; and the nurse's knowledge of psychopathology and skills available to guide the client (Fig. 2.1)
- Communication is intrapersonal (self-talk) or interpersonal (occurs between two or more individuals and contains both verbal and nonverbal messages)
- Communication is learned through the process of acculturation
- Communication is the avenue used to make needs known and to satisfy needs; it is the most important social link

FACTORS THAT AFFECT THERAPEUTIC COMMUNICATION

Cultural Considerations

- Culturally competent care requires effective communication
- Individuals from different cultures or generations often misunderstand and misinterpret slang phrases and idioms such as "double dipping," "my bad," and "sick"
  - It is necessary to periodically validate their interpretation
  - Examine cues that result from nonverbal responses

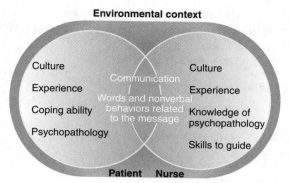

FIG. 2.1 A model of the communication process in psychiatric nursing, showing variables of the therapeutic environment. (From Keltner, N. L. & Steele, D. [2015]. *Psychiatric nursing* [7th ed.]. St. Louis, MO: Mosby/Elsevier.)

- Clear communication is even more important to overcome cultural or language barriers
- Listening is a key component to communication
- Consider the meanings of nonverbal (gestures, body positions, eye contact, etc.) and verbal variations (tone of voice, pace) in various cultures
- Realize that nodding may be a sign of respect and may not indicate understanding

Social Status

- The relationship between the two people in a conversation greatly influences the communication
- Consider your role as a nurse when communicating; clients look to you for accurate information and understanding

Gender

- Clients may not want to communicate personal information to you because of your or their gender or gender identity

Age

- Older patients
  - Consider any hearing or sight deficits and plan communication accordingly
  - Do not communicate messages of dependence and incompetence by using a style of speech that would be used to address a small child
  - Do not address older clients by their first names without permission
  - Communicate with the older client through the use of adult language that shows respect and caring and that maintains the client's autonomy, independence, and dignity
- Younger Clients
  - Rely on nonverbal skills when dealing with very young children by using kind and gentle facial expressions, a nurturing and caring attitude, and soothing voice tones
  - Having the parents participate in the child's care is helpful and will reduce the child's and the parents' anxiety
  - Ways to establish rapport with children and adolescents:
    - Take a personal interest in them by asking them about school, hobbies, and interests; be a skillful and active listener
    - Use simple language
    - Be nonjudgmental

- Appear relaxed; sit at eye level and establish good eye contact
- Communicate directly with the child to demonstrate interest
- Use broad, open-ended questions
- Welcome their thoughts and feelings

Developmental Level

- The level of communication must be adapted to the developmental age to match the client's ability to comprehend
  - Consider the client's developmental stage when communicating
- Stories, pictures, and examples may be needed to convey information

Barriers to Communication

- Variation in culture, language, and education
- Problems in hearing, speech, or comprehension (ineffective reception or perception)
  - Be sure client can hear and see you when you speak
- Refusal to listen to another point of view
- Use of selective inattention; may cause an interruption or distortion of messages
- Environmental considerations (eg, noise, lack of privacy, room temperature)
- Psychologic or physiologic discomfort (eg, anxiety, hunger, pain)

TYPES OF COMMUNICATION

Overview

- Modes include verbal and nonverbal
- Confusion arises from conflict between verbal and nonverbal message—lack of congruence in overt and covert messages
- Themes of communication: Recurring thoughts and ideas that give insight into what client is feeling and that tie communication together
  - Content: Conversation may appear superficial, but attention to underlying theme helps nurse identify problem areas and provides insight into client's self-concept
  - Mood: Emotion or affect that client communicates to nurse; includes personal appearance, facial expressions, and gestures that reflect client's mood and feelings
  - Interaction: How client reacts or interacts with nurse; includes how client relates and what role is assumed when communicating with nurse and others
- Communication can be categorized as social (not related to work; equal sharing of information), collegial (for professional collaboration), or therapeutic
- Therapeutic communication, the psychiatric nurse's single most important tool, has three purposes:
  - To allow clients to express thoughts, feelings, behaviors, and life experiences in a meaningful way
  - To understand the client's problems and how the client and people in the client's life perpetuate these problems
  - To assist with identification and resolution of health-related behaviors
    - An interactive process that occurs between the nurse (helper) and the client (recipient) in any health care setting
    - A learned skill that involves both nonverbal and verbal communication
    - Enhances client growth and supports health-promoting interventions
    - Client-focused, it involves the client disclosing personal information

- Sharing such feelings is extremely beneficial for the client because it allows the client to identify and discuss experiences and accompanying feelings in a safe, therapeutic setting
- The nurse provides a confidential and quiet setting in which the interaction takes place, encourages the client to openly discuss thoughts and feelings, and practices active listening, acceptance, and empathy
- Note that there is a difference between communication to gather information, such as while taking a history, versus therapeutic communication.

Verbal Communication

- Anything associated with spoken word
- Includes speaking, writing, use of language or symbols, and arrangements of words or phrases
- Hearing is essential to development of effective speech because one learns to form words by hearing words of others
- Includes pace, intonation, simplicity, clarity, brevity, timing, relevance, adaptability, credibility, and humor
  - Consider that tone can completely change the meaning of a message
- Precise verbal communication is important because spoken words often mean different things to different people
- Avoid medical jargon.
- Use of slang or idioms may be confusing
  - Many words or phrases have slang meanings or have developed new meanings
  - Some words and phrases also have different meanings for different groups
  - Figures of speech, jokes, clichés, colloquialisms, and other terms or special phrases carry a variety of meanings
- Telephone communication
  - Telephone orders/prescriptions from health care providers must be "read back" to ensure accuracy
  - Clarity is especially important for medication prescriptions received via telephone
  - Accessibility to telephone communication is especially important for clients with mental health disorders and can sometimes prevent an admission by handling situations on a telephone call
  - Having a phone contact for clients can help adherence
  - Text messaging can be used for client reminders
- Written communication
  - The nurse needs to clearly expresses ideas in written form, whether it is documentation in the medical record or in the form of statistical reports
  - The ability to write legibly, spell correctly, use proper grammar, and organize ideas clearly is critical for the nurse
  - The nurse must have the ability to document a client's behavior in objective, descriptive, clear, and concise terms
  - The nurse must be aware that the use of slang, emojis, and abbreviations can be misinterpreted.
- Electronic communication
  - Because most documentation is in the form of a computerized client record, the ability to navigate through and document within electronic records and templates is essential
  - Although e-mail can be fast and convenient, privacy must be ensured
  - Extra care must be taken to protect privacy of electronic health records
  - Although electronic communication makes sense in many instances, it may also become habitual and time-consuming, replacing face-to-face interpersonal interactions that are critical in meaningful relationships, therapeutic or otherwise

Nonverbal Communication

- Messages sent and received without use of words
- Expressed through appearance, body motions, use of space, nonverbal sounds, personal appearance, posture, gait, facial expression, gestures, and eye contact
- More accurately conveys feelings, because behavior is less consciously controlled than verbal communication
- Body language includes facial expressions, reflexes, body posture, hand gestures, eye movement, mannerisms, touch, and other body motions
  - Body posture and facial expressions, including eye movements, are two of the most important cues to determine how a person is responding to the message
  - Nonverbal behavior is an excellent index of feelings because it is less likely to be consciously controlled; relaxation of muscles and facial expression are examples of nonverbal behavior
  - A slumped or stooped posture sometimes means that a client is depressed or, at the very least, feeling sad or dejected
  - A closed posture with arms folded often indicates that a client is withdrawing or possibly feeling some anger
  - An erect posture with the shoulders back means that the client feels more confident or is trying to appear confident
  - The gait or way that an individual walks also indicates the client's self-concept
  - Nurses need to carefully observe hand gestures because they also signal anger, restlessness, frustration, hopelessness, relaxation, or apathy
  - Be aware of contradictions between the verbal and nonverbal cues
  - Body language is affected by culture.
- Paralinguistic (paralanguage) behavior includes any sound that is not a spoken word, such as voice tone, inflection, word spacing, rate, emphasis, intensity, groaning, coughing, laughing, crying, grunting, moaning, and other audible sounds
- Space (proxemics): Each person has a comfort zone or space boundary that invisibly surrounds him or her during interactions with others; the boundary varies depending on the relationship
  - *Intimate space* is the closest distance between two individuals
  - *Personal space* is for close relationships within touching distance
  - *Consultative space* is larger than personal space and requires louder speech
  - *Public space* is for public gatherings; it usually applies to individuals in a large hall or auditorium
  - The nurse and the client need to respect the distance that each one needs; for successful communication, both parties need to feel safe
    - Some clients have problems with boundaries and invade other clients' own safe zones; clients who perceive this as threatening react aggressively
    - The nurse may need to help the client understand an appropriate distance by stating the specific boundary for the client
    - When the client violates the nurse's own comfortable space, the nurse needs to set a limit for the client
    - Consider that clients who are actively psychotic may require more distance
- Touch is a nonverbal message that involves both action and personal space
  - It typically conveys a message to the receiver that the sender wants to connect with him or her
  - Nurses have used touch to send messages of concern and empathy
  - Use caution when deciding whether to touch a client with a psychiatric disorder; not all clients want to be touched—some perceive it as a threat and respond with aggression, or

they may interpret it as an intimate move and respond with withdrawal or an inappropriate sexual response
  - For some patients with a history of mental health concerns, touch has been associated with negative experiences
- Appearance refers to the way an individual uses clothing, makeup, hairstyle, jewelry, and other items such as hats, purses, or eyeglasses as well as grooming and hygiene
  - Nonverbally communicates a particular image as well as clues to mental status
  - These nonverbal cues often show how the person wishes to be viewed by others
- Try to interpret a client's nonverbal behavior while evaluating the verbal content and incorporate this evaluation into the assessment of the client and the plan of care
- Nurses need to be aware of their own nonverbal cues; for effective communication, make sure that nonverbal messages are congruent with verbal messages and communicate genuine interest and respect

NURSE'S ROLE IN THERAPEUTIC COMMUNICATION

Attributes of Therapeutic Communication

- Positive regard: Respect and acceptance; includes being nonjudgmental
- Empathy: Ability to see things from the client's viewpoint and communicate this understanding to the client
  - Empathy is not sympathy; sympathy is overinvolvement and sharing your own feelings, and its primary purpose is to decrease your own personal distress
  - Two stages of empathy: First, the nurse is receptive to and understanding of the client's problem by seeing situations from the client's viewpoint; second, the nurse communicates understanding to the client (Box 2.1)

BOX 2.1 Skills That Help Nurses Develop Empathic Responses

- *Attending to the client physically* by sitting in front of the client at a slight angle and leaning slightly forward with hands and arms in an open stance
- *Attending to the client emotionally* by clearing your mind of other thoughts and focusing your full attention on the client
- *Focusing on the client's strengths*
- *Expressing caring, warmth, interest, and concern* with the use of nonverbal behaviors
- *Determining the most important point* of what the client is trying to say
- *Demonstrating consistency* between your own nonverbal and verbal communication
- *Active listening,* a central element of understanding, is closely associated with empathy; it incorporates nonverbal and verbal behaviors necessary for therapeutic communication
  - Nonverbally, the nurse leans slightly forward and faces the client, uses eye contact, nods, and uses verbal phrases such as "I see" or "I understand"
  - Active listening is a dynamic and interactive nonjudgmental process; it requires listening for facts, trying to determine the underlying meaning of the client's communication, accurate interpretation of meaning, and providing the client with feedback regarding understanding the message
  - Clients need to know that the nurse is there to help and wants to help
  - A nurse who listens actively is displaying interest and is engaged
  - The result is full understanding of the meaning of the communication
- *Checking your* empathic *responses* for effectiveness by observing verbal and nonverbal clues

Adapted from Fortinash, K.M. & Holoday, P.A. (2012). *Psychiatric mental health nursing* (5th ed.). St. Louis, MO: Mosby.

- Trustworthiness
  - Trustworthy nurses are responsible and dependable by keeping commitments and promises and are consistent in approach and response to clients
  - Trustworthy nurses respect client privacy, rights, and need for confidentiality
- Responsibility
  - Responsible communication involves being accountable for the outcome of professional interactions
  - Responsible language involves the use of "I" statements when being assertive
- Assertiveness (Box 2.2)
- Congruence: Verbal and nonverbal communication match
- Feedback confirms effective therapeutic communication

Support of Therapeutic Communication

- Maintenance of a nonjudgmental attitude and responses
- Implementation of actions that support dignity and worth
  - Maintaining eye contact when communicating when culturally appropriate
  - Using names rather than labels such as room numbers or diagnoses; approach client as a person with difficulties, not as a "difficult person"
  - Providing privacy
  - Maintaining confidentiality
  - Being courteous toward client, family, visitors, and members of the health team
  - Permitting personal possessions when practical and safe
  - Providing explanations at client's level of understanding
- Encouragement of participation in problem solving and decision making
- Spending time with client
- Fostering trust through honesty, consistency, reliability, and competence
- Answering client call bell immediately

BOX 2.2 **Behaviors of Assertive Communication**

Assertive
Stands up for own rights and respects those of others; uses expressive, directive, and self-enhancing speech; chooses relevant words and actions

Aggressive
Stands up for own rights but abuses those of others; speaks in demeaning or attacking manner; fails to monitor or control words or actions

Passive
Does not stand up for own rights; accepts the domination and bullying of others; performs unwanted tasks; feels victimized

Examples of Assertive Behaviors
- "I" messages (eg, "I need," "I feel," "I will")
- Eye contact (eg, looking directly into the eyes of the person when making or refusing a request)
- Congruent verbal and facial expressions (ie, making certain that the facial expression matches the intent of the spoken message; a serious message accompanied by laughter negates the credibility of the message)

From Fortinash, K. M. & Holoday, P. A. (2012). *Psychiatric mental health nursing* (5th ed.). St. Louis, MO: Mosby.

Use of Therapeutic Techniques to Facilitate Communication

- Reflection of feelings, attitudes, and words: Helps client identify feelings
- Open-ended questions and comments: Permit client to focus on issues that most concern them and encourage communication
- Paraphrasing: Rephrasing of feeling or thought in similar words to convey that a message was understood or to provide an opportunity for clarification if necessary
- Silence: Provides nurse and client with necessary time for reflecting about what is being discussed and allows time to formulate a response
- Touch: Conveys caring, but its effectiveness can vary among individuals and cultures
- Clarification: Helps ensure that a message is understood as intended
- Direct questions: Facilitate collection of objective data but may block expression of feelings
- Offering self to listen or just "be" with the patient is therapeutic.

Avoidance of Nontherapeutic Communication

- Any overt/covert response conveys a judgmental (approval or disapproval) or superior attitude
- Direct personal questions are probing or invasive
- Ridicule conveys a hostile attitude
- Talking about one's own problems (self-disclosure) and not listening convey a self-serving attitude and loss of interest in the client
- Stereotyping devalues uniqueness of the client
- Changing the subject conveys a lack of interest in the client's concerns
- False reassurance eventually results in lack of trust
- Minimizing concerns is demeaning
- Asking for explanations using the word "why" may put client on the defensive
- Using clichés minimizes concerns
- Using terms of endearment such as "honey" is demeaning
- Defensive responses shut off communication
- Giving advice, agreeing, and disagreeing interfere with the client's ability to problem-solve
- Challenging client to defend a position/feeling may put client on the defensive

APPLICATION AND REVIEW

1. A nurse considers that communication links people with their surroundings. What should the nurse identify as the **most** important function of communication?
   1. Social
   2. Physical
   3. Materialistic
   4. Environmental
2. How can a nurse **best** evaluate the effectiveness of communication with a client?
   1. Client feedback
   2. Medical assessments
   3. Health care team conferences
   4. Client's physiologic responses
3. An older client whose family has been visiting on the psychiatric unit is visibly angry and states to the nurse, "My daughter-in-law says they can't take me home until the doctor lets me go. She doesn't understand how important this is to me; she is not from our culture." What should the nurse do?
   1. Ignore the statement for the present
   2. Say, "You feel she doesn't want you at home"
   3. Reflect on the client's feelings about the cultural differences
   4. State, "The health care provider makes decisions about discharge"

4. A 6-year-old child is diagnosed with type 1 diabetes. Considering the child's cognitive developmental level, which explanation of the illness is **most** appropriate?
   1. "Diabetes is caused by not having any insulin in your body"
   2. "Diabetes will require you to take insulin shots for the rest of your life"
   3. "You will be taught how to give yourself insulin now that you have diabetes"
   4. "Taking insulin for your diabetes is like getting new batteries for your superhero toys"

5. A parent of a 13-year-old adolescent who was recently diagnosed with Hodgkin disease tells a nurse, "I don't want my child to know the diagnosis." How should the nurse respond?
   1. "It is best if your child knows the diagnosis"
   2. "Did you know the cure rate for Hodgkin disease is high?"
   3. "Would you like someone with Hodgkin disease to talk with you?"
   4. "Let's talk about your feelings regarding your child's diagnosis"

6. A male nurse is caring for a client. The client states, "You know, I've never had a male nurse before." What is the nurse's **best** reply?
   1. "Does it bother you to have a male nurse?"
   2. "How do you feel about having a male nurse?"
   3. "There aren't many male nurses; we are a minority"
   4. "You sound upset; I will get a female nurse to care for you"

7. As depression begins to lift, a client is asked to join a small discussion group that meets every evening. The client is reluctant to join and says, "I have nothing to talk about." What is the **best** response by the nurse?
   1. "Maybe tomorrow you will feel more like talking"
   2. "Could you start off by talking about your family?"
   3. "A person like you has a great deal to offer the group"
   4. "You feel you will not be accepted unless you have something to say"

8. The parent of a child with a tentative diagnosis of attention deficit hyperactivity disorder (ADHD) arrives at the pediatric clinic insisting on receiving a prescription for medication that will control the child's behavior. What is the nurse's **best** response?
   1. "It must be frustrating to deal with your child's behavior"
   2. "Have you considered any alternatives to using medication?"
   3. "Perhaps you are looking for an easy solution to the problem"
   4. "Let me teach you about the side effects of medications used for ADHD"

9. A client diagnosed with bipolar disorder, depressed, is being admitted to the mental health unit. The client avoids eye contact, responds in a very low voice, and is tearful. Which comment is **most** therapeutic for a nurse to make during the assessment interview?
   1. "You'll find that you'll get better faster if you try to help us to help you"
   2. "Hold my hand; I know you are frightened; I will not allow anyone to harm you"
   3. "I'm your nurse; I'll take you to the day room as soon as I get some information"
   4. "I know this is difficult, but as soon as we are finished, I'll take you to your room"

10. When admitting a client who is in labor to the birthing unit, a nurse asks the client about her marital status. The client refuses to answer and becomes very agitated, telling the nurse to leave. How should the nurse respond?
    1. Question the family about the client's marital status
    2. Try to obtain this information to complete the client's history
    3. Refer the client to the social service department for counseling
    4. Ask questions that relate to the client's present clinical situation

11. A pregnant client in the third trimester tells the nurse, "I want to be unconscious for the birth." How should the nurse respond?
    1. "You are worried about too much pain"
    2. "You don't want to be awake during the birth?"
    3. "I can understand that because labor is uncomfortable"
    4. "I will tell your health care provider about this request"

12. A client becomes hostile when learning that amputation of a gangrenous toe is recommended. After the client's outburst, what is the **best** indication that the nurse-client interaction has been therapeutic?
    1. Increased physical activity
    2. Absence of further outbursts
    3. Relaxation of tensed muscles
    4. Denial of the need for further discussion

13. When awaiting the biopsy report before removal of a tumor, the client reports being afraid of a diagnosis of cancer. How should the nurse respond?
    1. "Worrying is not going to help the situation"
    2. "Let's wait until we hear what the biopsy report says"
    3. "It is very upsetting to have to wait for a biopsy report"
    4. "Operations are not performed unless there are no other options"

14. "But you don't understand" is a common statement associated with adolescents. What is the nurse's **best** response when hearing this?
    1. "I don't understand what you mean"
    2. "I do understand; I was a teenager once too"
    3. "It would be helpful to understand; let's talk"
    4. "It's you who should try to understand others"

15. A client is hospitalized with a tentative diagnosis of pancreatic cancer. On admission the client asks the nurse, "Do you think I have anything serious, like cancer?" What is the nurse's **best** reply?
    1. "What makes you think you have cancer?"
    2. "Your test results are incomplete at this time; let's talk about your feelings"
    3. "Why don't you discuss this with your health care provider?"
    4. "You needn't worry now; we won't know the answer for a few days"

16. A client asks the nurse, "Should I tell my partner that I just found out I'm HIV positive?" What is the nurse's **most** therapeutic response?
    1. "This is a decision you alone can make"
    2. "Do not tell your partner unless asked"
    3. "You are having difficulty deciding what to say"
    4. "Tell your partner that you don't know how you became sick"

17. A client becomes anxious after being scheduled for a colostomy. What is the **most** effective way for the nurse to help the client?
    1. Administer the prescribed prn sedative
    2. Encourage the client to express feelings
    3. Explain the postprocedure course of treatment
    4. Reassure the client that there are others with this problem

18. When receiving a preoperative enema, a client starts to cry and says, "I'm sorry you have to do this messy thing for me." What is the nurse's **best** response?
    1. "I don't mind it"   3. "This is part of my job"
    2. "You seem upset"   4. "Nurses get used to this"

19. A client is hospitalized with a diagnosis of metastatic cancer. The client has a temperature of 100.4° F, a distended abdomen, and abdominal pain. The client asks the nurse, "Do you think that I'm going to have surgery?" How should the nurse respond?
    1. "You seem concerned about having surgery"
    2. "Some people with your problem do have surgery"
    3. "I'll find out for you; your record will show if surgery is scheduled"
    4. "I don't know about any surgery; you'll have to ask your health care provider"
20. After a therapy session with a health care provider in the mental health clinic, a client tells the nurse that the therapist is uncaring and impersonal. What is the nurse's **best** response?
    1. "Your therapist is really very good"
    2. "I hope that the rest of the staff is caring"
    3. "The therapist is there to help you; try to cooperate"
    4. "You have strong feelings about your therapy session and your therapist"

See Answers on pages 30-33.

ANSWER KEY: REVIEW QUESTIONS

1. **1 Without some form of communication there can be no socialization**

   2 People interact with other social beings, not with inanimate objects. **3** People interact with other social beings, not with inanimate objects. **4** People interact with other social beings, not with inanimate objects in the environment

   Client Need: Psychosocial Integrity; **Cognitive Level:** Comprehension; **Integrated Process:** Communication/Documentation; **Nursing Process:** Assessment/Analysis

2. **1 Feedback permits the client to ask questions and express feelings and allows the nurse to verify client understanding**

   2 Medical assessments do not always include nurse-client relationships. **3** Team conferences are subject to all members' evaluations of a client's status. **4** Nurse-client communications should be evaluated by the client's verbal and behavioral responses

   Client Need: Psychosocial Integrity; **Cognitive Level:** Comprehension; **Integrated Process:** Communication/Documentation; **Nursing Process:** Evaluation/Outcomes

3. **2 Identifying and accepting feelings help to open lines of communication**

   1 Ignoring the statement does not allow the client to explore feelings with an accepting person. **3** Reflecting on the client's feelings focuses on only one aspect of the statement; it does not allow exploration of feelings. **4** Stating that the health care provider makes the decisions about discharge is avoiding the real issue

   Clinical Area: Mental Health Nursing; **Client Needs:** Psychosocial Integrity; **Cognitive Level:** Analysis; **Nursing Process:** Planning/Implementation

4. **4 The child is in Piaget's stage of preoperational thought, which is manifested by magical thinking; therefore, teaching should also use magical thinking**

   1 Explaining about insulin is too technical and does not take into account the child's preoperational stage of development; this statement is appropriate for an adolescent in the formal operational stage of cognitive development. **2** Discussing the lifelong need for insulin is too direct and does not consider the child's cognitive developmental stage of preoperational thought; this statement is appropriate for an adolescent in the formal operational stage of cognitive development; also, the use of the word "shots" may precipitate anxiety. **3** Explaining that the client will be taught to give himself or herself insulin is too direct and does not consider the child's cognitive developmental stage of preoperational thought; this statement is appropriate for an adolescent in the formal operational stage of cognitive development

   Client Need: Psychosocial Integrity; **Cognitive Level:** Analysis; **Integrated Process:** Communication/Documentation; **Nursing Process:** Planning/Implementation

5. **4 Asking after the parent's feelings regarding the child's diagnosis does not prejudge the parent; it encourages communication**
   1 Telling the parent that the child should know the diagnosis disregards the parent's feelings and cuts off further communication. 2 Discussing the cure rate may stop communication and does not recognize the parent's concerns. 3 Suggesting that someone with Hodgkin disease talk with the parent is premature and does not recognize the parent's concerns
   Client Need: Psychosocial Integrity; **Cognitive Level:** Analysis; **Integrated Process:** Caring, Communication/Documentation; **Nursing Process:** Planning/Implementation

6. **2 Asking after the client's feelings encourages the client to express and explore feelings; also, it is open and nonjudgmental**
   1 Asking the client if having a male nurse bothers him or her puts the client on the defensive rather than encouraging verbalization of feelings. 3 Stating that male nurses are a minority does not encourage further conversation, and the client will not have the opportunity to express feelings; this response focuses on the nurse rather than on the client. 4 Stating that the client sounds upset puts the client on the defensive rather than encouraging verbalization of feelings
   Client Need: Psychosocial Integrity; **Cognitive Level:** Application; **Integrated Process:** Caring, Communication/Documentation; **Nursing Process:** Planning/Implementation

> **Memory Aid:** To remind yourself of the attributes of therapeutic communication, and in particular to be nonjudgmental, use the memory aid "PERFACT." After all, you don't expect anyone to be perfEct!
> **P:** Positive regard
> **E:** Empathy
> **R:** Responsible communication
> **F:** Feedback
> **A:** Assertiveness
> **C:** Congruence
> **T:** Trustworthiness

7. **4 Inquiring into the client's feelings of acceptance allows the client to either validate or correct the nurse**
   1 Suggesting the client will feel like talking tomorrow delays addressing the problem and avoids exploring feelings. 2 Suggesting the client talk about his or her family is a response that gives advice and does not allow the client to explore feelings. 3 Telling the client they have something to offer the group denies the client's statement and does not allow the exploration of feelings
   Client Need: Psychosocial Integrity; **Cognitive Level:** Analysis; **Integrated Process:** Communication/Documentation; **Nursing Process:** Planning/Implementation

8. **1 Stating that the parents must be frustrated acknowledges the parent's distress and encourages a verbalization of feelings**
   2 Asking the parents if they have considered alternatives is insensitive to the parent's feelings; it may be more appropriate later when the parent's stress has diminished. 3 Although it may be true that the parents are looking for an easy solution, this response is confrontational and may close off communication. 4 Telling the parents you will teach them about side effects of medications for ADHD is insensitive to the parent's feelings; it may be more appropriate later if medication is prescribed and health teaching is started
   Client Need: Psychosocial Integrity; **Cognitive Level:** Application; **Integrated Process:** Caring, Communication/Documentation; **Nursing Process:** Planning/Implementation

9. **4 Acknowledges the difficulty, recognizes feelings, and explains what is expected when the interview is over**
   1 Suggesting that the client is not trying to get better fast enough is threatening and gives false reassurance; it puts the responsibility on the client and does not allow for expression of feelings. 2 Telling the client to hold your hand and that you will protect them may lead the client to think that the environment is unsafe, which may increase insecurity and anxiety. 3 Being with other people in a strange situation will add more stress to the new and already frightening experience of hospitalization

Client Need: Psychosocial Integrity; **Cognitive Level:** Analysis; **Integrated Process:** Caring, Communication/Documentation; **Nursing Process:** Planning/Implementation

10. **4 The nurse has invaded the client's right to privacy; the client's marital status has no bearing on the needs of the client at this time**
   1 Questioning the family about the client's marital status action is an invasion of privacy. 2 Trying to obtain the information is an invasion of privacy. 3 There is no indication at this time that the client requires this referral
   Client Need: Psychosocial Integrity; **Cognitive Level:** Analysis; **Integrated Process:** Communication/Documentation; **Nursing Process:** Planning/Implementation

11. **2 Paraphrasing encourages the client to express the rationale for this request**
   1 Suggesting that the client is worried about pain is making an assumption without enough information. 3 Reminding the client that labor is uncomfortable may increase the client's anxiety. 4 Although the client's request should be forwarded to the health care provider, the reason for the choice of general anesthesia should be explored
   Client Need: Psychosocial Integrity; **Cognitive Level:** Application; **Integrated Process:** Communication/Documentation; **Nursing Process:** Assessment/Analysis

12. **3 Relaxation of muscles and facial expression are examples of nonverbal behavior; nonverbal behavior is an excellent index of feelings because it is less likely to be consciously controlled**
   1 Increased activity may be an expression of anger or hostility. 2 Clients may suppress verbal outbursts despite feelings and become withdrawn. 4 Refusing to talk may be a sign that the client is just not ready to discuss feelings
   Client Need: Psychosocial Integrity; **Cognitive Level:** Application; **Integrated Process:** Communication/Documentation; **Nursing Process:** Evaluation/Outcomes

13. **3 Reflecting the client's feelings addresses the fact that the client's feelings of anxiety are valid**
   1 Telling the client that worrying does not help does not address the client's concerns and may inhibit the expression of feelings. 2 Telling the client to wait for the biopsy does not address the client's concerns and may inhibit the expression of feelings. 4 Whether operations are performed is irrelevant and does not address the client's concerns
   Client Need: Psychosocial Integrity; **Cognitive Level:** Application; **Integrated Process:** Caring; **Nursing Process:** Planning/Implementation

14. **3 Letting an adolescent know it would be helpful to understand and requesting to talk attempts to open the communication process**
   1 Reflecting the words, not the feelings, serves to entrench the communicant's position and does little to open the flow of communication. 2 Talking about when you were a teenager shifts the focus away from the client. 4 Authoritative language closes the flow of communication
   Client Need: Psychosocial Integrity; **Cognitive Level:** Application; **Integrated Process:** Communication/Documentation; **Nursing Process:** Planning/Implementation

15. **2 The nurse has demonstrated recognition of the verbalized concern and a willingness to listen**
   1 The client did not state that he or she thinks that cancer is the diagnosis; this response puts the client on the defensive. 3 Avoiding the question indicates that the nurse is unwilling to listen. 4 Suggesting that the client wait to worry cuts off communication and denies feelings
   Client Need: Psychosocial Integrity; **Cognitive Level:** Application; **Integrated Process:** Caring, Communication/Documentation; **Nursing Process:** Planning/Implementation

16. **3 Reflecting the client's feelings is a response that promotes an exploration of the client's dilemma; it encourages further communication**
   1 Although true, telling the client that only he or she can make the decision is not supportive and abandons the client. 2 It is inappropriate for the nurse to give advice. 4 It is inappropriate for the nurse to give advice
   Client Need: Psychosocial Integrity; **Cognitive Level:** Application; **Integrated Process:** Caring, Communication/Documentation; **Nursing Process:** Planning/Implementation

17. **2 Communication is important in relieving anxiety and reducing stress**

    1 Administering a sedative does not acknowledge the client's feelings and does not address the source of the anxiety. **3** Learning is limited when anxiety is too high. **4** The focus should be on the client, not others; reassurance may cut off communication and deny emotions

    Client Need: Psychosocial Integrity; **Cognitive Level:** Application; **Integrated Process:** Caring, Communication/Documentation; **Nursing Process:** Planning/Implementation

18. **2 The nurse should identify clues to a client's anxiety and encourage verbalization of feelings**

    1 Telling the client you don't mind the task negates the client's feelings and presents a negative connotation. **3** Telling the client that the task is part of your job focuses on the task rather than on the client's feelings. **4** Telling the client that you are accustomed to the task negates the client's feelings and presents a negative connotation

    Client Need: Psychosocial Integrity; **Cognitive Level:** Application; **Integrated Process:** Caring, Communication/Documentation; **Nursing Process:** Planning/Implementation

19. **1 Reflecting the client's concern is open-ended and encourages the client to verbalize concerns**

    2 Making a generalized statement about other people cuts off communication. **3** Nothing in the situation indicates that surgery is planned; referring to the client's record may increase anxiety. **4** Stating your lack of information and referring the client to the health care provider cuts off communication

    Client Need: Psychosocial Integrity; **Cognitive Level:** Application; **Integrated Process:** Caring, Communication/Documentation; **Nursing Process:** Planning/Implementation

---

Memory Aid: *It is important to reflect on the "products" of your communication.* Use the memory aid "PRODuCTS" to recall how important it is for YOU to use the therapeutic communication techniques:

P: Paraphrasing

R: Reflection

O: Open-ended questions

D: Direct questions

u: YOU!

C: Clarification

T: Touch

S: Silence

---

20. **4 The use of reflection assists the client in expressing feelings, which is the major goal of therapy**

    1 Telling the client that the therapist is good is a defensive response by the nurse that tends to cut off communication and limit the expression of feelings. **2** Giving a response about the rest of the staff avoids discussion of the client's feelings about the therapist. **3** Putting the responsibility on the client to cooperate is a defensive response by the nurse that tends to cut off communication and limit the expression of feelings

    Client Need: Psychosocial Integrity; **Cognitive Level:** Application; **Integrated Process:** Caring, Communication/Documentation; **Nursing Process:** Planning/Implementation

3 Standards of Practice and Nursing Process

STANDARDS OF PRACTICE IN MENTAL HEALTH NURSING

Overview
- The nursing process is a systematic, analytic approach to health care that encompasses critical thinking, specific actions, and decision making (Fig. 3.1). It is a sequence of steps used to meet the client's needs.

Assessment
- Purpose: To gather and organize a database with the eventual goal to develop a client-centered treatment plan and prioritize problems to be addressed to meet the client's needs
- Includes client's mental status, psychosocial state, physical health, pain level, cultural and spiritual preferences, and verbal/nonverbal behaviors with the use of various methods of data collection:
  - Types of data: Objective (overt, measurable, detected by physical assessment); subjective (covert, feelings, sensations, and symptoms verbalized by client)
  - Sources of data: Client (primary), family and friends, health care team members, clinical record, and other documents
  - Methods of data collection: Interviewing, observation of nonverbal cues, congruency between verbal and nonverbal data, physical assessment (eg, observation, palpation, auscultation, percussion)
- Assessment includes management of data: Screening, organizing, and grouping or clustering significant defining characteristics and related information
- Three stages of assessment: Initial assessment, assessment, and ongoing assessments
  - Initial assessment covers demographic data, reason for and date of admission, previous psychiatric history, current medical problems and medications, any substance use or abuse, disturbances in daily living, culture and spirituality, current or history of substance use disorder, and support systems
  - Assessment: The mental status examination (MSE) and the psychosocial assessment are essential parts of every nursing assessment
    - The MSE helps the nurse collect objective data about the client's appearance, behavior, activity, attitude, speech, mood, affect, perceptions, thoughts, thought content and process, sensorium, cognition, insight, and reliability
    - Psychosocial assessment collects criteria that include the client's stressors; coping skills; relationships; *and* cultural, spiritual, and work-related issues
  - Ongoing assessments continue throughout care as client behavior is observed, allowing for follow-up questions
    - Important steps of the nursing assessment include:
      - Consider the client's age: Use observation of play as part of assessment of children and consider sensory deficits common in the older adult
      - Assess for behaviors or risk factors that threaten the safety of the client or others (eg, suicide, self-harm, assault or violence, withdrawal from alcohol or other substances, allergic reactions, command hallucinations)

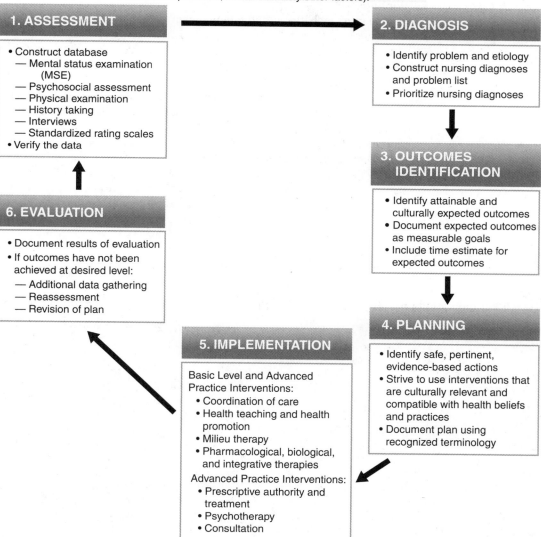

NURSING ASSESSMENT

The assessment interview requires culturally effective communication skills and encompasses a large database (e.g., significant support system; family; cultural and community system; spiritual and philosophical values, strengths, and health beliefs and practices; as well as many other factors).

1. ASSESSMENT

- Construct database
  — Mental status examination (MSE)
  — Psychosocial assessment
  — Physical examination
  — History taking
  — Interviews
  — Standardized rating scales
- Verify the data

2. DIAGNOSIS

- Identify problem and etiology
- Construct nursing diagnoses and problem list
- Prioritize nursing diagnoses

3. OUTCOMES IDENTIFICATION

- Identify attainable and culturally expected outcomes
- Document expected outcomes as measurable goals
- Include time estimate for expected outcomes

6. EVALUATION

- Document results of evaluation
- If outcomes have not been achieved at desired level:
  — Additional data gathering
  — Reassessment
  — Revision of plan

5. IMPLEMENTATION

Basic Level and Advanced Practice Interventions:
- Coordination of care
- Health teaching and health promotion
- Milieu therapy
- Pharmacological, biological, and integrative therapies

Advanced Practice Interventions:
- Prescriptive authority and treatment
- Psychotherapy
- Consultation

4. PLANNING

- Identify safe, pertinent, evidence-based actions
- Strive to use interventions that are culturally relevant and compatible with health beliefs and practices
- Document plan using recognized terminology

FIG. 3.1   The nursing process in psychiatric mental health nursing. Note the cyclic and interactive nature of the nursing process. (From Varcarolis, E. M., & Halter, M. J. [2010]. *Psychiatric mental health nursing: A clinical approach* [6th ed.]. St. Louis, MO: Saunders.)

- Review physical status, perform a review of systems, and obtain baseline vital signs *with the knowledge that some physical conditions mimic psychiatric illness*
- Assess for physical pain on a scale of 1 to 10 and for medical problems that may affect client functioning, mood state, or overall well-being
- Establish trust, rapport, and respect throughout client contact; rapport can be defined as feelings of warmth, acceptance, trust, and nonjudgmental attitude between the client and the nurse that ideally takes place at the beginning of a therapeutic relationship
- Maintain a calm, empathetic, and nonjudgmental attitude
- Consider the age, ethnicity, culture, sexuality, and language of client and the family
- Determine the client's current level of mental, emotional, and psychosocial functioning; include cognition, mood, affect, coping, relatedness, recent stress or trauma, hygiene, and posture
- Recognize aspects of the client's behaviors, vulnerabilities, beliefs, or other areas that require attention to affect a positive outcome. In addition, determine the importance of religion to the client
- Conduct an MSE (Box 3.1); the completion of the MSE sometimes involves several interviews, because the client is not always immediately responsive to all parts of the examination during the acute phase of illness; therefore patience and persistence are important
  - Behavioral rating scales can be used to assess various disorders such as anxiety, depression, mania, schizophrenia, cognitive disorders, eating disorders, and substance use disorders
- Ask the client and family what outcomes they expect to obtain from treatment; family expectations may differ from realistic outcomes
- Assess coping skills, resources, motivation, and supportive relationships

---

BOX 3.1 **Components of Assessment: Mental Status Examination and Psychosocial Criteria**

Mental Status Examination

Appearance
Dress, grooming, hygiene, cosmetics, age, posture, and facial expression

Behavior/Activity
Hypoactivity or hyperactivity; rigid, relaxed, restless, or agitated motor movements; gait (way of walking) and coordination; facial grimacing; gestures or mannerisms that are passive, combative, or bizarre (eg, odd repetitive gestures, abnormal movements)

Attitude
Interactions with the interviewer: Cooperative, resistive, friendly, hostile, or ingratiating

Speech
Quantity: Poverty of speech (few words), poverty of content (lack of content), or voluminous (too many words)
Quality: Articulate (well spoken), congruent (makes sense), monotonous (monotone), talkative, repetitious, spontaneous, circumlocutory (circular), confabulation (fabrication), tangential (superficial), pressured (rapid, urgent), stereotypic (repetitive), disorganized (unstructured), or fragmented (broken speech)
Rate: Slowed, rapid, or normal

Mood and Affect
Mood (intensity, depth, and duration): Sad, fearful, depressed, angry, anxious, ambivalent (opposing feelings), happy, ecstatic, or grandiose (feeling of greatness)
Affect (intensity, depth, and duration): Appropriate, sad, apathetic (indifferent), constricted (narrowed), blunted (little expression), flat (no expression), labile (changing expressions), euphoric (exaggerated happiness), or bizarre (odd or abnormal)

Perceptions
Hallucinations (experiences an unreal presence; can be auditory, visual, tactile, or olfactory), illusions (misinterprets reality; can be auditory, visual, tactile, or olfactory), depersonalization (detachment), derealization (disconnects from reality), or distortions (views objects out of proportion)

BOX 3.1	Components of Assessment: Mental Status Examination and Psychosocial Criteria—cont'd

Thoughts

Form and content: Logical versus illogical, loose associations (fragmented), flight of ideas (rapid thoughts), autistic (internally stimulated thoughts), blocking, broadcasting, neologisms (new words), word salad (mixed-up words), obsessions (persistent thoughts), ruminations (rethinking the same thought), delusions (fixed beliefs), or abstract (conceptual) versus concrete (literal)

Sensorium/Cognition

Levels of consciousness, orientation (awareness of person, place, time, and situation), attention span, recent and remote memory (can recall current and past events), and concentration; ability to comprehend and process information; intelligence, fund of knowledge (sufficient amount of knowledge), and insight (awareness of situation such as of own illness and reason for hospitalization); and ability to abstract and use proverbs (understands meanings of common sayings and expressions)

Judgment

Ability to assess and evaluate situations, make rational decisions, understand consequences of behavior, and take responsibility for actions

Insight

Ability to perceive and understand the cause and nature of own and others' situations; aware of his or her mental illness and its effects and symptoms

Reliability

Interviewer's impression that individual reported information accurately and completely

Risk Assessment

Suicide ideation, homicide (or violence) ideation; self-harm ideation

Psychosocial Criteria

Stressors

Internal: Psychiatric or medical illness, including pain and perceived loss (eg, loss of self-concept or self-esteem)

External: Actual loss (eg, death of a loved one, divorce, lack of support system, job or financial loss, retirement, dysfunctional family system)

Coping Skills

Adaptation to internal and external stressors, the use of functional and adaptive coping mechanisms and techniques, the management of activities of daily living, and the ability to solve problems associated with daily life

Relationships

Attainment and maintenance of satisfying interpersonal relationships congruent with developmental stage, including sexual relationships as appropriate for age and status

Cultural

Ability to adapt and conform to prescribed norms, rules, ethics, and mores of an identified group

Spiritual (Value Belief)

Presence of a self-satisfying value-belief system that the individual regards as right, desirable, worthwhile, and comforting

Occupational

Engagement in useful and rewarding activity that is congruent with developmental stage and societal standards (ie, work, school, and recreation)

Modified from Fortinash, K.M. & Holoday, P.A. (2012). *Psychiatric mental health nursing* (5th ed.). St. Louis: Mosby.

Nursing Diagnosis

- The nurse develops a nursing diagnosis based on subjective and objective data that are analyzed during the assessment phase
- Nursing diagnoses are statements that describe a person's health state and responses to actual or potential health problems; they are based on reliable clinical judgments made by the nurse after an *extensive* nursing assessment
- It is critical for the nurse to select nursing diagnoses that are based on accurate assessment of the client's immediate needs because these diagnoses determine the selection of therapeutic outcomes and interventions

- Diagnoses requiring emergent care and focused on safety get priority
- Format of nursing diagnoses: Three parts include
  - Actual problem, unmet need, or "risk for"
  - Contributing or etiologic factors
  - Defining characteristic or behavioral outcome
- Note: Nursing diagnoses do <u>not</u> include medical diagnoses in any of the three parts
- Nursing diagnoses are based on client responses and needs that the nurse is able to treat; they differ from medical diagnoses in that the medical diagnosis names the disease
- Although nurses are knowledgeable about mental health disorders and treatments, they focus mainly on the client's responses to the disorder and the effects that the disorder has on the client
- Nurses also manage the client's vulnerabilities, coping methods, risk factors, and other responses related to the mental disorder
- NANDA-I includes health promotion and wellness diagnoses as categories that are less commonly used in acute care settings; these types of diagnoses are often one-part only.
- DSM-5 is the source for medical psychiatric diagnoses, released in 2013
  - This approach is consistent with the World Health Organization (WHO) and the International Classification of Diseases (ICD) guidelines that consider the individual's functional state separately from his or her diagnosis or symptom status
- Because nursing diagnoses describe client's responses to illness and because there are many more nursing diagnoses than psychiatric diagnoses, nurses have every opportunity to assess a client's overall functioning status through the steps of the nursing process

Outcome Identification

- The nurse identifies goals for client behaviors (outcomes) that will indicate resolution of a problem on the basis of nursing diagnosis statements and as the result of nursing interventions
- Outcome statements are *specific, measurable* indicators that nurses use to evaluate the results of their interventions (Table 3.1)
  - Outcomes are desired changes in client's behavior, activity, or physical state
  - Outcomes must be objective, achievable, and measurable, and include a realistic period for accomplishment to determine whether outcome has been achieved

TABLE 3.1   Correct vs. Incorrect Outcome Statements

Nursing Diagnosis	Incorrect Outcome Statement	Correct Outcome Statement
Anxiety	Exhibits decreased anxiety; engages in stress reduction	Verbalizes feeling calm and relaxed, with an absence of muscle tension and diaphoresis; practices deep breathing
Ineffective coping	Demonstrates effective coping abilities	Makes own decisions to attend groups; seeks staff for interactions rather than remaining isolated in room
Hopelessness	Expresses increased feelings of hope	Makes plans for the future (eg, to continue therapy after discharge); states, "My kids need me to be well"

- Nurses collaborate with client, family or significant others, and appropriate health care team members to formulate a plan to reach identified outcomes
- Outcomes are measured along a continuum, and they describe the best health state that the client can realistically achieve
- Outcomes come from nursing diagnosis statements and are projections or estimates of what nurses expect to happen as a result of their interventions
- The term *behavioral goals* is often used interchangeably with *outcomes* to describe the effectiveness of nursing interventions in replacing dysfunctional behaviors
- The Nursing Outcomes Classification (NOC) was the first standardized language for describing client outcomes that are most responsive to nursing care or that are most influenced by the actions or interventions of nurses
  - NOC outcomes contain indicators that are rated on a five-point continuum, which allows the nurse to measure a client's mental or physical state in relation to an outcome
  - Outcomes reflect the client's actual health state at the time of achievement and are met at any place along the continuum
  - Some outcomes are achieved in less time than others, and the nurse continues to intervene with the client until the client reaches all outcomes at the highest possible level
  - Outcome statements are the opposite of defining characteristics or risk factors; for example, "client exhibits proper hygiene" as an outcome statement instead of "body odor" as a defining characteristic
- Outcomes should be stated so that they clearly describe client behaviors and use the client's own words to describe his or her feelings and thoughts, as appropriate
- It is important to include some type of measurement tool or limits for predicting client progress or problem resolution

APPLICATION AND REVIEW

1. A nurse is explaining the nursing process to a nursing assistant. Which step of the nursing process should include interpretation of data collected about the client?
   1. Analysis
   2. Assessment
   3. Nursing interventions
   4. Proposed nursing care
2. Which of these parts is included in a nursing diagnosis? *Select all that apply.*
   1. Actual problem
   2. Associated DSM-5 diagnosis
   3. Contributing or etiologic factors
   4. Defining characteristic or behavioral outcome
3. Which of these are the *specific, measurable* indicators that nurses use to evaluate the results of their interventions?
   1. Data from assessment
   2. Evidence-based practices
   3. Concept maps
   4. Nursing outcomes
4. Why is review of physical status part of the nursing assessment for psychiatric clients?
   1. To confirm relationships the client has with others
   2. In case the client is at the wrong location for treatment
   3. In case there is a physical etiology to the mental condition
   4. To complete the standard form

5. Which of these is a type of data?
   1. Health promotion
   2. Interviewing
   3. Subjective
   4. Client
6. Which tool does the nurse use to collect objective data about the client's activity, attitude, speech, mood, affect, perceptions, thoughts, sensorium, cognition, insight, and reliability?
   1. Mental status examination
   2. Psychosocial assessment
   3. Nursing outcomes
   4. Initial assessment

See Answers on pages 44-45.

Planning

- The nurse plans and prioritizes client care with the client, the health care provider, and the interdisciplinary team
- The planning of client care builds on the previous three phases of the nursing process
- The ultimate selection of nursing interventions should help provide successful client outcomes
- The planning phase consists of the total planning of the client's treatment to achieve quality outcomes in a safe, effective, and timely manner
- Nursing interventions with rationales are selected during the planning phase on the basis of the client's identified risk factors and defining characteristics
- The nurse's planning process includes:
  - Meeting and working with clients, family members, and treatment team members
    - Identifying priorities of care
    - Coordinating and delegating responsibilities according to the treatment team's expertise as it relates to client needs
    - Making clinical decisions about the use of psychotherapeutic scientific principles with the use of evidence-based practice
- Evidence-based practice is practice that is based on evidence and scientific principles that have been developed through research
- It is vital to include empiric methods in clinical practice when relevant rather than use only intuitiveness, experience, fashion, or ideology, because many research findings conflict with public beliefs about mental health
- *Clinical Pathways* are standardized multidisciplinary planning tools that monitor client care through projected caregiver interventions and expected client outcomes and that are based on the client's DSM mental health disorder
  - They are tools that promote cost-effectiveness, interdisciplinary care, and accessible client status reports among staff
  - A pathway is mapped along a continuum of chronologic targets
  - It usually includes an estimate of the client's length of stay based on the designated related group of mental illnesses and the need for continued treatment
  - Client progress is measured daily along the timelines
  - Nurses primarily initiate pathways, and they involve other disciplines in planning and implementation
  - A pathway may be extended to include the client's transfer to home care or to another treatment facility
  - Pathway variances occur when the client did not respond to the interventions in the typical way; they can be positive or negative

- A concept map is a problem-solving plan that includes *all* of the relevant elements of the client's database: Medical diagnosis, nursing diagnosis, pathophysiology, risk factors, clinical manifestations, collaborative problems, expected outcomes, and interventions
  - Interventions include medication administration, therapeutic modalities, laboratory tests and other procedures, social skills training, and teaching and learning needs
  - It clarifies the *relationships* among concepts and topics and promotes an understanding of the client situation as a whole
  - The client is the focus of care, and data are arranged in a logical structure that shows the relationships among the elements via lines or arrows
    - They break down complex relevant data into manageable pieces that can be quickly absorbed
  - There is generally a brief case history or case study of the client's status (diagnosis, objective data, subjective data, orders) and a summary statement
  - A concept map can be the care plan or an adjunct to the care plan

Implementation

- Nursing interventions are critical action components of the implementation phase and the most powerful pieces of the nursing process
- Nursing interventions describe a specific course of action or a therapeutic activity that helps the client move toward a more functional state; they do not simply respond to health care provider orders
- Nursing interventions relate directly to planning: Safety, structure, support, and symptom management; for example:
  - Promoting health and safety
  - Monitoring medication schedules and effects
  - Providing adequate nutrition and hydration
  - Creating a nurturing and therapeutic environment
  - Continuing to build trust, self-esteem, and dignity
  - Participating in therapeutic groups and activities
  - Developing client strengths and coping methods
  - Improving communication and social skills
  - Connecting family and community support systems
  - Preventing relapse with the use of effective discharge planning
- In Nursing Interventions Classification (NIC), the authors define nursing interventions as "any treatment based upon clinical judgment and knowledge that a nurse performs to enhance patient/client outcomes"
- Care can be individualized from a standard intervention
- NIC interventions are linked to NOC outcomes, NANDA-I diagnoses, and other organizing structures to ensure clear and consistent language for nurses in all practice settings and locations
- Interventions have the greatest influence when they are focused toward etiologies (related factors) that accompany an actual diagnosis or when the nurse aims them at the risk factors of a risk diagnosis
- Etiologies and risk factors change from client to client, even when the diagnosis is the same, so it is important to select interventions that target each client's specific etiologies, risk factors, and defining characteristics (signs and symptoms)
- A rationale statement is the reason for the nursing intervention
  - Rationales are not always part of the written care plan in clinical practice, yet they are generally part of the overall discussion of treatment in team meetings
  - Rationales reflect nurses' accountability for their actions

Evaluation

- Overview
  - Assess client's response to care
  - Compare actual outcome to expected outcome
  - Evaluation reflects the success of nursing interventions
  - If outcome is not reached, previous steps must be examined to determine reason
  - Plan of care may need to be revised
  - Priorities may require reordering because process of evaluation is ongoing
- Evaluation of the client's progress and the nursing activities involved are critical because nurses are accountable for the standards of care in each discipline
- The evaluation of achieved outcomes occurs at various times during treatment as stated in the outcomes section, with the client's health state and capabilities being the primary considerations
- There are two steps in the evaluation phase:
  - The nurse compares the client's current mental health state or condition with the outcome statement
  - The nurse considers all of the possible reasons that the client did not achieve outcomes by asking questions
- The nurse makes recommendations on the basis of the conclusions drawn from these questions; this often includes a review of the previous steps of the nursing process
- When the implementation of a plan does not produce the desired outcome, it is necessary to revise the plan
- An informal evaluation of the client's progress takes place continually

Documentation

- It is mandatory for the nurse to record (in accordance with facility standards) an evaluation of the client's changing condition, informed consents (for medication and treatment), response to medication, ability to engage in treatment programs, signs and symptoms (with suicidal and homicidal tendencies being the most critical), concerns (in the client's words, as appropriate), and any other critical incidents that occur
- Documentation can be in narrative, checklist, or electronic (computerized) form
- Although the entire team is responsible for relating client progress, the nurse in charge is generally accountable for accurate record keeping. However, each discipline has standards for documentation; for insurance reimbursement, medical documentation is critical.
- Documentation is important for legal issues such as confidentiality and privacy acts, insurance reimbursement, accreditation, quality assurance, case management, utilization review, peer review, and research
  - The entire chart is a legal document
  - Different types of records (progress notes, shift reports, discharge summary, etc.) and different formats (written and electronic) are all legal documents
- Problem-oriented SOAP charting
  - The SOAP note is a problem-solving method that nurses use in all health care settings to analyze relevant client problems and to prevent long text.
  - *SOAP* is an acronym for *s*ubjective data (client statement), *o*bjective data (nurse's observations), assessment (nurse's analysis of S and O, which is often a problem statement or nursing diagnosis), and *p*lan (nurse's proposed actions)
    - SOAP notes are generally based on problems or diagnoses that are formulated by the multidisciplinary team

- SOAP notes become part of the client's care plan. Although this promotes consistency during problem solving, it also restricts entries to only identified problems; therefore recorders need to be aware of other client issues that happen and to report them as well
  - Two other letters were added later to the SOAP note: *I* (*i*nterventions, or nurse's response to problem) and *E* (*e*valuation of client outcomes)
- Other similar problem-oriented methods are DAR (for *d*ata, *a*nalysis, and *r*esponse) and PIE (for *p*roblem, *i*ntervention, and *e*valuation)
- The medical record should also include changes in client condition, informed consents (for medications and treatments), reaction to medication, documentation of symptoms (verbatim—using quotes around what the patient says—when appropriate), and the client's concerns
- All concerns in documentation for privacy, timeliness, completeness, and communication for other types of clients apply to psychiatric/mental health clients. There are additional privacy regulations that relate to privacy regarding substance abuse.
- Electronic documentation
  - Electronic health records (EHRs) are also be used for documentation
  - Some EHRs have software for nursing care plans
  - Components of electronic documentation are basically the same as written documentation, and all legal parameters apply equally to electronic documentation as they do to written documentation
  - Protect screens from inadvertent viewing by others; privacy regulations apply equally to electronic formats as they do to written formats

APPLICATION AND REVIEW

7. Place each step of the nursing process in the order that they should be used.
   1. _____ Identify goals for care
   2. _____ Develop a plan of care
   3. _____ State client's nursing needs
   4. _____ Obtain client's nursing history
   5. _____ Implement nursing interventions
8. A newly oriented home health nurse on a first visit checks the client's vital signs and obtains a blood sample for an international normalization ratio (INR). After completion of these tasks, the client asks the nurse to straighten the blankets on the bed. What is the nurse's **most** appropriate response?
   1. "I would, but my back hurts today"
   2. "OK. It will be my good deed for the day"
   3. "Of course. I want to do whatever I can for you"
   4. "I would like to, but it is not in my job description"
9. A nurse is reviewing a client's plan of care. What is the determining factor in the revision of the plan?
   1. Time available for care
   2. Validity of the problem
   3. Method for providing care
   4. Effectiveness of the interventions
10. Which of these are standardized multidisciplinary planning tools that monitor client care?
    1. Evidence-based practices
    2. NOC
    3. NIC
    4. Clinical pathways

11. Interventions have the greatest influence when they are focused toward _____ that accompany an actual nursing diagnosis or aimed at the risk factors of a risk nursing diagnosis.

    1. Etiologies (related factors)   3. Potential problems
    2. Defining characteristics   4. Concept maps

12. When does an informal evaluation of the client's progress take place?

    1. Never   3. Continually
    2. Part of MSE   4. In SOAPIE

See Answers on pages 44-45.

ANSWER KEY: REVIEW QUESTIONS

1. **1 An actual or potential client health problem is based on the analysis and interpretation of the data previously collected during the assessment phase of the nursing process**

   2 Gathering data is included in the client's assessment. **3** Nursing interventions are based on the earlier steps of the nursing process. **4** The plan of care includes nursing actions to meet client needs; the needs must first be identified before nursing actions are planned

   Client Need: Management of Care; **Cognitive Level:** Comprehension; **Integrated Process:** Teaching/Learning; **Nursing Process:** Planning/Implementation

2. **Answers: 1, 3, 4**

   1 The actual problem, unmet need, or "at risk for" condition is included in a nursing diagnosis. **3** Contributing or etiologic factors are included in a nursing diagnosis. **4** Defining characteristic or behavioral outcome are included in a nursing diagnosis.

   2 DSM diagnoses are medical diagnoses and not included in nursing diagnoses

   Client Need: Management of Care; **Cognitive Level:** Comprehension; **Nursing Process:** Diagnosis

3. **4 Nursing outcomes are the *specific, measurable* indicators that nurses use to evaluate the results of their interventions**

   1 Data from assessment are not the specific, measurable indicators used to evaluate the results of nursing interventions. **2** Evidence-based practices are not the specific, measurable indicators used to evaluate the results of nursing interventions. **3** Concept maps are not the specific, measurable indicators used to evaluate the results of nursing interventions

   Client Need: Management of Care; **Cognitive Level:** Comprehension; **Nursing Process:** Assessment/Analysis

4. **3 Review of physical status part of assessment for psychiatric clients is important because some physical conditions mimic psychiatric illness**

   1 Assessment of relationships occurs during the psychosocial assessment. **2** The initial assessment should confirm that the client is at the correct location. **4** Completing a standard form is not why the review of physical status is performed

   Client Need: Physiological Integrity; **Cognitive Level:** Comprehension; **Nursing Process:** Assessment/Analysis

5. **3 Subjective data is a type of data collected during assessment**

   1 Health promotion is not a type of data, but it can be included in a nursing diagnosis. **2** Interviewing is not a type of data; it is a method used to collect data. **3** The client is not a type of data, but data is collected from the client

   Client Need: Management of Care; **Cognitive Level:** Knowledge; **Nursing Process:** Assessment/Analysis

6. **1 The nurse uses the MSE to collect objective data about the client's appearance, behavior, activity, attitude, speech, mood, affect, perceptions, thoughts, sensorium, cognition, insight, and reliability**

   2 Psychosocial assessment collects information about the client's stressors, coping skills, relationships, and cultural, spiritual, and work-related issues. **3** Nursing outcomes are not a data assessment tool. **4** The initial assessment covers demographic data, reason for and date of admission, previous psychiatric history, current medical problems and medications, any substance use or abuse, disturbances in daily living, culture and spirituality, and support systems

Client Need: Management of Care; **Cognitive Level:** Knowledge; **Nursing Process:** Assessment/Analysis

7. **Answer: 4, 3, 1, 2, 5**

4 First the nurse should gather data. **3** Based on the data, the client's needs are assessed; **1** After the needs have been determined, the goals for care are established. **2** The next step is planning care based on the knowledge gained from the previous steps. **5** Implementation follows the development of the plan of care

Client Need: Management of Care; **Cognitive Level:** Application; **Nursing Process:** Planning/Implementation; **Reference:** Chapter 2, Nursing Process

8. **3 Helping the client meet physical needs is within the role of the nurse; arranging blankets on the client's bed is an appropriate intervention**

1 The nurse's comfort needs should not take precedence over the client's needs; the nurse should not assume responsibility for the role of care provider if incapable of providing care. **2** It is not a good deed but fulfills the expected role of the nurse; this response sounds grudgingly compliant. **4** Helping the client meet physical needs is within the nurse's job description

Client Need: Physiological Integrity; **Cognitive Level:** Application; **Integrated Process:** Caring; **Nursing Process:** Planning/Implementation

9. **4 When the implementation of a plan of care does not effectively produce the desired outcome, the plan should be changed**

1 Time is not relevant in the revision of a plan of care. **2** Client response to care is the determining factor, not the validity of the health problem. **3** Various methods may have the same outcome; their effectiveness is most important

Client Need: Management of Care; **Cognitive Level:** Comprehension; **Nursing Process:** Evaluation/Outcomes

10. **4 Clinical pathways are standardized multidisciplinary planning tools that monitor client care**

1 Evidence-based practices are practices based on evidence and scientific principles that have been developed through research. **2** NOC is standardized language for describing client outcomes that are most responsive to nursing. **3** NIC are treatments based on clinical judgment and knowledge that a nurse performs to enhance client/client outcomes

Client Need: Management of Care; **Cognitive Level:** Comprehension; **Nursing Process:** Planning/Implementation

11. **1 Interventions have the greatest influence when they are focused toward etiologies (related factors) that accompany an actual diagnosis or aimed at the risk factors of a risk diagnosis**

2 Focusing interventions on defining characteristics is not as effective as focusing toward etiologies. **3** Potential problems or risk diagnoses are not the focus of intervention for an actual diagnosis. **4** A concept map is a problem-solving plan that includes *all* of the relevant elements of the client's database; it is not the focus of an intervention for an actual nursing diagnosis

Client Need: Management of Care; **Cognitive Level:** Knowledge; **Nursing Process:** Planning/Implementation

12. **3 An informal evaluation of the client's progress takes place continually**

1 Informal evaluation of the client's progress takes place continually. **2** The MSE gathers data such as appearance, behavior, activity, attitude, speech, mood, affect, perceptions; it is not a form of evaluation; it is part of the assessment step. **4** SOAPIE is a form of charting by exception—*s*ubjective data (client statement), *o*bjective data (nurse's observations), *a*ssessment (nurse's analysis of S and O, which is often a problem statement or nursing diagnosis), *p*lan (nurse's proposed actions), *I* (*i*nterventions or nurse's response to problem), and *E* (*e*valuation of client outcomes); the "E" of SOAPIE is a formal evaluation, not an informal one

Client Need: Management of Care; **Cognitive Level:** Knowledge; **Nursing Process:** Evaluation

Legal and Ethical Issues

ETHICAL DILEMMAS

- Ethics is that body of knowledge that explores the moral problems surrounding specific issues
- Ethical dilemma: Situation with conflict between or among more than one course of action in which each option has advantages and disadvantages
  - The conflict arises because of differences in values or judgments
  - For example, a client's right to refuse treatment can seem like an ethical dilemma to a nurse
- Your value system can conflict with that of your workplace, which can create more stress for you; ethical problems occur in mental health law when statutes conflict with a nurse's personal beliefs
- You have a duty to examine your values so you are aware of them and prepared to handle situations
- Nurses working with mental health clients need to be prepared to confront ethical dilemmas and analyze issues that may conflict with personal beliefs as thoroughly as possible

ETHICAL PRINCIPLES

Terminology

- *Autonomy* (self-determination)
  - *Defined* as having respect for an individual's decisions or self-determination regarding health care issues
  - Especially important with problems such as the right to die and, in mental health, treatment with the use of the least restrictive alternative
  - When involuntary commitment is necessary, it is difficult for mental health providers to have to follow the law rather than to do what the client currently desires
  - The caregiver will want to allow the client to make decisions, but if the individual is demonstrating intent by threatening suicide with an active plan, proceeding against the wishes of the person is necessary for safety and compliance with the law
  - This kind of decision in ethical terms is called a *paternalistic decision,* which often causes anxiety for the health care professional
  - One loses autonomy when secluded or restrained
- *Beneficence* (promotion of or bringing about good)
  - Individuals in health care have a duty and responsibility to act in a manner that benefits rather than harms clients
- *Nonmaleficence* (avoidance of harm)
  - The moral rule of *primum non nocere* ("first do no harm") applies to psychiatric mental health nursing
- *Justice* (fairness)
- *Veracity* (truthfulness) and *fidelity* (faithfulness)
  - The nurse has a duty to be truthful with clients and to care faithfully for them
- *Accountability* (answerable for one's own actions) and *responsibility* (dependable role performance)
  - The nurse is responsible for his or her own actions and must be dependable in performing tasks
- *Confidentiality* (maintaining privacy)
  - The nurse has a duty to keep client records confidential (see Rights of Clients)

MAKING ETHICAL DECISIONS

Overview

- Code of ethics (American Nurses Association Code of Ethics for Nurses) guides professional practice and reflects moral values of group
  - Code of ethics is broader and more universal than laws but cannot override laws
  - Ethical issues become legal issues through court case decisions or by legislative enactment

Steps in Ethical Decision Making (Table 4.1)

- Gathering background information means finding information to understand and clarify any issues
- Identifying ethical components means determining the ethical dilemma
- Clarification of the rights of agents means understanding and clarification of the rights of all the parties involved
- Exploring options involves considering every possible choice in the situation
- The fifth step, applying principles, can be approached in differing manners, including the best choice for all (utilitarianism), the best choice for oneself (egoism), using a formal rule (formalism), or fairness based on justice
- Resolution into action means to execute the plan chosen

Ethical Issues in Psychiatric-Mental Health Nursing

- Innumerable situations arise that raise ethical issues, such as:
  - Potentially irreversible side effects of medications: Is it worth taking the medication for a psychiatric diagnosis considering the irreversible damage to other body systems
  - Effects of treatments such as ECT (potential memory loss)
  - The potential harm by a health care worker having a sexual relationship with a client
  - Health care cost constraints: Who will be treated
  - Whether physical health care should be prioritized over mental health care

TABLE 4.1	Steps and Questions in Ethical Decision Making	
Steps	**Relevant Questions**
Gathering background information	Does an ethical dilemma exist? What information is known? What information is needed? What is the context of the dilemma? What is the underlying issue?
Identifying ethical components	Who is affected by this dilemma? What are the rights of each involved party? What are the obligations of each involved party?
Clarification of agents	Who should be involved in the decision making? For whom is the decision being made? What degree of consent is needed by the client? What alternatives exist?
Exploration of options	What is the purpose or intent of each alternative? What are the potential consequences of each alternative? What criteria should be used?
Application of principles	What ethical theories are advocated? What scientific facts are relevant? What is the nurse's philosophy of life and nursing? What are the social and legal constraints and ramifications? What is the goal of the nurse's decision?
Resolution into action	How can the resulting ethical choice be implemented? How can the resulting ethical choice be evaluated?

From Stuart, G. W. (2013). *Principles and practice of psychiatric nursing* (10 ed.). St. Louis, MO: Mosby/Elsevier.

- How reimbursement for mental health care is structured by third-party payers for health care
- Role of the nurse as a client advocate: What if the client's will is in conflict with that of the health care provider
- When there is an annual cap (limit) on how much a third-party payer will pay, will there be resistance to treating a client with a severe and persistent mental illness
- Are all treatment sites equal; will some disorders only be treated in hospitals; which disorders will be covered by insurance for treatment at community centers

LEGAL CONSIDERATIONS

Nurse Practice Acts

- Specific to each of the 50 US states
- Establish scope of practice for nurses in that state

Sources of Law

- Three main sources: Common law from judicial decisions, statutory law from state and federal governments, and administrative law made by agencies authorized by federal and state governments
- *Common law* is derived from actual court cases; the judicial system helps interpret written laws because written laws cannot cover every possible situation
- *Statutory law* is written by legislation; the order of precedence of laws that override other laws is US Constitution, federal law, and federal treaties; those three override state and local laws
- *Administrative law* is in charge of administration of government such as state boards of nursing
- *Civil law* concerns relationships of individuals and is different from criminal or military law; these laws regulate private matters and deal with people's rights instead of crimes
  - *Torts* are acts (that are not contract breaches) that hurt someone but are not crimes; torts are handled by civil court (see Torts Important to Nurses later in the chapter)
- *Contracts* are legal, binding agreements between parties (people or companies, for example)
- *Criminal law is* the law of crimes and their punishments

APPLICATION AND REVIEW

1. A graduate nurse is preparing to apply to the State Board of Nursing for licensure to practice as a registered professional nurse. What group primarily is protected under the regulations of the practice of nursing?
   1. The public
   2. Practicing nurses
   3. The employing agency
   4. People with health problems
2. Which ethical principle means avoidance of harm?
   1. Veracity
   2. Autonomy
   3. Beneficence
   4. Nonmaleficence

See Answers on pages 61-64.

LEGAL ISSUES IN PSYCHIATRIC-MENTAL HEALTH NURSING

Overview

- A fundamental component of psychiatric nursing is to understand the legal framework used to regulate the care and treatment of clients diagnosed with mental illness
- Each state has its own mental health code that delineates the law in this area; therefore the mental health laws vary from state to state; case law may also set precedents that guide care

Rights of Clients

- Adherence to the Patient Care Partnership (formerly the Patient's Bill of Rights) is essential
- All civil rights are maintained by clients
- Many states require that all clients receive a written summary of their rights in their own language on admission to an inpatient facility
- Clients have the right to be treated in the least restrictive environment; any curtailment of autonomy must be substantiated by documentation supporting the need to limit the client's freedom; clients retain the right to a lawyer and the right to request a court hearing; clients may execute a psychiatric advance directive stating treatment preferences
- Statutory restrictions may be imposed on client's rights
- The United States government has set stringent rules about using human subjects in research
- Rights of clients include:
  - Right to be treated with the least restrictive environment
  - Right to confidentiality
  - Right to freedom from restraints and seclusion
  - Right to give or refuse consent to treatment

The Right to Be Treated with the Least-Restrictive Environment

- Mental health treatment must be provided in the least restrictive environment with the use of the least restrictive treatment
- Developing a treatment plan involves the consideration of all alternatives, including such options as inpatient treatment, partial hospitalization, intensive outpatient treatment, home health services, and foster and respite care; an individual who resides in a community that has developed many care options is the least likely to be hospitalized
- The cost of health care services is also an important factor; the nurse needs to select the least restrictive, most clinically appropriate, and most cost-effective intervention to assist the client

HIPPA

- The Health Insurance Portability and Accountability Act (HIPAA) of 1996 regulates the protection and privacy of health information
- It guarantees the security and privacy of health information and outlines standards for enforcement; it gives clients the rights to:
  - Be educated about HIPPA
  - Access their own medical records
  - Correct or add to their records
  - Demand their authorization before records are shared with others
- HIPPA applies to all health care providers (ie, individuals or organizations that send bills or that are paid for health care)
- The Privacy Rule defines protected health information as any individually identifiable health information that an organization keeps, files, uses, or shares in an oral, electronic, or written form
- Both civil and criminal penalties of fines and prison sentences were established under HIPAA for the knowing violation of client privacy

Confidentiality and Right to Privacy

- The American Nurses Association *Code of Ethics for Nurses* defines the importance of keeping a client's information confidential
- Client information regarding all clients, voluntary and involuntary, should be treated confidentially

- At the time of admission to a mental health facility, admission staff often requests that clients sign a release-of-information document; the release of information usually includes:
  - The information that will be released
  - The persons or parties that the information will be shared with such as other health care providers and insurance providers
  - The purpose of the release of the information
  - The period of time during which the information will be released
- The release of confidential client information even for the best-intended purposes is risky; even when presented with a subpoena for the release of protected health information, consulting with an attorney from the nurse's place of employment before information is released is advisable
- The confidentiality of the client's information and the necessity of having a signed release from the client before releasing information—even to family members who are closely involved with the client's daily care—present challenges for the nurse
  - For instance, a client experiencing paranoia who refuses to sign a release of information for his parents who are the caregivers will result in the nurse having to tell the parents when they telephone, "I'm sorry, but I'm not able to give you any information at this time"; however, it is possible to also say, "However, if you have information that you think it would be important for me to know, I can listen to you"; in this way, the family is able to communicate important medical or behavioral history to the treatment facility without the nurse releasing any information about the client without that client's permission
- *Privileged communication* differs from confidentiality
  - It is enacted by statute to designated professionals such as clergy, attorneys, psychologists, or physicians
  - Several states are now including nurses and other health care professionals under these conditions; this reflects a major change in direction
  - The provisions of these statutes allow certain information given to professionals by clients to remain secret during any litigation
  - The privilege belongs to the client, and only the client can assert or waive this privilege; these statutes exclude the mandatory reporting of child, elder, impaired adult, and (in some instances) domestic violence; some communicable diseases that affect public safety; and information that will prevent a felony (eg, murder) from occurring

Restraint and Seclusion

- Restraint is any limiting of a person's body movement; it can be physical or chemical
- Seclusion is isolation of a person in a room that the person cannot leave
- The right to be treated without restraint or seclusion protects the client and prevents injury or death from the restraints or seclusion
- Restraint and seclusion must not be used to substitute for appropriate treatment and management
- A client who is a threat to self or others may be placed in a seclusion room or in four-point restraint to prevent injury or harm. Laws vary by state and protocols by institution; consider the following as typical requirements:
  - A health care provider must give an order for seclusion or restraint for each incident and renew it every few hours as determined by state mental health law; prn seclusion and restraint orders are not acceptable
  - The nurse must document the initial and continued need for seclusion or restraints; the client must be observed constantly if in restraints and checked every 15 minutes if in seclusion; hourly physical assessment must be performed if the client's condition permits

- Hydration, nutrition, and elimination needs must be met when the client is in seclusion or restraint
- When it is determined that the client is no longer a threat to self or others, the client must be released from seclusion or restraints
- Chemical restraint: The nurse may administer a prescribed prn medication without the client's consent if the client is dangerous to self or others
- In inpatient settings, nurses play a primary role in maintaining or changing unit culture with regard to the use of seclusion and restraints; the leadership role of nurses in staff training, treatment planning, and performance improvement activities related to decreasing seclusion and restraint is critical

Right to Consent to or Refuse Treatment

- In psychiatric emergencies, medications can be given without consent to prevent harm to the client or to others
- If a client is capable of giving informed consent, that client has the right to refuse medication
- If the court finds that the person is not competent to understand the need for treatment, medication can be given against the client's will
  - How the determination of competence is applied varies from state to state in the United States
- Court-ordered medication: A client's right to refuse treatment may be overruled, and the client may be court mandated to take medication to decrease the threat of injury to self or others
  - This illustrates the ethical dilemma of the conflict about what is more important: the client's autonomy (in refusing treatment) or the potential harm to self or others if the client does not take the medication
- Nurses practicing in mental health facilities need to be aware of the state and case laws and policies and procedures for that jurisdiction regarding the administration of medication to voluntary and involuntary competent clients
  - Frequent nursing assessment for side effects and the careful documentation of clients' complaints related to side effects are essential for the adjustment or discontinuance of medication
  - Nurses need to carefully analyze and question the reason for the refusal of medication: Is it because of the client's denial of the illness or of the symptomatology of the condition, or is it because of side effects or resistance to authority or staff?

Informed Consent

- Consent is essential for any treatment, except in an emergency in which failure to institute treatment may constitute negligence; routine procedures are covered by a consent signed on admission
- In an emergency situation, two health care providers may sign consent for a client when failure to intervene may cause death or when common law permits administration of health care to unconscious or mentally incompetent persons in emergency situations; if family members voice opposition, a court order may be required. Note that there is a difference between involuntary commitment and mental incompetence.
- Informed consent must include an explanation of treatment to be done with presentation of advantages and disadvantages and description of possible alternatives; there must be time for decision making with an absence of undue pressure; the explanation and decision making must occur before sedation is given; clients have a right to be informed by their health care provider of all treatment options; the explanation of treatment is performed by the health care provider not the nurse; the health care provider must also determine whether the client's knowledge level is sufficient to give consent before asking for that consent.

- Legal consent requires that it be voluntary, that it authorizes the specific treatment or care and the person giving the treatment or care, and that it is given by a person with the legal and mental capacity to consent based on an informed decision; clients 18 years or older and emancipated minors are legally able to give consent; emancipated minors include individuals who are younger than 18 years of age and are either married, a parent, or legally emancipated by the courts

Duty to Warn

- Nurses have a duty to warn of threatened suicide or harm
- Mental health professionals, including nurses, have a duty to notify an intended and identifiable victim
- Many mental health treatment facilities have duty-to-warn policies (known as "Tarasoff" policies after the court case) and procedures in place that will guide nurses and other clinicians in the notification and documentation processes

Advance Directives

- Psychiatric advance directive: A client with a recurrent or severe and persistent psychiatric disorder may establish an advance directive to guide treatment during a future episode of mental illness when judgment is impaired
    - Some states have special provisions and have made psychiatric models that allow a competent person to describe warning signs of declining mental health and consent to or refuse a treatment method
    - These models also allow a competent person to agree to commitment in a psychiatric care facility for a determined period of time and to appoint a surrogate (substitute) decision maker
- Concepts
    - Living wills: Allow clients to state their wish to die in certain situations and not have life prolonged by using medications, artificial means, or heroic measures; living wills set forth clients' wishes regarding health care decisions and include which medical procedures are authorized or declined
    - Health care proxy: Designates an agent to make health care decisions according to client's plans or wishes; includes power to stop or withhold treatment necessary for life when client is unable to do so
- Advantages of living wills and health care proxies: Permit expression of a client's preferences; promote communication between client and caregivers; foster respect for a client as a person; and support belief that a client has rights to self-determination
- Client's Self-Determination Act of 1991: Mandates that health care agencies receiving Medicare and Medicaid reimbursement advise clients of their right to advance directives

Death with Dignity: Legal, Ethical, and Emotional Issues

- Death with dignity includes two fundamental factors: Individual has control over one's own life, and worth of individual as a unique being is demonstrated through respect even after death
- Laws empower clients to have as much control as possible over their care and activities, recognizing that pain, helplessness, and hopelessness lead to despair
- Public should be educated about advance directives through literature distribution and discussions; about appropriateness of care for terminally ill clients derived from continuous quality management; and about availability and accessibility of palliative care services

- Criteria of death: Every state has increasingly been forced to define death (many using signs of brain death as the indicator) and to define when death occurs
- Do not resuscitate (DNR) status
  - All health care agencies are required to have DNR procedures to meet accreditation standards
  - DNR orders must be included in clients' clinical records and be periodically updated
  - Most important factors considered are client's wishes, prognosis, ability to cope, and whether there is a reasonable possibility that an acceptable quality of life will be achieved through CPR
  - In many states, the right to request a DNR status is mandated within the Patient Care Partnership (Patient's Bill of Rights); health care agencies must provide education on the issue of DNR to clients and families
  - DNR orders require a team decision; client and family must be included in decision-making process

APPLICATION AND REVIEW

3. Among members of the nursing team, which functions are registered nurses legally permitted to perform in a mental health hospital? **Select all that apply.**
   1. Psychotherapy
   2. Health promotion
   3. Case management
   4. Prescribing medication
   5. Treating human responses
4. A health care provider orders "Restraints prn" for a client who has a history of violent behavior. What is the nurse's responsibility concerning this order?
   1. Ask that the order indicate the type of restraint
   2. Recognize that prn orders for restraints are unacceptable
   3. Implement the restraint order when the client begins to act out
   4. Ensure that the entire staff is aware of the order for the restraint
5. What is the nurse's specific responsibility when the rights of a client on a mental health unit are restricted by the use of seclusion?
   1. Inform the client's family
   2. Monitor all pharmacologic intervention
   3. Complete a rights denial form and forward it to the administrative officer
   4. Document the client's behavior and the reason why specific rights were denied
6. A client on the psychiatric unit is undergoing a pretreatment evaluation for electroconvulsive therapy (ECT). The nurse doubts that the client can provide an "informed consent" because of profoundly depressed behavior. What should be the nurse's initial intervention?
   1. Consult with the hospital's legal staff and follow their recommendation
   2. Have the client verbalize an understanding and outcomes of the procedure
   3. Ask the client to sign the consent form because the client has not been declared incompetent
   4. Suggest to the health care provider that a family member sign the consent form for the client
7. A toddler screams and cries noisily after parental visits, disturbing all the other children. When the crying is particularly loud and prolonged, the nurse puts the crib in a separate room and closes the door. The toddler is left there until the crying ceases, a matter of 30 or 45 minutes. Legally, how should this behavior be interpreted?
   1. Limits had to be set to control the child's crying
   2. The child had a right to remain in the room with the other children
   3. The child had to be removed because the other children needed to be considered
   4. Segregation of the child for more than half an hour was too long a period of time

8. A pregnant woman is admitted with a tentative diagnosis of placenta previa. The nurse implements orders to start an IV infusion, administer oxygen, and draw blood for laboratory tests. The client's apprehension is increasing, and she asks the nurse what is happening. The nurse tells her not to worry, that she is going to be all right, and that everything is under control. What is the **best** interpretation of the nurse's statement?
   1. Adequate, because the preparations are routine and need no explanation
   2. Effective, because the client's anxieties would increase if she knew the danger involved
   3. Questionable, because the client has the right to know what treatment is being given and why
   4. Incorrect, because only the health care provider should offer assurances about management of care

9. A client who has been told she needs a hysterectomy for cervical cancer is upset about being unable to have a third child. What is the **next** nursing action?
   1. Evaluate her willingness to pursue adoption
   2. Encourage her to focus on her own recovery
   3. Emphasize that she does have two children already
   4. Ensure that other treatment options for her will be explored

10. The family of an older adult who is aphasic reports to the nurse manager that the primary nurse failed to obtain a signed consent before inserting an indwelling catheter to measure hourly output. What should the nurse manager consider before responding?
    1. Procedures for a client's benefit do not require a signed consent
    2. Clients who are aphasic are incapable of signing an informed consent
    3. A separate signed informed consent for routine treatments is unnecessary
    4. A specific intervention without a client's signed consent is an invasion of rights

11. The spouse of a comatose client who has severe internal bleeding refuses to allow transfusions of whole blood because they are Jehovah's Witnesses. What action should the nurse take?
    1. Institute the ordered blood transfusion because the client's survival depends on volume replacement
    2. Clarify the reason why the transfusion is necessary and explain the implications if there is no transfusion
    3. Phone the health care provider for an administrative order to give the transfusion under these circumstances
    4. Give the spouse a treatment refusal form to sign and notify the health care provider that a court order can now be sought

12. A client is voluntarily admitted to a psychiatric unit. Later, the client develops severe pain in the right lower quadrant and is diagnosed as having acute appendicitis. How should the nurse prepare the client for the appendectomy?
    1. Have two nurses witness the client signing the operative consent form
    2. Ensure that the surgeon and the psychiatrist sign for the surgery because it is an emergency procedure
    3. Ask the client to sign the operative consent form after the client has been informed of the procedure and required care
    4. Inform the client's next of kin that it will be necessary for one of them to sign the consent form because the client is on a psychiatric unit

13. What should the nurse consider when obtaining an informed consent from a 17-year-old adolescent?
    1. If the client is allowed to give consent
    2. The client cannot make informed decisions about health care

3. If the client is permitted to give voluntary consent when parents are not available
4. The client probably will be unable to choose between alternatives when asked to consent

14. A client with rheumatoid arthritis does not want the prescribed cortisone and informs the nurse. Later, the nurse attempts to administer cortisone. When the client asks what the medication is, the nurse gives an evasive answer. The client takes the medication and later discovers that it was cortisone. The client states an intent to sue. What factors in this situation must be considered in a legal action? **Select all that apply.**
1. Clients have a right to refuse treatment
2. Nurses are required to answer clients truthfully
3. The health care provider should have been notified
4. The client had insufficient knowledge to make such a decision
5. Legally prescribed medications are administered despite a client's objections

See Answers on pages 61-64.

Americans with Disability Act

- The Americans with Disabilities Act is a substantial breakthrough in discrimination against people with mental illnesses; however, there are specific exclusions
  - The definition includes mental barriers that limit the ability of the individual in one or more major activities; enforcement of the statute depends on the person's limitations
- Courts have ruled that if a person's mental condition is stabilized, then there is no disability
  - However, such people are protected if the fact that they once had a mental disability (eg, depression) is used against them in the employment situation
  - Some exclusions include persons who use controlled substances for unlawful purposes and individuals who take prescribed drugs without the supervision of a health care professional; in addition, people who are a direct threat to others are excluded
  - However, it is important to recognize that this must be based on the actual behavior of the individual and not on the mental disability itself
- An employer cannot ask about history of mental health treatment as part of an application process for employment
  - The employer can only evaluate the individual regarding his or her ability to perform the job functions
  - Questions about the prior use of health care insurance coverage are also not permissible

Commitment Issues

- *Commitment* is a term that refers to the various ways that an individual enters mental health treatment
- States have varying terms and mechanisms associated with commitment, but in general, there are three common types: (1) voluntary commitment (admission); (2) emergency commitment (hospitalization); and (3) longer-term judicial or civil commitment
- Voluntary admission: Clients of lawful age may apply to be admitted for treatment to a mental health facility; written notice of intent to leave may be required with a waiting period during which the health care provider may choose to change admission status to involuntary
  - Clients who access treatment voluntarily consent to be admitted and treated
  - Nurses treat voluntarily admitted clients whose clinical conditions vary widely with regard to their psychiatric severity
  - However, voluntary clients who are seeking a discharge from the hospital but who are an immediate danger to themselves or others may be placed on an emergency commitment status pending further evaluation and treatment

- Involuntary admission (commitment) (Fig. 4.1): Clients who have not agreed to treatment are placed in a mental health facility; criteria for involuntary admission in some states are very circumscribed (danger to self or others); in other states requirements are more liberal (mentally ill and in need of treatment, gravely disabled, and/or unable to provide for own basic needs); most states have various routes for involuntary admission that may include:
  - Court-ordered observational admission: Used to assess the mental status of a person in relation to legal activities (eg, competency to stand trial)
  - Severe mental illness sometimes affects a client's cognitive functions so that he or she refuses treatment for a variety of reasons; some individuals with psychosis, paranoia, delusions, or hallucinations reject psychiatric treatment for fear of being harmed or on the basis of some strange rationale that only they understand; persons who suffer from severe mood disturbances and who are depressed and suicidal sometimes refuse to enter treatment because of a sense of hopelessness and a wish to die
  - Emergency hospitalization: Used to intervene when there is an immediate threat by a client to self or others; this short-term (48–72 hours) commitment is allowed for the assessment of the client and to determine whether more long-term commitment is needed or the client can be discharged to outpatient treatment; in some states, if the effect of the mental illness is such that the client is unable to provide food, clothing, or shelter for himself or herself (ie, "gravely disabled"), an emergency commitment is also appropriate
  - Emergency commitment differs from a judicial or indefinite commitment; emergency commitment is for a shorter period and generally has more restrictive criteria for admission; usually a state requires that a mental health official such as a physician, psychologist,

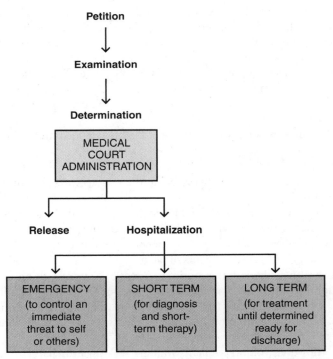

FIG. 4.1 Clinical algorithm for the involuntary commitment process. (From Stuart, G. W. [2013]. *Principles and practice of psychiatric nursing* [10 ed.]. St. Louis, MO: Mosby/Elsevier.)

social worker, or advanced practice nurse see the individual; some states require a licensed physician; after the individual is brought to the inpatient unit, a second mental health professional, usually a psychiatrist, has to make an examination; this procedure protects the rights of the individuals; usually within a short period (5 days or less, excluding weekends and holidays), a probable cause hearing must occur to continue the person's hospitalization
- Taking away an individual's freedom through a commitment procedure is a serious matter; the US Supreme Court has established the standard of clear and convincing evidence as the standard of proof that must be met for commitment
- Civil or judicial commitment is for a longer amount of time than an emergency commitment
  - The legal basis for the extended detention of an individual for treatment lies in the *parens patriae* power of the state to protect and care for individuals with disabilities and the police power of the state to protect the community from persons who are a threat
  - For a judicial commitment, the individual has to be given time to prepare a defense that states why hospitalization is not necessary
  - The client has the right to have his or her attorney cross-examine the mental health professionals regarding the necessity for continued inpatient treatment
- At least 35 states have passed legislation for mandatory outpatient treatment
  - The purpose of mandating outpatient mental health treatment is to break the cyclic pattern of clients who, when discharged from an inpatient treatment facility, discontinue their medications, deteriorate, exhibit dangerous behavior, and subsequently require readmission to the acute psychiatric care setting
  - Nurses need to acknowledge their advocate role and yet balance clients' need for progressive mental health treatment
  - This includes activating clients' participation in outpatient treatment programs that effectively address the recurring nature of severe and persistent mental illness
- Other commitment terms:
  - Formal commitment: Used to treat clients with chronic mental illnesses over a prolonged period; periodic reviews may be made at 3, 6, or 12 months
  - Two health care provider commitment: two health care providers document that the client has met the state's criteria for involuntary care; most states provide for an intermediate length of time (1–6 weeks) admission
  - Physician's emergency certificate: allows the facility to keep people against their will

Nurses' Rights and Responsibilities

- Performs within standards of practice for the profession
- Licensure required to practice as a nurse; each state defines scope of professional practice
  - Independent interventions: Nurse-initiated actions based on nursing's body of knowledge and scope of practice that do not require a health care provider's order (eg, teaching, assessment, meeting hygienic needs)
  - Dependent interventions: Health care provider–directed interventions or health care provider–established protocols that require specific nursing responsibilities and technical knowledge (eg, administration of medications, tube feedings, and dressing changes)
  - Collaborative interventions: Nursing actions that require cooperation and coordination with other health professionals (eg, coordinating intervention from physical therapist and social workers to meet needs of a client before discharge)
- Intervenes to protect clients from incorrect, unethical, and/or illegal actions by any person delivering health care
- Participates in and promotes growth of the nursing profession and individual competence

- Reports any suspected child abuse to appropriate authority; reporting is mandatory and does not incur legal liability
- See code of ethics (previously mentioned)
- Obtains professional liability insurance; *note that personal liability insurance will represent a nurse before the State Board of Nursing,* whereas employee liability insurance will not

NURSING LIABILITY

Overview

- Implement care that meets the scope and standard of psychiatric-mental health clinical nursing practice as described by the American Nurses Association (ANA) and nursing practice laws of the state where practicing (eg, health promotion, case management, treatment of human responses)
- Remain current with skills and knowledge base
- Keep accurate and concise client records
- Maintain client and family confidentiality; an exception must be made to notify others (eg, police, intended victim) if a credible threat against another person is made by the client
- Know the laws governing practice within the state, the rights and duties of the nurse, and the rights of the client
- Maintain current malpractice liability insurance coverage (per state or institution requirement)

Torts Important to Nurses

- Torts are violations of civil law against a person or person's property
  - Commission: Inappropriate action
  - Omission: Lack of appropriate action
- Unintentional torts
  - Negligence: Measurement of negligence is "reasonableness"; involves exposure of person or property of another to unreasonable risk for injury by acts of commission or omission
  - Malpractice is a type of negligence during professional practice; any unreasonable lack of skill in professional duties or illegal or immoral conduct that results in injury to or death of a client; involves violation of standards of nursing practice
  - Examples of malpractice or negligence: Leaving surgical sponges inside a client; causing burns; medication errors; failure to prevent falls; incompetent assessment leading to subsequent inappropriate actions; improper identification of clients; carelessness in caring for a client's property
- Tort is different from crime, but a serious tort can be tried as both a civil and criminal action
- Reasonableness and prudence usually are determining factors in a judgment
- Nurses are responsible for their own acts; also, employers may be held responsible under doctrine of *respondeat superior*; when responsibility is shared, nursing actions must lie within the scope of employment and legislation relating to nursing practice (eg, Nurse Practice Acts)
- Elements essential to prove negligence
  - Legally recognized duty of care to protect others against unreasonable risk
  - Failure to perform according to an established standard of conduct and care, which equals breach of duty
  - Damage to client, which can be physical, emotional, and/or mental; physical harm is not necessary to establish liability for intentional torts
  - Proximate cause or causation requires a causative relationship to exist between the failure to provide a standard of care and the damages suffered

- Good Samaritan laws protect health care professionals who administer first aid as volunteers in an emergency unless there is gross negligence or willful misconduct; it is presumed that nurses meet a level of care expected of a reasonably prudent professional with the same education
- Intentional torts occur when a person does damage to another person in a willful way and without just cause and/or excuse
  - *Assault:* A mental or physical threat; knowingly *threatening or attempting* to do violence to another without touching the person; forcing a medication or treatment on a person who does not want it
  - *Battery:* Touching or wounding a person in an offensive manner with or without intent to do harm
  - *Fraud:* Purposeful false presentation of facts to create deception; includes presenting false credentials for licensure or employment
  - *Invasion of privacy:* Involves privileged communication and unreasonable intrusion
    - *Encroachment or trespass on another's body* includes any unwarranted operation, unauthorized touching, and unnecessary exposure or discussion of client's case unless authorized
    - *False imprisonment,* even without force or malicious intent, includes intentional confinement without authorization, as well as threat of force or confining structures and/or clothing; it is not false imprisonment when it is necessary to protect an emotionally disturbed person from harming self or others
    - *Defamation* involves communications, even if true, that cause a lowering of opinion of the person; includes slander (oral) and libel (written, pictured, telecast), both of which are dependent on communication to a third party

Crimes Important to Nurses

- Crime: An intentional wrong that violates societal law punishable by the state; the state is the complainant
  - Felony: Serious crime, such as murder, punishable by prison term
  - Misdemeanor: Less serious crime that is punishable by a fine and/or short-term imprisonment
- Commission of a crime requires committing a deed contrary to criminal law or failing to act when there is legal obligation to act
- Criminal conspiracy occurs when two or more persons agree to commit a crime
- Giving aid to another in the commission of a crime makes the person equally guilty if there is awareness that a crime is being committed
- Ignorance of the law usually is not an adequate defense
- Administration of opioids by a nurse is legal only when prescribed by a licensed health care provider; possession or sale of controlled substances by a nurse is illegal
- If a nurse knowingly administers a drug that causes major disability or death, a crime may be charged

APPLICATION AND REVIEW

15. A family member brings a relative to the local community hospital because the relative "has been acting strange." Which statements meet involuntary hospitalization criteria? **Select all that apply.**
    1. "I cry all the time, I am so sad"
    2. "Since I retired I have been so depressed"
    3. "I would like to end it all with sleeping pills"
    4. "Voices say it is okay for me to kill all prostitutes"
    5. "My boss makes me so angry by always picking on me"

16. A client on the psychiatric unit is noisy, loud, and disruptive. The nurse informs the client, "Unless you are quiet, you will be isolated and put in restraints, if necessary." Legally,
    1. The information given to the client is actually an assault
    2. The client's behavior is to be expected and should be ignored
    3. Clients who are hyperactive need to be restrained for their own protection
    4. Clients who are disruptive and hyperactive cannot be expected to understand instructions

17. Nurses are held responsible for the commission of a tort. The nurse understands that a tort is:
    1. The application of force to the body of another by a reasonable individual
    2. An illegality committed by one person against the property or person of another
    3. Doing something that a reasonable person under ordinary circumstances would not do
    4. An illegality committed against the public and punishable by the law through the courts

18. A client is placed on a stretcher and restrained with straps when being transported to the x-ray department. A strap breaks, and the client falls to the floor, sustaining a fractured arm. Later, the client shows the strap to the nurse manager, stating, "See, the strap is worn just at the spot where it snapped." What is the nurse's accountability regarding this incident?
    1. Exempt from any lawsuit because of the doctrine of *respondeat superior*
    2. Totally responsible for the obvious negligence because of failure to report defective equipment
    3. Liable, along with the employer, for misapplication of equipment or use of defective equipment that harms the client
    4. Exonerated, because only the hospital, as principal employer, is responsible for the quality and maintenance of equipment

19. When being interviewed for a position as a registered professional nurse, the applicant is asked to identify an example of an intentional tort. What is the appropriate response?
    1. Negligence
    2. Malpractice
    3. Breach of duty
    4. False imprisonment

20. Several recently licensed registered nurses are discussing whether they should purchase personal professional liability insurance. Which statement indicates the **most** accurate information about professional liability insurance?
    1. "If you have liability insurance, you are more likely to be sued"
    2. "Your employer provides you with the liability insurance you will need"
    3. "Liability insurance is not available for nursing professionals working in a hospital"
    4. "Personal liability insurance offers representation if the State Board of Nursing files charges against you"

21. A 3-year-old child with eczema of the face and arms has disregarded the nurse's warnings to "stop scratching, or else!" The nurse finds the toddler scratching so intensely that the arms are bleeding. The nurse then ties the toddler's arms to the crib sides, saying, "I'm going to teach you one way or another." How should the nurse's behavior be interpreted?
    1. These actions can be construed as assault and battery
    2. The problem was resolved with forethought and accountability
    3. Skin must be protected, and the actions taken were by a reasonably prudent nurse
    4. The nurse had tried to reason with the toddler and expected understanding and cooperation

22. Which nursing behavior is an intentional tort?
    1. Miscounting gauze pads during a client's surgery
    2. Causing a burn when applying a wet dressing to a client's extremity
    3. Divulging private information about a client's health status to the media
    4. Failing to monitor a client's blood pressure before administering an antihypertensive

23. A client is hospitalized because of severe depression. The client refuses to eat, stays in bed most of the time, does not talk with family members, and will not leave the room. The nurse attempts to initiate a conversation by asking questions but receives no answers. Finally, the nurse tells the client that if there is no response, the nurse will leave and the client will remain alone. How should the nurse's behavior be interpreted?
1. A system of rewards and punishment is being used to motivate the client
2. Leaving the client alone allows time for the nurse to think of other strategies
3. This behavior indicates the client's desire for solitude that the nurse is respecting
4. This threat is considered assault, and the nurse should not have reacted in this manner

See Answers on pages 61-64.

ANSWERS TO REVIEW QUESTIONS

1. **1 Each state or province protects the health and welfare of its populace by regulating nursing practice**
   2 Although the members of the profession can also benefit from a clear description of their role, it is not the primary purpose of the law. **3** The employing agency does assume responsibility for its employees and therefore benefits from maintenance of standards, but it is not the purpose of the law. **4** People with health problems is too limited; they are just one portion of the population that is protected
   Client Need: Management of Care; **Cognitive Level:** Comprehension; **Nursing Process:** Assessment/Analysis

2. **4 Nonmaleficence means avoidance of harm**
   1 Veracity is truthfulness. **2** Autonomy is self-determination. **3** Beneficence is promotion of or bringing about good
   Client Need: Management of Care; **Cognitive Level:** Knowledge; **Nursing Process:** Assessment/Analysis

> **Memory Aid:** Consider the word parts to help you remember the meaning of nonmaleficence: Think "no bad"! You know that **mal**ware is bad for your computer, so **mal**eficence is bad; adding "non" is a negation. So "nonmal" at the beginning of the word nonmaleficence means "no bad"!

3. **Answers: 2, 3, 5**
   2 Health promotion is within the legal scope of nursing practice. **3** Case management is within the legal scope of nursing practice. **5** Treating human responses is within the legal scope of nursing practice
   1 Registered nurses may use counseling interventions but may not perform psychotherapy; the members of the nursing team permitted to perform psychotherapy are psychiatric-mental health clinical nurse specialists and psychiatric-mental health nurse practitioners.
   4 Only those who are legally licensed to prescribe medications, such as psychiatric nurse practitioners, may do so
   Client Need: Management of Care; **Cognitive Level:** Comprehension; **Nursing Process:** Planning/Implementation

4. **2 New orders must be written each time a client requires restraints; when a client is acting out, the nurse may use restraints or a seclusion room and then obtain the necessary order**
   1 PRN restraint orders are not permitted. **3** Less restrictive interventions should be used when the client begins to act out; restraints are used as a last resort. **4** PRN restraint orders are not permitted
   Client Need: Management of Care; **Cognitive Level:** Comprehension; **Nursing Process:** Planning/Implementation

> **Memory Aid:** Use the letters P-R-N to help you remember that prn Restraints are Not Permitted. The Latin meaning is actually *pro re nata,* meaning "as needed," but this abbreviation is not applicable to orders for restraints!

5. **4 Seclusion and restraints are special procedures for dealing with acting-out, aggressive behavior for the protection of the client and others; clear documentation is essential when the client's rights are restricted**

   1 Informing the client's family is not necessary because the use of seclusion and/or restraints is included in the general consent form that is signed on admission. **2** Pharmacologic intervention should be monitored for all clients. **3** There is not a typical rights denial form; however, documentation is required to justify the need for seclusion or the use of restraints

   Client Need: Management of Care; **Cognitive Level:** Comprehension; **Nursing Process:** Planning/Implementation; **Integrated Process:** Communication/Documentation

6. **2 The client's understanding should be assessed first. Depressed clients often are cognitively stable and capable of providing legal consent**

   1 Consulting with the hospital's legal staff and following their recommendation eventually may have to be done, but it is not the initial intervention. **3** The client's rights are not protected if the nurse elicits consent for a procedure when the nurse believes that the client does not comprehend the information; in this situation, just because the client is not legally determined to be incompetent, it does not mean that the client is competent; further assessment is necessary. **4** Unless the client has legally granted the family member authority to make decisions or the family member has been appointed as the client's guardian by the court, suggesting to the health care provider that a family member sign the consent form for the client is illegal

   Client Need: Management of Care; **Cognitive Level:** Application; **Nursing Process:** Assessment/Analysis; **Integrated Process:** Communication/Documentation

7. **2 Legally, a person cannot be locked in a room (isolated) unless there is a threat of danger either to the self or to others**

   1 Limit setting in this situation is not warranted; the child's behavior is a reaction to separation from the parent, which is common at this age. **3** Crying, although irritating, will not harm the other children. **4** A child should never be isolated

   Client Need: Management of Care; **Cognitive Level:** Application; **Nursing Process:** Evaluation/Outcomes

8. **3 The client's rights have been violated; all clients have the right to a complete and accurate explanation of treatment based on cognitive ability**

   1 All interventions should be explained because they are not routine to the client. **2** When administering treatment, the nurse is responsible for explaining what the treatment is and why it is being given. **4** The Patient Care Partnership (the Patient's Bill of Rights) states that the client should be informed

   Client Need: Management of Care; **Cognitive Level:** Comprehension; **Nursing Process:** Evaluation/Outcomes

9. **4 Although a hysterectomy may be performed, conservative management may include cervical conization and laser treatment that do not preclude future pregnancies; clients have a right to be informed by their health care provider of all treatment options**

   1 Evaluating her willingness to pursue adoption currently is not the issue for the client. **2** Encouraging her to focus on her own recovery negates the client's feelings. **3** Emphasizing that she has two children already negates the client's feelings;

   Client Need: Management of Care; **Cognitive Level:** Application; **Integrated Process:** Communication/Documentation; **Nursing Process:** Planning/Implementation

10. **3 Inserting an indwelling catheter is considered a routine procedure to meet basic physiologic needs and is covered by a consent signed at the time of admission**

    1 The need for consent is not negated because the procedure is beneficial. **2** The treatment does not require special consent. **4** The treatment does not require special consent

    Client Need: Management of Care; **Cognitive Level:** Analysis; **Integrated Process:** Communication/Documentation; **Nursing Process:** Evaluation/Outcomes

11. **4 The client is unconscious; although the spouse can give consent, there is no legal power to refuse a treatment for the client unless previously authorized to do so by a power of attorney or a health care proxy; the court can make a decision for the client**

  1 Instituting the ordered blood transfusion is without legal basis, and the nurse may be held liable. **2** Explanations will not be effective at this time and will not meet the client's needs. **3** Phoning the health care provider for an administrative order is without legal basis, and the nurse may be held liable

  Client Need: Management of Care; **Cognitive Level:** Analysis; **Integrated Process:** Communication/Documentation; **Nursing Process:** Planning/Implementation

12. **3 Because the client is not certified as incompetent, the right of informed consent is retained**

  1 The client can sign the consent, but the client's signature requires only one witness. **2** Because there is no evidence of incompetence, the client should sign the consent. **4** Because there is no evidence of incompetence, the client should sign the consent

  Client Need: Management of Care; **Cognitive Level:** Application; **Integrated Process:** Communication/Documentation; **Nursing Process:** Planning/Implementation

13. **1 A person is legally unable to sign a consent until the age of 18 years unless the client is an emancipated minor or married; the nurse must determine the legal status of the adolescent**

  2 Although the adolescent may be capable of intelligent choices, 18 is the legal age of consent unless the client is emancipated or married. **3** Parents or guardians are legally responsible under all circumstances unless the adolescent is an emancipated minor or married. **4** Adolescents have the capacity to choose but not the legal right in this situation unless they are legally emancipated or married

  Client Need: Management of Care; **Cognitive Level:** Application; **Integrated Process:** Communication/Documentation; **Nursing Process:** Planning/Implementation

14. **Answers: 1, 2, 3**

  1 Clients who are mentally competent have the right to refuse treatment; the nurse must respect this right. **2** Client's questions must always be answered truthfully. **3** The health care provider should be notified when a client refuses an intervention so that an alternate treatment plan can be formulated; this is done after the nurse explores the client's reasons for refusal.

  4 The client had a discussion with the nurse that indicated that the client had sufficient information to make the decision to refuse the medication. **5** The client has a right to refuse treatment; this right takes precedence over the health care provider's prescription

  Client Need: Management of Care; **Cognitive Level:** Analysis; **Integrated Process:** Communication/Documentation; **Nursing Process:** Evaluation/Outcomes

15. **Answers: 3, 4**

  3 The statement "I would like to end it all with sleeping pills" indicates a suicide threat; it is a direct expression of intent but without action. **4** The threat to harm others must be heeded; the client must be protected from self harm as well as harming others

  1 The statement, "I cry all the time, I am so sad" does not indicate that the client plans to harm self or others. **2** The statement "Since I retired I have been so depressed" does not indicate that the client plans to harm self or others. **5** The statement "My boss makes me so angry by always picking on me" reflects the client's feelings of anger and the cause but does not indicate a threat to self or others

  Client Need: Psychosocial Integrity; **Cognitive Level:** Analysis; **Nursing Process:** Assessment/Analysis

16. **1 A threat is considered a type of assault (legally, an intentional tort)**

  2 The client's behavior may be expected, but it should be dealt with directly; behavior should never be ignored. **3** Restraints are unnecessary for this client; restraints are used only when the client's behavior escalates to the point that it is a threat to the client or others. **4** The generalization, "Clients who are disruptive and hyperactive cannot be expected to understand instructions," may not be true; they may respond to calm limit setting

  Client Need: Management of Care; **Cognitive Level:** Application; **Nursing Process:** Evaluation/Outcomes

17. **2 An individual is held legally responsible for actions committed against another individual or an individual's property**
    1 The application of force to the body of another by a reasonable individual is battery, which involves physical harm. 3 Doing something that a reasonable person under ordinary circumstances would not do is the definition of negligence. 4 An illegality committed against the public and punishable by the law through the courts is the definition of a crime.
    Client Need: Management of Care; **Cognitive Level:** Knowledge; **Nursing Process:** Assessment/Analysis

18. **3 Using a stretcher with worn straps is negligent; this oversight does not reflect the actions of a reasonably prudent nurse**
    1 The nurse is responsible and must ascertain the adequate functioning of equipment. 2 The hospital shares responsibility for safe, functioning equipment. 4 The nurse is responsible and must ascertain the adequate functioning of equipment
    Client Need: Management of Care; **Cognitive Level:** Application; **Nursing Process:** Evaluation/Outcomes

19. **4 False imprisonment is a wrong committed by one person against another in a willful, intentional way without just cause and/or excuse**
    1 Negligence is an unintentional tort. 2 Malpractice, which is professional negligence, is classified as an unintentional tort. 3 Breach of duty is an unintentional tort
    Client Need: Management of Care; **Cognitive Level:** Comprehension; **Nursing Process:** Planning/Implementation

20. **4 Personal liability insurance will represent a nurse before the State Board of Nursing, whereas employee liability insurance will not**
    1 A nurse can be sued whether or not the nurse has liability insurance. 2 Employer liability insurance will represent the nurse in charges related to employment but not charges brought by the State Board of Nursing. 3 Liability insurance is available for all nurses
    Client Need: Management of Care; **Cognitive Level:** Comprehension; **Nursing Process:** Evaluation/Outcomes

21. **1 Assault is a threat or an attempt to do violence to another, and battery means touching an individual in an offensive manner or actually injuring another person**
    2 The nurse's behavior demonstrates anger and does not take into account the growth and developmental needs of children in this age group. 3 Although the behavior (scratching) needs to be decreased, this can be done with mittens, not immobilization. 4 A 3-year-old child does not have the capacity to understand cause (scratching) and effect (bleeding)
    Client Need: Management of Care; **Cognitive Level:** Application; **Nursing Process:** Evaluation/Outcomes

22. **3 Divulging private information about a client's health status to the media is an invasion of privacy, which is an intentional tort**
    1 Miscounting gauze pads during a client's surgery is an example of professional negligence (malpractice). 2 Causing a burn when applying a wet dressing to a client's extremity is an example of professional negligence (malpractice). 4 Failing to monitor a client's blood pressure before administering an antihypertensive is an example of professional negligence (malpractice)
    Client Need: Management of Care; **Cognitive Level:** Comprehension; **Nursing Process:** Evaluation/Outcomes

23. **4 This response is a threat (assault) because the nurse is attempting to put pressure on the client to speak or be left alone**
    1 The response is not a reward and punishment technique that is used in behavior modification therapy. 2 Clients in emotional crisis should not be left alone. 3 Clients in emotional crisis should not be left alone
    Client Need: Management of Care; **Cognitive Level:** Analysis; **Nursing Process:** Evaluation/Outcomes

MAJOR DIVISIONS OF THE NERVOUS SYSTEM

Central Nervous System (CNS)

- Brain: the most complex and vital of human organs
- Spinal cord

Peripheral Nervous System (PNS)

- Cranial nerves
- Spinal nerves
- Autonomic nervous system (ANS)
  - Conducts impulses from brainstem or cord out to visceral effectors (eg, cardiac muscle, smooth muscle, and glands)
  - Consists of two divisions
    - *Sympathetic* (adrenergic fibers) secretes norepinephrine: Influences heart, smooth muscle of blood vessels and bronchioles, and glandular secretion
    - *Parasympathetic* (cholinergic fibers) secretes acetylcholine: Influences digestive tract and smooth muscle to promote digestive gland secretion, peristalsis, and defecation; influences heart to decrease rate and contractility
- Autonomic antagonism and summation: Sympathetic and parasympathetic impulses tend to produce opposite effects (Fig. 5.1; Table 5.1)
- Under conditions of stress, sympathetic impulses to visceral effectors dominate over parasympathetic impulses; however, in some individuals under stress, parasympathetic impulses, via the vagus nerve, increase to glands and smooth muscle of the stomach, stimulating hydrochloric acid secretion and gastric motility

CENTRAL NERVOUS SYSTEM

Overview

- An understanding of the anatomy and physiology of the central nervous system is essential

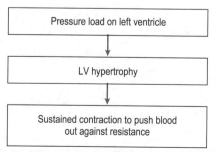

FIG. 5.1 The autonomic nervous system's two components, the parasympathetic and sympathetic divisions, have opposite effects on the body. (From Varcarolis, E. M., & Halter, M. J. [2010]. *Psychiatric mental health nursing: A clinical approach* [6th ed.]. St. Louis, MO: Saunders.)

| TABLE 5.1 | Autonomic Functions |

Autonomic Effector	Effect of Sympathetic Stimulation (Neurotransmitter: Norepinephrine Unless Otherwise Stated)	Effect of Parasympathetic Stimulation (Neurotransmitter: Acetylcholine)
Cardiac Muscle	Increased rate and strength of contraction (beta receptors)	Decreased rate and strength of contraction
Smooth Muscle of Blood Vessels		
Skin blood vessels	Constriction (alpha receptors)	No effect
Skeletal muscle blood vessels	Dilation (beta receptors)	No effect
Coronary blood vessels	Constriction (alpha receptors) Dilation (beta receptors)	Dilation
Abdominal blood vessels	Constriction (alpha receptors)	No effect
Blood vessels of external genitals	Constriction (alpha receptors)	Dilation of blood vessels causing erection
Smooth Muscle of Hollow Organs and Sphincters		
Bronchioles	Dilation (beta receptors)	Constriction
Digestive tract, except sphincters	Decreased peristalsis (beta receptors)	Increased peristalsis
Sphincters of digestive tract	Constriction (alpha receptors)	Relaxation
Urinary bladder	Relaxation (beta receptors)	Contraction
Urinary sphincters	Constriction (alpha receptors)	Relaxation
Reproductive ducts	Contraction (alpha receptors)	Relaxation
Eye		
Iris	Contraction of radial muscle; dilated pupil	Contraction of circular muscle; constricted pupil
Ciliary	Relaxation; accommodates for far vision	Contraction; accommodates for near vision
Hairs (pilomotor muscles)	Contraction produces goose pimples, or piloerection (alpha receptors)	No effect
Glands		
Sweat	Increased sweat (neurotransmitter: acetylcholine)	No effect
Lacrimal	No effect	Increased secretion of tears
Digestive (salivary, gastric, etc.)	Decreased secretion of saliva; not known for others	Increased secretion of saliva
Pancreas, including islets	Decreased secretion	Increased secretion of pancreatic juice and insulin
Liver	Increased glycogenolysis (beta receptors); increased blood glucose level	No effect
Adrenal medulla*	Increased epinephrine secretion	No effect

*Sympathetic preganglionic axons terminate in contact with secreting cells of the adrenal medulla. Thus the adrenal medulla functions, to quote someone's descriptive phrase, as a "giant sympathetic postganglionic neuron."
From Patton, K. T. & Thibodeau, G. A. (2016). *Anatomy and physiology* (9th ed.) St. Louis, MO: Mosby/Elsevier.

- The brain weighs about 3 lbs and is composed of trillions of cells, 100 billion neurons, and the cells that support their function
- Neurons (nerve cells) do not touch each other but communicate across synapses that separate them via chemical messengers called neurotransmitters
- Neurons are receptive to some neurotransmitters and not to others
- Major excitatory and inhibitory neurotransmitters include dopamine, norepinephrine, serotonin, acetylcholine, and gamma-aminobutyric acid (GABA)
- The level of neurotransmitters that excite or inhibit neural activity is influenced by their production, metabolism/inactivation, and reuptake/storage
- Abnormalities in the level of various neurotransmitters have been linked to many psychiatric illnesses (eg, excess of dopamine to schizophrenia; decreased serotonin levels to depression); most psychotropic medications alter levels of neurotransmitters

The Brain

- Major divisions: Brainstem, cerebellum, diencephalon, cerebrum (Fig. 5.2)
- Has large blood supply and high oxygen consumption
- Uses glucose for energy metabolism, so hypoglycemia can alter brain function
- Protected by blood-brain barrier, a selective filtration system that isolates the brain from certain substances in the general circulation
- Basic tissue types: Neuron cell aggregations (gray matter) and tracts of myelinated fibers (white matter)

Brainstem

- Consists of medulla, pons, and midbrain
- Conducts impulses between spinal cord and brain; most motor and sensory fibers decussate (cross over) in medulla
- Contains reflex centers for heart, respirations, vomiting, coughing, and swallowing; controls blood vessel diameter
- Cranial nerves III through XII originate in brainstem

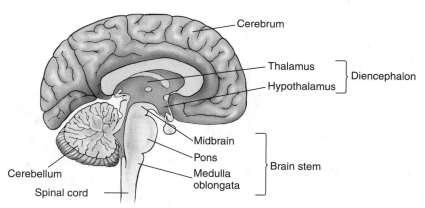

FIG. 5.2 Midsagittal section of the main structures of the brain. The brainstem consists of the midbrain, pons, and medulla, which is continuous with the spinal cord inferiorly. The diencephalon is above the brainstem and consists of the thalamus and hypothalamus. The cerebrum comprises most of the brain and spreads over the diencephalon. The cerebellum is beneath to the cerebrum and behind the brainstem. (From Leonard, P. [2018]. *Building a medical vocabulary* [10th ed.]. St. Louis, MO: Saunders.)

Cerebellum

- Exerts synergic control over skeletal muscles, producing smooth, precise movements; coordinates skeletal muscle contractions; promotes posture, equilibrium, and balance

Diencephalon

- Divided into thalamus and hypothalamus (di- means two; two main parts)
- Thalamus
  - Crudely translates sensory impulses into sensations but does not localize them
  - Processes motor information from cerebral cortex and cerebellum and projects it back to motor cortex
  - Contributes to emotional component of sensations (pleasant or unpleasant)
- Hypothalamus
  - Part of neural path by which emotions and other cerebral functions can alter vital, automatic functions (eg, heartbeat, blood pressure, peristalsis, and secretion by glands)
  - Secretes neuropeptides that influence secretion of various anterior pituitary hormones
  - Produces antidiuretic hormone (ADH) and oxytocin, which are secreted by the posterior pituitary
  - Contains appetite center and satiety center
  - Serves as a heat-regulating center by relaying impulses to lower autonomic centers for vasoconstriction, vasodilation, and sweating, and to somatic centers for shivering
  - Maintains waking state; part of arousal or alerting neural pathway
- Located on the inferior surface of the hypothalamus is the optic chiasm, the point of crossing over (decussation) of optic nerve fibers

Cerebrum

- Cerebral cortex: Consists of multiple lobes (frontal, parietal, temporal, occipital) divided into two hemispheres covered by gray matter forming folds (convolutions) composed of hills (gyri) and valleys (sulci) (Figs. 5.3, 5.4)

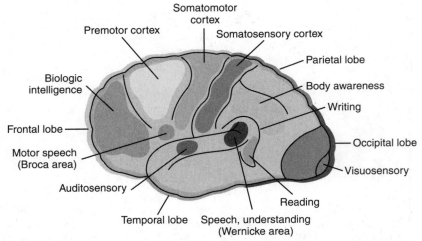

FIG. 5.3   Cerebral cortex. (Modified from Monahan F. D., Sands, J. K., Neighbors, M. Marek, J. F., & Green, C. [2007]. *Phipps' medical-surgical nursing: Health and illness perspectives* [8th ed.]. St. Louis, MO: Mosby.)

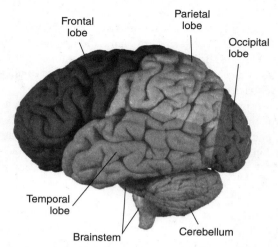

FIG. 5.4   Lateral view of the left cerebral hemisphere of the brain. Note sulci and gyri present in all cerebral lobes. (From Nolte, J., & Angevine, J. B., Jr [2000]. *The human brain: In photographs and diagrams* [2nd ed.]. St Louis, MO: Mosby.)

- Frontal lobe
  - Influences abstract thinking, sense of humor, and uniqueness of personality
  - Controls contraction of skeletal muscles and synchronization of muscular movement
  - Exerts control over hypothalamus; influences basic biorhythms
  - Controls muscular movements necessary for speech (Broca's area, usually in dominant hemisphere)
  - Prefrontal area controls executive functioning (higher level cognitive skills)
  - Uniqueness of personality
- Parietal lobes
  - Translate nerve impulses into sensations (eg, touch, temperature)
  - Interpret sensations; provide appreciation of size, shape, texture, and weight
  - Interpret sense of taste
- Temporal lobes
  - Translate nerve impulses into sensations of sound and interpret sounds (Wernicke's area; usually in dominant hemisphere)
  - Interpret sense of smell
  - Control behavior patterns
- Occipital lobe
  - Interprets sense of vision
  - Provides appreciation of size, shape, and color

Brain and Spinal Cord Protection

- Vertebrae around cord; cranial bones around brain
- Meninges
  - Dura mater: White fibrous tissue, outer layer
  - Arachnoid: "Cobwebby" middle layer
  - Pia mater: Innermost layer; adheres to outer surface of cord and brain; contains blood vessels

- Spaces
  - Subarachnoid space: Around brain and cord between arachnoid and pia mater
  - Subdural space: Between dura mater and arachnoid
  - Epidural space: Between dura mater and cranial bones
- Ventricles and cerebral aqueduct inside brain; four cavities known as first, second, third, and fourth ventricles
  - Cerebrospinal fluid (CFS) formed by plasma filtering from network of capillaries (choroid plexus) in each ventricle
  - CFS circulates throughout ventricles in the brain and subarachnoid space and returns to blood via venous sinuses of brain

Spinal Cord

- Structure
  - Inner core of gray matter shaped like a three-dimensional H
  - Long columns of white matter surround cord's inner core of gray matter—namely, right and left anterior, lateral, and posterior columns; composed of numerous sensory and motor tracts
- Functions
  - Sensory tracts conduct impulses up cord to brain (eg, spinothalamic tracts, two of the six ascending tracts, conduct sensations of pain, temperature, vibration, and proprioception)
  - Motor tracts (pyramidal and extrapyramidal tracts) conduct impulses down cord from brain (eg, the two corticospinal tracts decussate, controlling voluntary movement on side of body opposite the cerebral cortex from which the impulse initiated; three vestibulospinal tracts are involved with some autonomic functions)
  - Gray matter of cord contains reflex centers for all spinal cord reflexes

Spinal Nerves

- Thirty-one pairs, each containing a dorsal root and a ventral root
- Branches of spinal nerves form intricate networks of fibers (eg, brachial plexus) from which nerves emerge to supply various parts of skin, mucosa, and skeletal muscles
- All spinal nerves are composed of both sensory dendrites (dorsal root) and motor axons (ventral root)

Brain Cells

- *Neurons:* Basic structural and functional units
  - Sensory (afferent) neurons: Transmit impulses to spinal cord or brain
  - Motor neurons (efferent): Transmit impulses away from brain or spinal cord to muscles or glands
    - Upper motor neurons: Located in CNS; destruction causes loss of voluntary control, muscle spasticity, and hyperactive reflexes
    - Lower motor neurons: Cranial and spinal efferent neurons that lie in gray matter of spinal cord and extend into the peripheral nervous system and end at myoneural junctions in muscles; destruction causes loss of voluntary control, muscle flaccidity, and loss of reflexes
- Impulse transmission (Fig. 5.5)
  - Cell body: Contains a nucleus and other cytoplasmic matter
  - Dendrite: Carry impulses toward cell body
  - Axon: Carries impulse away from cell body

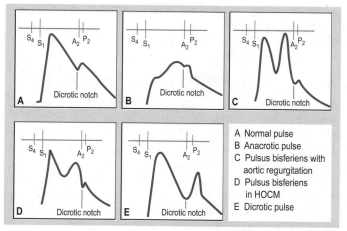

A Normal pulse
B Anacrotic pulse
C Pulsus bisferiens with aortic regurgitation
D Pulsus bisferiens in HOCM
E Dicrotic pulse

FIG. 5.5 Impulse transmission along a nerve. When conduction reaches the synapse, a neurotransmitter is released. Attachment of the neurotransmitter on the receptor can stimulate or inhibit the postsynaptic cell. (From Varcarolis, E. M., & Halter, M. J. [2010]. *Psychiatric mental health nursing: A clinical approach* [6th ed.]. St. Louis, MO: Saunders.)

- Myelin: Multiple, dense layers of membrane around an axon or dendrite; myelinated nerve fibers transmit nerve impulses more rapidly than nonmyelinated fibers
- Nerve impulses are excitatory or inhibitory
- Synapse
  - Point of contact between axon of one cell and dendrites of another
  - Axons enlarge to form synaptic terminals that secrete neurotransmitters
- Nerve impulse conduction
  - Sodium-potassium pump: Transports sodium out and potassium into cells; requires adenosine triphosphate (ATP) to function
  - Resting potential: Exists when cells are in an unstimulated or resting state
  - Action potential: Composed of depolarization and repolarization; known as the nerve impulse
  - Reflex arc: Pathway to spinal cord and back to effector organ that elicits a single, specific response; primitive nerve activity

NEUROTRANSMITTERS

Function

- Communication between one neuron and another depends on (1) the release of neurotransmitters by the presynaptic cell and (2) their reception on the postsynaptic membrane
- Although neurotransmitter movement is much slower than that of action potentials, it is effective for sending and regulating signals from one neuron to the next
- The specificity of neurotransmitter receptor sites on the postsynaptic membrane forms the basis of the chemical control of all neurologic functions
- After an action potential reaches the synaptic knob, the neurotransmitter leaves the area via the natural diffusion of a substance from an area of high concentration to one of low concentration

- A neurotransmitter is attracted to the postsynaptic membrane at receptor sites that are specific for the particular neurotransmitter
- It is typically deactivated by enzymatic degradation and reassimilated within the presynaptic cell; this process is repeated over and over

Types of Neurotransmitters (there are at least 30 types)

- Monoamines (eg, norepinephrine, epinephrine, dopamine, serotonin, acetylcholine, histamine); axons that release acetylcholine are called cholinergic; those that release norepinephrine are called adrenergic
- Amino acids (gamma-aminobutyric acid [GABA], glutamate, glycine, taurine); GABA is most common inhibitory transmitter in the brain
- Neuropeptides (eg, vasopressin, enkephalins, and endorphins); some influence hormone levels and others affect perception and integration of pain and emotional experience
- Prostaglandins: Some inhibit and some excite; may moderate actions of other transmitters by influencing the neuronal membrane

Dopamine

- Localized in several brain regions, including the substantia nigra, the midbrain, and the hypothalamus
- Dopamine-containing cells in the midbrain project into the limbic cortex; researchers think that these areas malfunction in clients with schizophrenia
- Dopamine antagonists are prescribed for the treatment of some psychoses

Serotonin

- Helps regulate a constant internal environment in relation to the maintenance of a normal body temperature, normal eating and sleep-rest patterns, and normal moods; all of these depend on adequate levels of serotonin
- Serotonin has a pattern of action similar to norepinephrine; is made from tryptophan, another amino acid
- Serotonin production occurs in the brainstem, and it is also widely dispersed throughout the cerebral cortex and the spinal cord
- Current thought is that clinically significant problems occur when clients have low levels of serotonin, and many behavioral symptoms related to depression occur when available serotonin is low or depleted

Histamine

- Involved in wakefulness, the inflammatory response (including allergies), and stimulates gastric secretion
- Histamine-1 receptor blockers are used in antipsychotic medications; side effects include sedation and weight gain; sedation may be useful in agitated clients
- Tricyclic antidepressants also block histamine-1 receptors in the brain, causing weight gain and sedation
- Antihistamines are used as sleep aids

Acetylcholine (ACh)

- Located throughout the brain, but particularly high concentrations occur in the basal nuclei and the motor cortex of the brain
- Neurons that use ACh as a neurotransmitter are often called "cholinergic"
  - Two types of acetylcholine receptors: muscarinic and nicotinic

- Many drugs interact with ACh and its receptor sites to produce anticholinergic side effects, which occur when muscarinic acetylcholine receptors are blocked; side effects include dry mouth, blurred vision, constipation, tachycardia, and urinary retention; these side effects are a common reason why clients stop using their medications; in severe cases, muscarinic receptor blockade produces confusion and delirium, especially among older clients
- Acetylcholine is the neurotransmitter at neuromuscular junctions
  - Axon terminal, containing synaptic vesicles, forms a junction with sarcolemma of muscle fiber; tiny synaptic cleft separates presynaptic membrane (axon) from postsynaptic membrane (sarcolemma)
  - When a nerve impulse reaches an axon terminal, acetylcholine is released from synaptic vesicles into the synaptic cleft; when acetylcholine binds to receptor sites on the sarcolemma, a channel opens and sodium and potassium ions flow down their concentration gradients; the sarcolemma is depolarized, and electrical energy flows into the muscle fiber; cholinesterase inactivates acetylcholine to prevent static contraction

Norepinephrine

- Norepinephrine or noradrenaline is concentrated in a small area of the brain known as the *locus coeruleus*
- Norepinephrine-producing neurons are sometimes referred to as "adrenergic"
- Many studies indicate that clients with mood disorders, particularly major depression, have a deficiency of norepinephrine
- Sympathetic nerves that innervate smooth muscles in the blood vessels have a heavy concentration of norepinephrine, which helps explain norepinephrine's role in the elevation of blood pressure during the fight-or-flight response (Fig. 5.6); when it is released directly into the bloodstream, norepinephrine acts as a hormone that enhances the effect of locally released norepinephrine at neuromuscular junctions
- Both norepinephrine and its chemical relative epinephrine are synthesized from the amino acid tyrosine; foods that are high in tyrosine and tyramine are avoided by clients who are taking certain psychotropic medications

Glutamate (Glutamic Acid) and GABA

- Most common *excitatory* neurotransmitter in the brain
- The brain's most common *inhibitory* neurotransmitter, γ-aminobutyric acid (GABA), is chemically derived from glutamate; a decrease in GABA is linked to anxiety disorders
- Nerve cells stimulated by inhibitory neurotransmitters such as GABA will be turned off, which slows or stops actions completely in the postsynaptic neurons
- Glutamate may have a role in schizophrenia; a decrease in glutamate is involved in psychotic thinking
- Glutamate may be involved in memory and learning
- Glutamate and GABA are the subjects of extensive research in disorders such as Alzheimer's disease and schizophrenia

Genetics

- Genes are the hereditary units in chromosomes that determine specific characteristics in an organism; the Human Genome Project identified all genes contained on the 23 pairs of human chromosomes

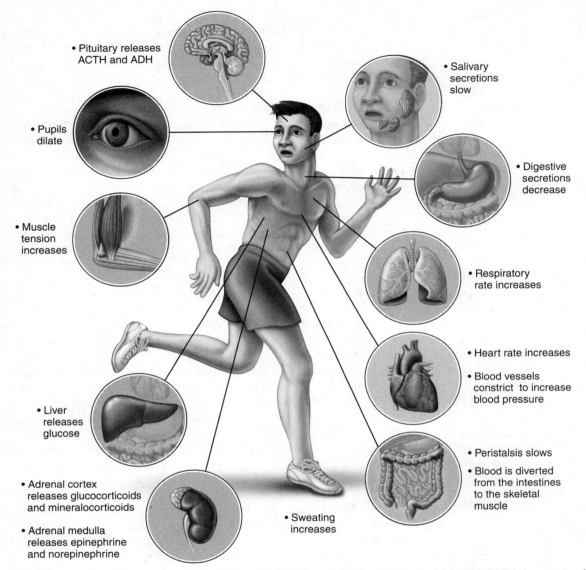

- Pituitary releases ACTH and ADH
- Salivary secretions slow
- Pupils dilate
- Digestive secretions decrease
- Muscle tension increases
- Respiratory rate increases
- Heart rate increases
- Blood vessels constrict to increase blood pressure
- Liver releases glucose
- Peristalsis slows
- Blood is diverted from the intestines to the skeletal muscle
- Adrenal cortex releases glucocorticoids and mineralocorticoids
- Adrenal medulla releases epinephrine and norepinephrine
- Sweating increases

FIG. 5.6 Fight-or-flight response. (From Harkreader, H., Hogan, M. A., & Thobaben, M. [2007]. *Fundamentals of nursing: Caring and clinical judgment* [3rd ed.]. St. Louis, MO: Saunders.)

- Genes only determine the *potential* to develop any normal or abnormal condition, which complicates the problem of identifying genetic causes of specific psychiatric disorders
- In theory, defective genes code for the incorrect synthesis of neurotransmitters or their deactivating enzymes or for other factors that interfere with the proper transmission of vital chemical agents
- A few neurologic disorders have identified genetic markers, including Huntington disease and Parkinson's disease; both diseases have been linked to genes found on chromosome number 4, but evidence for the genetic causes of some other specific neurologic disorders is not as clear

- Research has identified genes that are linked to bipolar disorder and substance addiction
- Researchers are attempting to specify schizophrenia genes; there are as many as 150 genes on nearly a dozen different chromosomes that contribute to the causes of schizophrenia; research indicates that schizophrenia results from the interaction of multiple genes rather than from a single gene
- Genetics help explain why certain psychiatric disorders recur in families and why the first degree-relatives of individuals with psychiatric disorders have an increased risk for developing the same or similar disorders
- Although few researchers believe that any one single gene causes a psychiatric illness, genetics clearly plays a significant role in development of mental health disorders; the interaction of genes is highly complex, and the link of genes to behavior remains controversial
- It appears that many genes influence psychiatric illness and the dysfunctional behaviors that are symptomatic of those illnesses
- There is increased evidence that environmental and developmental conditions in utero contribute to the expression of these genes that subsequently manifests as abnormal behavior

APPLICATION AND REVIEW

1. A nurse identifies which clinical indicator of parasympathetic dominance in a client under stress?
   1. Constipation
   2. Goose bumps
   3. Excess epinephrine secretion
   4. Increased gastrointestinal secretions
2. When caring for a client with a head injury that may involve the medulla, the nurse bases assessments on the knowledge that the medulla controls a variety of functions. Which ones apply? **Select all that apply.**
   1. Breathing
   2. Pulse rate
   3. Fat metabolism
   4. Blood vessel diameter
   5. Temperature regulation
3. A nurse is caring for an anxious, fearful client. Which client response indicates sympathetic nervous system control?
   1. Dry skin
   2. Skin pallor
   3. Constriction of pupils
   4. Pulse rate of 60 beats/min
4. Soon after admission to the hospital with a head injury, a client's temperature increases to 102.2° F (39°C). The nurse considers that the client has sustained injury to what structure?
   1. Thalamus
   2. Hypothalamus
   3. Temporal lobe
   4. Globus pallidus
5. A nurse is caring for a client who is experiencing a crisis. Which nervous system is primarily responsible for the clinical manifestations that the nurse is likely to identify?
   1. Central nervous system
   2. Peripheral nervous system
   3. Sympathetic nervous system
   4. Parasympathetic nervous system
6. An adult has panic attacks. Which neurotransmitter is most likely to be implicated in this problem?
   1. Norepinephrine
   2. Ach
   3. Serotonin
   4. GABA
7. Which statement made by a family member of a person with schizophrenia demonstrates effective learning about the disease?
   1. "The disease was probably caused by problems with several genes; these genes cause changes in how certain brain chemicals work"

2. "The disease could be cured if our politicians and laws allowed for more stem cell research; adult stem cells hold so much promise"
3. "The disease probably resulted from the mother's smoking during pregnancy; nicotine is actually a neurotransmitter"
4. "If our family had more money, we could afford the promising psychoneuroimmunologic treatments available in other countries"

See Answers on pages 82-86.

CONCEPTS OF PSYCHOBIOLOGY

Personality Development

- Overview
  - Sum of all traits that differentiate one individual from another
  - Total behavior pattern of an individual through which inner interests are expressed
  - Unique and distinctive way of perceiving, behaving, and interacting with the environment and other people
  - Constellation of defense mechanisms for coping with inner and outer pressures
  - Influenced by the functional role within a family system
  - Emergence of personality occurs at about 2 years of age
- Factors involved in personality development
  - Behavior is a learned response that develops as a result of past experiences and genetic, environmental, and psychologic factors
  - To protect the individual's emotional well-being, these experiences are organized in the psyche on three different levels
    - *Conscious:* Composed of past experiences, easily recalled; everything in one's awareness
    - *Subconscious:* Composed of material that has been pushed out of the conscious but can be recalled with some effort
    - *Unconscious:* Contains the largest body of material and greatly influences behavior; this material cannot be intentionally brought back into awareness because usually it is unacceptable and painful to the individual; if recalled, usually it is disguised or distorted, as in dreams or slips of the tongue; however, it is still capable of producing high levels of anxiety
  - According to Freud, the personality consists of three parts: id, ego, and superego
    - *Id* is the inborn unconscious instincts, impulses, and urges; it is totally self-centered
    - *Ego* is the conscious self, the "I" that deals with reality; the part of the personality that is revealed to the environment; ego strengths enable an individual to cope with frustration and delay gratification; it begins to develop during infancy
    - *Superego* is the part of the personality that, mainly on an unconscious level, controls, inhibits, and regulates impulses and instincts whose uncontrolled expression would endanger the emotional well-being of the individual and the stability of society; incorporates parental, religious, and societal values; it develops between the ages of 3 to 6 years

Formation of the Personality

- Develops in overlapping stages that shade and merge together
  - Particular conflicts and tasks must be mastered during each stage of development from infancy to maturity if needs are to be met and mental health maintained or enhanced
  - Successful resolution of the conflicts and acquisition of the tasks associated with each stage is essential to development

- If these tasks are not acquired at specific periods, the basic structure of the personality is weakened
- Factors in each stage persist as a permanent part of the personality
- Childhood identifications are integrated with basic drives, native endowments, and opportunities offered in social roles
- Unresolved conflicts remain in the unconscious and may, at times, result in maladaptive behavior
- Personality is capable of change throughout life; as one ages, there may be a decreased ability to cope
- Psychodynamic theory (Freud)
  - Psychodynamic theories propose that human behavior is largely governed by motives and drives that are internal and often unconscious
  - Freud believed that development proceeds best when children's psychosexual needs at each stage are met, but not exceeded; the stages are:
    - *Oral (birth to 1 year)*—psychosexual needs gratified orally; unable to delay gratification; begins to develop self-concept from the responses of others
    - *Anal (1–3 years)*—bladder and bowel training occurs; this interferes with instinctual impulses; struggle of giving of self and breaking the symbiotic ties to mother; as the ties are broken, the child learns independence; struggle with toilet training creates conflict between child's needs and parents' desires
    - *Phallic (3–5 years)*—psychosexual energy directed to genitals (oedipal); values and rules learned from parents; guilt and self-esteem develop; incestuous desire for opposite sex parent develops and creates fear and guilt feelings; desires are repressed, and introjection and role identification with parent of the same sex occurs
    - *Latency (6–12 years)*—mastery of learning; relationships with same-sex peers develop; sexual instincts are relatively quiet
    - *Genital (12 years and beyond)*—period of sexual maturity in which psychosexual needs are directed toward sexual relationships; sexual activity increases; sexual identity is strengthened or attacked
- Psychosocial theory (Erikson)
  - Psychosocial theory attributes development to social interactions and relationships that occur throughout the life span; failure to master a developmental stage may leave a person more susceptible to mental illness
  - Erikson believed that development results from social aims or conflicts arising from feelings, parent-child interactions, and social relationships
  - Eight major crises or conflicts need to be faced during a lifetime; each stage is marked by a struggle between two opposing tendencies, both of which are experienced by the individual; stages are:
    - *Trust versus mistrust (birth to 1 year)*—infant develops a sense of whether the world can be trusted; learns to depend on satisfaction that is derived from attention to needs; trust develops when needs are met; psychosocial strength—hope; failure to consistently meet the needs of the infant can lead to difficult interpersonal relationships
    - *Autonomy versus shame and doubt (1–3 years)*—child develops first sense of self as independent or as shameful and doubtful; the struggle of holding on to or letting go; an internal struggle for self-identity; love versus hate; psychosocial strength—will; if not provided the opportunity for some independence in activity, the child will lack self-confidence
    - *Initiative versus guilt (3–6 years)*—child learns ability to try new things and learns how to handle failure; period of intensive activity, play, and consuming fantasies, in which

child interjects parents' social consciousness; psychosocial strength—purpose; if outlets for creativity and exploration are not provided, child blames self for lack of initiative

- *Industry versus inferiority (6–12 years)*—child learns how to make things with others and strives to achieve success; psychosocial strength—self-worth; if not provided with mastery experiences and realistic positive feedback about performance, low self-esteem will occur
- *Identity versus role confusion (puberty to young adulthood)*—adolescent determines own sense of self; psychosocial strength—fidelity; if overly restricted in the exploration of interests and independent growth, discouragement and confusion about the direction to take in life will occur
- *Intimacy versus isolation (young adulthood)*—person makes commitment to another; moves from the relative security of self-identity to the relative insecurity involved in establishing intimacy with another; psychosocial strength—love; if there has been a lack of intimacy in the family of origin and previous developmental stages are not achieved successfully, the development of intimacy is unlikely to occur and the individual may become isolated and self-absorbed
- *Generativity versus stagnation (middle adulthood)*—person seeks to guide the next generation or risks feelings of personal incompleteness; psychosocial strength—care; if previous developmental stages were unsuccessfully completed and there is a continued lack of self-confidence or preoccupation with self, the adult fails to engage in meaningful activities that help support others
- *Integrity versus despair (late life)*—older adult seeks a sense of personal accomplishment, adapts to triumphs and disappointments with a certain ego integrity and accepts death, or falls into despair; psychosocial strength—wisdom; if this stage is not achieved, there is a feeling of being unfulfilled and sad
- Interpersonal theory (Sullivan)
  - Development results from interpersonal relationships with others in maximizing satisfaction of needs and minimizing insecurity
  - Development results from interpersonal relationships in the infancy, childhood, juvenile, preadolescent, adolescent, and late adolescent stages:
    - *Infancy (0–2 years)*—learns to differentiate self from others; learns through trial and error; learns from parental interactions to rely on others to gratify needs and satisfy wishes; develops a sense of basic trust, security, and self-worth; ends with language development; if needs are not met anxiety and emotional withdrawal occur
    - *Childhood (2–6 years)*—language development allows for education; development of body image and self-perception; self-esteem develops with sublimation; child learns to communicate needs through the use of words and to accept delayed gratification and interference with wish fulfillment; expresses impulses in socially acceptable ways or develops a feeling of living among enemies
    - *Juvenile (6–10 years)*—relations with peers allow child to see self objectively; develops conscience; behavior is connected to others' opinions; organizes and uses experiences in terms of approval and disapproval received; begins using selective inattention and disassociates those experiences that cause physical or emotional discomfort and pain; difficulty with this stage results in ineffective social interaction and social isolation
    - *Preadolescent (10–13 years)*—develops same-sex friends; moves from egocentrism to love; able to form satisfying relationships and work with peers; uses competition, compromise, and cooperation; difficulty with this stage results in a lack of reciprocity in interpersonal relationships

- *Adolescent (13–17 years)*—interest in sexual activity; learns how to establish satisfactory relationships with members of the opposite sex; if attractions are severely discouraged or thwarted, insecurity and loneliness develop
- *Late adolescent (17–19 years)*—personality integration; able to integrate the needs of society without becoming overwhelmed with anxiety; inability to achieve personality integration results in regression and egocentrism for life
- Cognitive development theory (Piaget)
  - *Sensorimotor stage (infancy-toddler)*—infant develops physically with a gradual increase in the ability to think and use language; progresses from simple reflex responses through repetitive behaviors to deliberate and imaginative activity
  - *Preoperational thought stage (preschool)*—child learns to imitate and play; begins to use symbols and language although interpretation is literal
  - *Preoperational thought stage continues (school age)*—child begins to understand relationships and develops basic conceptual thought and intuitive reasoning
  - *Concrete operational thought stage (preadolescent)*—thinking is more socialized and logical with increased intellectual and conceptual development; begins problem-solving by use of inductive reasoning and logical thought
  - *Formal operational stage (adolescent)*—develops true abstract thought by application of logical tests; achieves conceptual independence and problem-solving ability

Adaptation to Stress

- Human beings must be able to perceive and interpret stimuli to interact with the environment
  - Perception and cognitive functioning influenced by
    - Nature of stimuli
    - Culture, beliefs, attitudes, and age
    - Past experiences
    - Present physical and emotional needs
  - Personality development is influenced by ability to perceive and interpret stimuli
    - External world is internalized through these processes
    - External world may in turn be distorted by perceptions
- Selye's general adaptation syndrome (GAS) is body's nonspecific physiologic response to stress; occurs in three stages: alarm, resistance, and exhaustion
  - Stress produces wear and tear on body; can be internal or external, beneficial or detrimental, and always elicits some response from or change in the individual
  - First: Alarm phase—sympathetic nervous system prepares body's physiologic defense for fight or flight by stimulating adrenal medulla to secrete epinephrine and norepinephrine; adrenocortical hormones (aldosterone and cortisol) are secreted (Fig. 5.6)
    - Heartbeat increases to pump more blood to muscles
    - Peripheral blood vessels constrict to provide more blood to vital organs
    - Bronchioles dilate and breathing becomes rapid and deep to supply more oxygen to cells
    - Pupils dilate to increase vision
    - Liver releases glucose for quick energy
    - Prothrombin time is shortened to protect body from loss of blood in event of injury
    - Sodium is retained to maintain blood volume
  - Second: Resistance stage—when stress continues, increased secretion of cortisone enables body to cope with stress
  - Third: Exhaustion—if stress continues and responses are no longer effective, the last stage is exhaustion and death

- Local inflammatory response: Body's nonspecific response of tissue to injury or infection
  - Erythema (redness): Histamine is released at site of injury, causing vasodilation (hyperemia)
  - Heat: Vasodilation brings more core-warmed blood to area
  - Edema (swelling): Histamine causes increased capillary permeability, allowing fluid, protein, and white blood cells (WBCs) to move into interstitial space
  - Pain: Nerve endings are irritated by chemical mediators (eg, serotonin, prostaglandin, and kinins) and pressure from edema
  - Loss of function: A protective response because of pain and edema

Neurobiology

- Feelings, thoughts, physiology, and behaviors are interactive, and each influences the others
- There is general acceptance that there is no real division between mind and body, mental and physical, brain and thought
- Research into the neurophysiologic basis for behavior focuses on anatomy and physiology of the brain and nervous system and their relationship to health and illness
  - Structural differences, such as ventricle size or cerebral atrophy, are identified by neuroimaging methods such as magnetic resonance imaging (MRI) and computed tomography (CT) scans
  - Physiologic differences, such as hyperactivity in certain areas of the brain, are identified by electroencephalogram (EEG) studies and positron emission tomography (PET) scans
- Neuroplasticity is the ability of the brain to change its structure and function
  - Brain cell regeneration is possible in some conditions

Biologic Basis of Mental Health Disorders

- Overview
  - Much of the stigma attached to psychiatric illness had been due to a lack of understanding of the biologic basis of these disorders
  - Effective client, family, and public teaching is an important function of the role of the psychiatric mental health nurse as researchers discover new information regarding the structures and functioning of the CNS
  - Considerable knowledge gaps exist as to the specific pathophysiology of most psychiatric disorders, but research continues to shed light, especially in the area of neurotransmitters (Table 5.2)
  - Research is examining the importance of other factors such as genetics, infections, sleep deprivation, toxins, nutrition, hormonal shifts, trauma, and stress (consider cortisol's effects) as influences on neurobiology and behavior
- Specific conditions
  - Depression is linked with a decrease in norepinephrine and serotonin and possibly other neurotransmitters
    - Hypothyroidism can present as depression
  - Anxious clients can be calmed with drugs that activate GABA
  - Research shows that schizophrenia has a multifactorial origin, with genetics, heredity, increased ventricle size, altered neurotransmitter function, and neuroanatomic differences all playing roles, as biologic changes interact with psychosocial elements
  - Brains of those with Alzheimer disease have atrophied, have altered topography, and contain specific microscopic changes

TABLE 5.2   Relationship of Neurotransmitter Dysfunction to Mental Health Disorders*

Neurotransmitter	Dysfunction	Disorder
Dopamine	Increase (in some areas; decrease in others)	Schizophrenia
Serotonin	Decrease	Depression
Norepinephrine	Decrease	Depression
γ-Aminobutyric acid (GABA)	Decrease	Anxiety disorders
Acetylcholine	Decrease	Alzheimer's disease
Glutamate	Decrease	Psychotic thinking

*This is a simplified explanation.
Adapted from Fortinash, K. M., & Holoday, P. A. (2012). *Psychiatric mental health nursing* (5th ed.). St. Louis, MO: Mosby and Keltner, N. L., & Steele, D. (2015). *Psychiatric nursing* (7th ed.). St. Louis, MO: Mosby.

- In Parkinson's disease, the substantia nigra (where dopamine is primarily synthesized) deteriorates; reduction of dopamine impedes the normal balance of dopamine and acetylcholine
- Anorexia nervosa appears to have hypothalamic dysfunction
- See also the Genetics section

APPLICATION AND REVIEW

8. Which relationship is of **most** concern to the nurse because of its importance in the formation of the personality?
   1. Peer
   2. Sibling
   3. Spousal
   4. Parent-child
9. On which generally accepted concept of personality development should a nurse base care?
   1. By 2 years of age the personality is firmly set
   2. The personality is capable of modification throughout life
   3. The capacity for personality change decreases rapidly after adolescence
   4. By the end of the first 6 years of life the personality has reached its adult parameters
10. Which individual is coping with issues concerning dependence versus independence?
    1. Infant
    2. Toddler
    3. School-age child
    4. Preschool-age child
11. A 17-year-old teenager is diagnosed with leukemia. Which statements by the teenager reflect Piaget's cognitive processes associated with adolescence? **Select all that apply.**
    1. "My smoking pot probably caused the leukemia"
    2. "I'm going to do my best to fight this terrible disease"
    3. "Now I can't go to the prom because I have this stupid illness"
    4. "I know I got sick because I've been causing a lot of problems at home"
    5. "This illness is serious, but with treatment I think I will have a chance to get better"
12. A person mowing the lawn is badly disfigured by the lawn mower blade. According to Erikson's theory, a person at which age will demonstrate the greatest risk of long-term psychological effects?
    1. 11-year-old
    2. 35-year-old
    3. 55-year-old
    4. 70-year-old

13. A nurse is interviewing an 8-year-old girl who was admitted to the pediatric unit. Which statement by the child warrants additional assessment?
    1. "Wow—this place has bright colors"
    2. "Are my parents allowed to visit me tonight?"
    3. "Those boys are so cute; I hope their room is next to mine"
    4. "I am scared about being here; can you stay with me awhile?"

14. A nurse must consider a child's cognitive level of development when providing preoperative teaching. At which stage of Piaget's cognitive theory should the nurse anticipate a child will experience the greatest fear of surgery?
    1. Sensorimotor
    2. Preoperational
    3. Formal operational
    4. Concrete operational

15. A nurse is assessing a young adult for evidence of achievement of the age-related developmental stage based on Erikson's developmental theory. What developmental crisis is associated with this age group?
    1. Trust versus mistrust
    2. Intimacy versus isolation
    3. Industry versus inferiority
    4. Generativity versus stagnation

16. According to Erikson, a person's adjustment to the period of senescence will depend largely on the adjustment the individual made to which previous developmental stage?
    1. Trust versus mistrust
    2. Industry versus inferiority
    3. Identity versus role confusion
    4. Generativity versus stagnation

17. A client who retired a year ago tells the nurse in the community health center, "I don't have any hobbies or interests, and since I retired, I feel useless and unneeded." According to Erikson's developmental theory, with which developmental conflict is the client faced?
    1. Initiative versus guilt
    2. Integrity versus despair
    3. Intimacy versus isolation
    4. Identity versus role confusion

18. To provide appropriate psychosocial support to clients, a nurse must understand development across the life span. What theory is the nurse using when relationships and resulting behaviors are considered the central factors that influence development?
    1. Cognitive theory
    2. Psychosocial theory
    3. Interpersonal theory
    4. Psychosexual theory

19. Using Piaget's theory of cognitive development, what should the nurse expect a 6-month-old infant begin to demonstrate?
    1. Early traces of memory
    2. Beginning sense of time
    3. Repetitious reflex responses
    4. Beginning of object permanence

20. What should the nurse assist the older adult to accomplish to successfully complete Erikson's major task of this stage?
    1. Invest creative energies in promoting social welfare
    2. Feel a sense of satisfaction when considering past achievements
    3. Develop deep, lasting relationships with other people or institutions
    4. Look to recapture opportunities that were not started or were not completed

See Answers on pages 82-86.

ANSWER KEY: REVIEW QUESTIONS

1. **4 Parasympathetic nerves increase peristalsis and GI secretion**
   1 The parasympathetic nervous system increases intestinal motility, which may cause diarrhea. **2** Goose bumps (piloerection), caused by contraction of the *musculi arrectores pilorum*, are under sympathetic control; vasoconstriction is also under sympathetic control. **3** Epinephrine is a sympathomimetic
   Client Need: Physiologic Adaptation; **Cognitive Level:** Comprehension; **Nursing Process:** Assessment/Analysis

> 🔑 **Memory Aid:** You can think of the parasympathetic division as the "rest and digest" division; it has opposing effects to the sympathetic system. To remember that pa**r**asympathetic is the "**r**est and digest" division (instead of sympathetic, which is the "fight-or-flight" division), notice the "r" in **r**est and in pa**r**a.

2. **Answers: 1, 2, 4**

   1 The medulla, part of the brainstem just above the foramen magnum, is concerned with vital functions such as respirations. **2** The medulla is concerned with vital functions such as the heart rate. **4** The medulla is concerned with vital functions such as blood pressure by controlling blood vessel diameter.

   3 Fat metabolism is not controlled by the CNS. **5** Temperature regulation is controlled by the hypothalamus
   Client Need: Physiologic Adaptation; **Cognitive Level:** Analysis; **Nursing Process:** Assessment/Analysis

> 🔑 **Memory Aid:** Consider that the **m**e**dull**a performs the "**dull**, **m**aintenance" tasks of your biological unit, such as respiration, heart rate, and blood pressure control, as opposed to the more interesting cerebral tasks of reasoning, voluntary motor ability, or humor.

3. **2 The sympathetic nervous system constricts the smooth muscle of blood vessels in the skin when a person is under stress**

   1 The sympathetic system stimulates, rather than inhibits, secretion by the sweat glands. **3** Constriction of pupils is not under sympathetic control; the parasympathetic system constricts the pupils. **4** The parasympathetic system (vagus nerve) slows the pulse, and the sympathetic system increases it
   Client Need: Physiologic Adaptation; **Cognitive Level:** Application; **Nursing Process:** Assessment/Analysis

4. **2 The hypothalamus connects with the autonomic area for vasoconstriction, vasodilation, and perspiration and with the somatic centers for shivering; therefore it is an important area for regulating body temperature**

   1 The thalamus receives all sensory stimuli, except taste, for transmission to the cerebral cortex; it is also involved with emotions and instinctive activities. **3** The temporal lobe is concerned with auditory stimuli; it may also be involved with the sense of smell. **4** The globus pallidus is part of the basal ganglia; it is also called the pallidum; together with the putamen, it comprises the lenticular nucleus; it is concerned with muscle tone, which is required for specific body movements
   Client Need: Physiologic Adaptation; **Cognitive Level:** Comprehension; **Nursing Process:** Assessment/Analysis

5. **3 The sympathetic nervous system reacts to stress by releasing epinephrine, which prepares the body to fight or flee by increasing the heart rate, constricting peripheral vessels, and increasing oxygen supply to muscles**

   1 Although the brain responds to stress, it is the sympathetic nervous system that is primarily affected. **2** The sympathetic and parasympathetic nervous systems are both part of the peripheral nervous system; the sympathetic nervous system primarily is affected; the parasympathetic nervous system does not play a role in the fight-or-flight reaction. **4** The parasympathetic nervous system has an effect opposite to that of the sympathetic nervous system
   Client Needs: Psychosocial Integrity; **Cognitive Level:** Comprehension; **Nursing Process:** Assessment/Analysis

6. **4 A decrease in GABA is involved in anxiety disorders**

   1 Decreased norepinephrine is seen in depression. **2** Decreased ACh is seen in Alzheimer's. **3** Decreased serotonin is seen in depression
   Client Need: Psychosocial Integrity; **Cognitive Level:** Comprehension; **Nursing Process:** Assessment/Analysis

7. **1 It is clear that several genes are implicated in the origins of schizophrenia**

   2 Although stem cells do hold promise for many diseases, there is no support for them to cure schizophrenia. **3** Although nicotine is a neurotransmitter, it has not been linked to the development of schizophrenia. **4** No psychoneuroimmunology treatment exists to cure schizophrenia in any country at this time
   Client Need: Psychosocial Integrity; **Cognitive Level:** Analysis; **Integrated Process:** Communication/Documentation; **Nursing Process:** Assessment/Analysis

8. **4 Children view their own worth by the response received from their parents; this sense of worth sets the basic ego strengths and is vital to the formation of the personality**

   1 Peer groups come later in a child's development, but the parent-child relationship is still the most important. **2** Although important, sibling relationship is not as important as the parent-child relationship. **3** Spousal relationship comes later in life, after the basic personality has been formed

   Client Need: Health Promotion and Maintenance; **Cognitive Level:** Comprehension; **Nursing Process:** Assessment/Analysis

9. **2 New methods of coping with situations require modifications of approach and attitudes; hence personality is always capable of change**

   1 Certain personality traits are established by age **2** but not the total personality. **3** The capacity for change exists throughout the life cycle. **4** Accepting that theory (that by the end of the first 6 years of life the personality has reached its adult parameters) denies the fact that the personality is capable of change throughout life

   Client Need: Health Promotion and Maintenance; **Cognitive Level:** Comprehension; **Nursing Process:** Assessment/Analysis

10. **2 The toddler is learning autonomy, but because of the nature of development, there is still physical and emotional dependence on the parents**

    1 The major task during infancy is the development of trust. **3** School-age children cope with the task of industry and developing skills for working in and relating to the world. **4** Preschool-age children cope with developing a sense of initiative

    Client Need: Health Promotion and Maintenance; **Cognitive Level:** Comprehension; **Nursing Process:** Assessment/Analysis

11. **Answers: 2, 3, 5**

    2 At 17 years of age the adolescent is in the formal operational stage of cognitive development and therefore is able to understand the seriousness of leukemia. **3** At 17 years of age the adolescent is in the formal operational stage of cognitive development and therefore understands the seriousness of the illness; the statement also reflects an adolescent's preoccupation with peer socialization. **5** At 17 years of age the adolescent is in the formal operational stage of cognitive development and therefore is able to comprehend the seriousness of leukemia and the need for treatment

    1 At 2 to 7 years of age children are in the preoperational stage of cognitive development; they believe that external, unrelated, concrete phenomena cause illness. **4** At 7 to 10 years of age children are in the concrete operational stage of cognitive development; because of their egocentrism, they believe that they are responsible for situations, such as illnesses, and are being punished

    Client Need: Psychosocial Integrity; **Cognitive Level:** Analysis; **Integrated Process:** Communication/Documentation; **Nursing Process:** Assessment/Analysis

12. **1 An 11-year-old child generally is in Erikson's stage of industry versus inferiority, which involves the mastery of skills; the child did not master the skill of lawn mowing; also, the child will be entering adolescence (stage of identity versus confusion) when major physical and emotional changes occur in relation to how one is perceived by the self and by others**

    2 A 35-year-old adult generally is in Erikson's stage of intimacy versus isolation and thus is less concerned about proving industriousness and has moved through the stage of identity versus confusion. **3** A 55-year-old adult generally is in the stage of generativity versus stagnation and is therefore less concerned about being industrious and has moved through the stage of identity versus confusion. **4** A 70-year-old adult generally is in Erikson's stage of ego integrity versus despair and is less concerned about becoming industrious and has moved through the stage of identity versus confusion

    Client Need: Health Promotion and Maintenance; **Cognitive Level:** Application; **Nursing Process:** Assessment/Analysis

13. **3 A 7-year-old child should be more concerned with same-gender relationships; a child demonstrating a strong attraction to opposite-gender relations should be questioned further regarding the possibility of sexual abuse**

1 Noticing the colors in the environment is not unusual because 7-year-old children usually are attracted to a colorful environment. **2** Asking about whether the mother can visit is not unusual because 7-year-old children will want the presence of a trusted parent when experiencing stress. **4** Expressing fear and asking about the nurse staying is not unusual because 7-year-old children will want the support of a trusted person when experiencing stress

Client Need: Psychosocial Integrity; **Cognitive Level:** Analysis; **Integrated Process:** Communication/Documentation; **Nursing Process:** Assessment/Analysis

14. **2 (Preoperational) Children 2 to 7 years of age have difficulty distinguishing reality from fantasy, which may increase fears**

1 Children from birth to 1 year of age (Sensorimotor) focus on "in the moment" thinking; preoperative preparation most likely will not be recalled. **3** Children 12 to 16 years of age (Formal operational) can think in the abstract and have the ability to solve complex problems; children in this stage usually do not pose difficulties in preoperative teaching. **4** Children 7 to 11 years of age (Concrete operations) have the ability to comprehend and visualize a series of events and can think about the past and present; this stage provides less of a challenge to absorb preoperative teachings

Client Need: Health Promotion and Maintenance; **Cognitive Level:** Application; **Integrated Process:** Teaching/Learning; **Nursing Process:** Assessment/Analysis

15. **2 The major task of young adulthood (intimacy versus isolation) is centered on human closeness and sexual fulfillment; lack of love results in isolation**

1 Trust versus mistrust is associated with infancy. **3** Industry versus inferiority is associated with middle childhood (school age). **4** Generativity versus stagnation is associated with middle adulthood

Client Need: Health Promotion and Maintenance; **Cognitive Level:** Knowledge; **Nursing Process:** Assessment/Analysis

16. **4 Erikson theorized that how well people adapt to the present stage depends on how well they adapted to the stage immediately preceding it—in this instance adulthood**

1 Although Erikson believed that the strengths and weaknesses of each stage are present in some form in all succeeding stages, their influence decreases with time. **2** Although Erikson believed that the strengths and weaknesses of each stage are present in some form in all succeeding stages, their influence decreases with time. **3** Although Erikson believed that the strengths and weaknesses of each stage are present in some form in all succeeding stages, their influence decreases with time

Client Need: Health Promotion and Maintenance; **Cognitive Level:** Comprehension; **Nursing Process:** Assessment/Analysis

17. **2 Integrity versus despair is the task of the older adult; this client has not adapted to triumphs and disappointments, so there is no acceptance of what life is and was; this results in feelings of despair and disgust**

1 Initiative versus guilt is the task of the preschool period. **3** Intimacy versus isolation is the task of the young adult. **4** Identity versus role confusion is the task of the adolescent

Client Need: Health Promotion and Maintenance; **Cognitive Level:** Application; **Nursing Process:** Assessment/Analysis

18. **3 The interpersonal theory of human development by Harry Stack Sullivan highlights interpersonal behaviors and relationships as the central factors influencing child and adolescent development across six "eras"; the need to satisfy social attachments and a longing to meet biologic and psychologic needs are two dimensions associated with this theory**

1 Cognitive theory is associated with Jean Piaget; cognitive theory explains how thought processes develop, are structured, and influence behavior. **2** Psychosocial theory is associated with Erik Erikson; psychosocial theory identifies social interaction as the source that influences human development; Erikson identified eight stages of human life, with each stage built on the previous stages and influenced by past experiences. **4** Psychosexual theory is associated with Sigmund Freud; psychosexual theory views child development as a biologically driven series of conflicts and gratifying internal needs

Client Need: Psychosocial Integrity; **Cognitive Level:** Comprehension; **Nursing Process:** Assessment/Analysis

19. **4 The concept of object permanence begins to develop at about 6 months of age because of brain development and experience**

    1 Early traces of memory occur between 13 and 24 months. **2** Beginning sense of time occurs between 13 and 24 months. **3** Repetitious reflex responses occur during the first several months of life; these diminish as the newborn grows

    Client Need: Health Promotion and Maintenance; **Cognitive Level:** Application; **Nursing Process:** Assessment/Analysis

20. **2 Feeling a sense of satisfaction when considering past achievements allows the client to accept what life is or was and helps** avoid **feelings of despair**

    1 Investing creative energies in promoting social welfare is the major task of middle adulthood (30–65 years). **3** Developing deep, lasting relationships with other people or institutions is the major task of the young adult (20–30 years). **4** Feeling a need to make up for past failings is a negative resolution of the major task of the older adult

    Client Need: Health Promotion and Maintenance; **Cognitive Level:** Analysis; **Nursing Process:** Planning/Implementation; **Integrated Process:** Caring

Crisis Theory and Intervention 6

CHARACTERISTICS OF CRISES

- A crisis is an acute, time-limited, emotional response to a stressful event or series of stressful events that can be real, potential, or imagined; a crisis can overwhelm a person's coping abilities
- A crisis is defined as a situation in which the client's previous methods of adaptation are inadequate to meet present needs
- Crises progress through four distinct phases (Table 6.1)
- Continuing stress increases vulnerability, causes anxiety and physical discomfort, and threatens the person's self-esteem, integrity, and safety
- The response to a stressor varies from person to person and will be determined by perception of the situation, prior coping skills, the client's support system, and psychologic and physical health (eg, some may experience a midlife crisis or empty-nest syndrome and others may not)
- Crises are usually self-limiting and last between 4 and 6 weeks
- Ineffective coping during a crisis can lead to personality disorganization and long-term maladaptive behaviors
- Crisis intervention is a focused short-term therapy for clients in situations in which their usual coping has been overwhelmed
- The goal is to return the client to *precrisis* level of functioning, but as the individual tries to regain psychologic equilibrium, there is the opportunity for personal growth by learning new coping skills and developing additional resources

TYPES OF CRISES (Table 6.2)

Situational Crisis

- Also called an external crisis
- Results from actual events or circumstances in the environment that upset an individual's psychologic balance
- Examples: Job loss, divorce, loss of a loved one, unwanted pregnancy, onset or worsening of a medical illness, school problems, and witnessing a crime

Subjective Crisis

- Also called an internal crisis
- Subjectively perceived and experienced
- Examples: Betrayal, fear, response to aging, loss, abandonment, loss of loyalty, and a threat to a deeply held belief or value

Phase-of-Life Crisis

- Also called a maturational crisis
- Occurs when developmental events require a role change
- May occur during the course of normal growth and developmental phases and milestones

TABLE 6.1	Caplan's Phases of Crisis Development
Phase	**Description**
Phase 1	Exposure to stressor (can be real or imagined) causes increasing anxiety as usual coping skills do not bring resolution to the problem.
Phase 2	Previous coping and problem-solving strategies fail to bring relief. Utilization of more dysfunctional coping behaviors occurs as high level of anxiety impedes problem-solving.
Phase 3	Resources from within and outside of the individual are mobilized to resolve the problem and to alleviate the discomfort caused by the stressor. Anxiety reaches panic level when effective coping is lost.
Phase 4	The absence of resolution of the crisis leads to anxiety overwhelming the individual, who feels immobilized or acts out with violence and self-destructive behaviors; personality disorganization occurs.

Data from: Nugent, P. M., Green, J. S., Hellmer Saul, M. A., & Pelikan, P. K. (2012). *Mosby's comprehensive review of nursing for the NCLEX-RN examination* (20th ed.). St Louis, MO: Mosby.
Fortinash, K. M., & Holoday, P. A. (2012). *Psychiatric mental health nursing* (5th ed.). St. Louis, MO: Mosby.

TABLE 6.2	Types of Crises
Type of Crisis	**Description**
Maturational	Transitions in development require new behaviors and skills (basis of Erikson's theory); considered normal and often are predictable so that preventive strategies can be implemented (eg, retirement planning)
Situational	Specific common external events that are not anticipated and create stress (eg, job loss, amputation of a limb)
Adventitious	Disaster-type events that affect groups (eg, tornado) or unpredictable, unusual, individual event (eg, rape) Some theorists believe that crisis intervention immediately after an adventitious crisis can reduce the incidence of posttraumatic stress disorder

From Nugent, P. M., Green, J. S., Hellmer Saul, M. A., & Pelikan, P. K. (2012). *Mosby's comprehensive review of nursing for the NCLEX-RN examination* (20th ed.). St Louis, MO: Mosby.

- Transitions between life stages are common triggers for phase-of-life crises: Moving from early to middle childhood, moving from adolescence to adulthood, marriage, parenthood, midlife, and retirement
- Erikson's developmental crises are typical flashpoints for crises: Trust versus mistrust; intimacy versus isolation; industry versus inferiority; generativity versus stagnation
- Nature of crises is influenced by role models—both positive and negative viewpoints

Disasters

- Also called adventitious crises, caused by events not part of ordinary life as a result of extraordinary events
- Can be natural (such as an earthquake) or man-made (such as a fire or violent crime)

Psychiatric Emergencies

- Sudden and serious psychologic disturbance that requires intervention to prevent a life-threatening or psychologically damaging consequence

- Client poses danger to self or others (for example, use of a weapon) or is gravely disabled psychologically
- Client can be detained involuntarily for evaluation and treatment (see Chapter 4)
- Can occur in any setting
- Includes suicide attempts (see "Suicide" section)
- Can result from violence, substance use disorder, biopsychosocial stressors, and many other causes
- Anxiety is common in client and family/friends during the emergency and can spread to the health care team; requires the nurse to remain calm and focused
- Acts of violence, self-harm, and development of psychosis are other psychiatric emergencies that arise from unsuccessful resolution of a crisis

HUMAN RESPONSES TO CRISIS

Nurse's Role (*see also* Nursing Care of Clients in Crisis)

- Identify individuals with risk factors for crisis as a result of nurses' daily interactions with individuals and families who are experiencing life disruptions
- Use risk factors assessment criteria to identify individuals and families who are at high risk for crises and then intervene to prevent those crises from occurring

Risk Factors for Crises

- The presence of concurrent or multiple biopsychosocial stressors
- Multiple losses, unexpected life changes, and unresolved problems
- Limitations in adaptive ability and coping skills
- Chronic physical or psychologic pain or disability
- Concurrent psychiatric disorders, substance use disorder, and suicidality
- Poor social support networks
- Limited access to health care services

Signs and Symptoms of Critical Incident Stress

- Physical: Fatigue, sleep disturbance, headache, dizziness, elevated blood pressure, rapid heart rate, muscle tension or tremors, nausea, chest pain, shortness of breath, grinding of teeth, and changes in appetite
- Cognitive: Difficulty focusing or concentrating, trouble making decisions or problem-solving, negative thought patterns, flashbacks, intrusive thoughts, nightmares, and altered awareness of surroundings
- Emotional: Anxiety, grief, anger, irritability, depression, panic attacks, guilt, hopelessness, psychologic numbness, decreased stress tolerance, failure of usual coping strategies, and difficulty regulating emotional responses
- Behavioral: Withdrawal, restlessness, changes in social activity, changes in speech patterns, alterations in awareness of surroundings (ie, increased or decreased awareness or distortions), suspiciousness, use of recreational substances, and engaging in high-risk behavior

Coping

- Stress or distress can be physical, emotional, social, or spiritual
- Stressors activate the person's sympathetic (fight-or-flight) nervous system in response
- Coping abilities are conscious and unconscious ways to deal with stress
- Coping is a change in behavior in reaction to an actual or perceived threat in an attempt to maintain psychological integrity (Fig. 6.1)

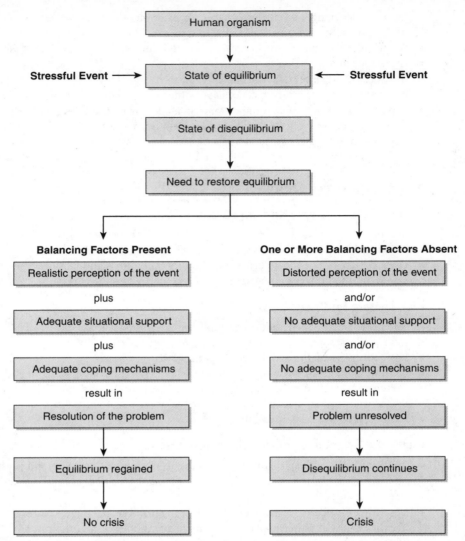

FIG. 6.1   **Paradigm: The effect of balancing factors in a stressful event.** (From Aguilera, D. C. [1998]. *Crisis intervention: Theory and methodology* [8th ed.]. St Louis, MO: Mosby.)

APPLICATION AND REVIEW

1. A child in the first grade is murdered, and counseling is planned for the other children in the school. What should a nurse identify **first** before assessing a child's response to a crisis?
    1. Developmental level of the child
    2. Quality of the child's peer relationships
    3. Child's perception of the crisis situation
    4. Child's communication patterns with family members

2. How should a nurse characterize a sudden terrorist act that causes the deaths of thousands of adults and children and effects negatively on their families, friends, communities, and the nation?
   1. Recurring
   2. Situational
   3. Maturational
   4. Adventitious
3. A 44-year-old client is unable to function since her husband asked for a divorce 2 weeks ago. What type of crisis reflects this situation?
   1. Social
   2. Situational
   3. Maturational
   4. Developmental

See Answers on pages 104-107.

NURSING CARE OF CLIENTS IN CRISIS

Overview

- Crisis intervention is short-term therapy with the major goal of restoring clients to their precrisis state of psychologic equilibrium. Roberts' seven-stage crisis intervention model overlaps with nursing steps:
  1. Plan and conduct a thorough biopsychosocial-spiritual assessment that addresses the individual's dangerousness to himself or herself and others
  2. Establish rapport and rapidly establish a collaborative relationship with the individual or family in crisis
  3. Identify major problems, including those that may have triggered the crisis
  4. Encourage the expression of feelings and emotions with active listening and validation
  5. Generate and explore alternatives for coping
  6. Collaboratively develop an action plan that serves to empower the client and that restores functioning
  7. Develop a follow-up plan to assess postcrisis status and the need for further intervention
- Assess the client's developmental level, perception of the event, past and current coping skills, resources and support systems, and potential for violence/suicide
- Implement interventions that are directive and goal oriented because of the short time frame; focus on present problem and immediate crisis issues only
- Progress through stages: Intervening immediately, stabilizing the client, facilitating a realistic understanding of the event, facilitating use of resources, encouraging self-reliance, developing and utilizing healthy support systems
- Encourage the client to express feelings and develop healthier coping skills
- Refer the client for more long-term care treatment, to support groups, and to social services as needed
- Perform self-assessment to ensure you are acting within the nurse-client relationship; use these techniques yourself to cope:
  - *Talk it out:* Find a trusted other to share your feelings with and who will allow you to express fears and frustrations
  - *Set limits:* Learning to say "no" is a challenge for many professional helpers, including nurses; having the motivation to care for others in crisis can also precipitate a crisis for the nurse who has trouble setting limits with regard to taking on more than is possible or healthy
  - *Nurture relationships:* Maintaining meaningful relationships both at work and at home can support crisis nurses in both their personal and professional lives

- *Develop positive stress management patterns:* Nurses need to find meaningful ways to manage daily stressors so that they can "recharge," both physically and psychologically
- *Recruit a mentor:* Forming a developmental relationship with a more experienced crisis/intervention practitioner can help a less experienced practitioner learn valuable survival skills for ongoing work in the specialty of crisis nursing
- *Cultivate a sense of humor:* Humor can be one of the most adaptive and powerful strategies to help provide perspective through crisis as well as for the professional who is working with individuals in crisis

Nursing Assessment

- Can occur in the field (on site) or in controlled environment (hospital)
- For situations with traumatic physical and emotional threats, see Box 6.1
- The nurse should assume an active role in assessing the current situation and facilitate the interview with authority
- Assess client's perception of the event, support systems, and coping skills
  - The most significant factor in either precipitating or avoiding a crisis is not the events, *but how the individual perceives them*
- Assess client's ability to perform activities of daily living
- It is essential to assess lethality (suicide , homicide, self-harm ideation)

Nursing Diagnosis

- Nursing diagnoses are varied, but the client's abilities to maintain self-esteem, resume prior effective role function or ideally master new roles, work effectively with others, and maintain safety are key to nursing diagnoses

---

BOX 6.1 The 10 Stages of Acute Traumatic Stress Management

1 *Assess for danger and for the safety of yourself and others.* Are there factors that will compromise your safety or the safety of others?

2 *Consider the mechanism of injury.* How did the event physically and perceptually affect the individual?

3 *Evaluate the level of responsiveness.* Is the individual alert and responsive? Is he or she under the influence of a substance?

4 *Address medical needs.* This should be done by individuals who are specifically trained to manage acute medical conditions.

5 *Observe and identify.* Who has been exposed to the event? Who is showing signs of traumatic stress?

6 *Connect with the individual.* Introduce yourself and state your title or position. After the individual has had a medical evaluation, move him or her away from the stressor. Begin to develop rapport.

7 *Ground the individual.* Discuss the facts, ensure safety, and have individuals tell their own story. Discuss behavioral and physiologic responses.

8 *Provide support.* Be empathic. Communicate a desire to understand the feelings that lie behind the words.

9 *Normalize the response.* Normalize, validate, and educate; understand that this is a normal person trying to cope with an abnormal event.

10 *Prepare for the future.* Review the event, bring the person to the present, describe events that will occur in the future, and provide referrals.

From Lerner M. D., & Shelton, R. F. (2001). *Acute traumatic stress management* (www.atsm.org). New York: American Academy of Experts in Traumatic Stress

Nursing Interventions

- The primary goal is restoring the client's psychologic equilibrium
- During crisis intervention, the nurse should be active and goal-directed to assist the client with coping with the crisis
- Tasks:
  - Help client explore feelings and describe the situation; accept the client's feelings
  - Help client identify coping mechanisms and support systems
  - Help client develop a plan for coping and focus on the present situation
  - Support coping measures and assign tasks from the developed plan
  - Encourage self-reliance
- When helping a child, consider the child's developmental stage as the first step

APPLICATION AND REVIEW

4. Which approaches should a nurse use during crisis intervention? **Select all that apply.**
   1. Active
   2. Passive
   3. Reflective
   4. Interpretive
   5. Goal-directed

5. Which action should a nurse implement first when initially helping clients resolve a crisis situation?
   1. Encourage socialization
   2. Meet dependency needs
   3. Support coping behaviors
   4. Involve clients in a therapy group

6. A nurse provided crisis intervention for a client who recently left her husband because he was beating her. Which client behaviors indicate to the nurse that the therapy was successful? **Select all that apply.**
   1. Is able to cry
   2. Sleeps half the day
   3. Utilizes healthier coping skills
   4. Refuses a referral to supportive services
   5. Describes the current situation realistically

7. A nurse works in a crisis intervention center. A woman who experienced sexual abuse comes in and says, "I've got to talk to someone or I'll go crazy. I should not have dated him." What is **most** important for the nurse to identify after initially assessing the client's physical condition?
   1. Support network
   2. Sexual background
   3. Ability to relate the facts
   4. Knowledge of sexual assault terminology

8. A 24-year-old secretary who is pregnant for the first time receives a letter from her boyfriend with a check for $500 and the news that he has left town. The client is upset, feels hopeless, and calls the crisis intervention center for help. What reason does the nurse identify for the client to be experiencing a crisis?
   1. Client is under a great deal of stress
   2. Client is going to have to raise her child alone
   3. Client's boyfriend left her when she was pregnant
   4. Client's past methods of adapting are ineffective for this situation

9. A single, pregnant client who is attending a crisis intervention group has decided to go through with the pregnancy and keep the baby. What is the nurse's **primary** responsibility at this time?
   1. Confirm that this really is what the client wants to do
   2. Explore other problems that the client may be experiencing
   3. Select a health care provider that the client can visit for prenatal care
   4. Provide information about resources from which the client may receive assistance

10. A nurse is intervening with a client who is having a crisis. What is the nurse's concern after the initial crisis issues are addressed?
    1. Nature of the precipitating factor
    2. Effect of the situation on significant others
    3. Client's ability to cope with successive crises
    4. Client's potential to perform activities of daily living
11. A client who was involved in a near-fatal automobile collision arrives at the mental health clinic with complaints of insomnia, anxiety, and flashbacks. The nurse determines that the client is experiencing symptoms of crisis. What is the nurse's **initial** intervention?
    1. Focus on the present
    2. Identify past stressors
    3. Discuss a referral for psychotherapy
    4. Explore the past history of mental health problems
12. A nurse is conducting the sixth and final session of crisis intervention with a client in a community health center. Evaluation demonstrates that the client has not yet fully resolved crisis issues. What is the **most** acceptable intervention by the nurse?
    1. Discharge the client on time whether or not the crisis is fully resolved
    2. Agree to continue the treatment until the client feels the crisis has resolved
    3. Provide additional information and referral regarding other community resources
    4. Focus on underlying personality conflicts in preparation for referral to long-term therapy
13. A nurse educator is leading a class on supporting middle-aged adults who are experiencing midlife crisis. What should the nurse include as the **most** significant factor in the development of this type of crisis?
    1. The perception of their life situation
    2. Many role changes that alter their experiences at this time
    3. The anticipation of negative changes associated with old age
    4. Lack of support from family members who are busy with their own lives
14. What is the **priority** goal when planning care for a client in crisis?
    1. Referring the client for occupational therapy
    2. Restoring the client's psychologic equilibrium
    3. Scheduling the client for follow-up counseling
    4. Having the client gain insight into the problem
15. Which is the **most** important assessment data for a nurse to gather from the client in crisis?
    1. The client's work habits
    2. Any significant physical health data
    3. A history of emotional problems in the family
    4. The client's perception of the circumstances surrounding the crisis

See Answers on pages 104-107.

SUICIDE

Overview

- Suicide is a major public health and mental health problem in the United States
- The most vulnerable groups for suicide are adults over 60 years and youths between the ages of 15 and 24 years; Caucasians, Native Americans, and men are more likely to be at risk for suicide; suicide crosses all socioeconomic levels

- Suicidal behavior is strongly associated with the occurrence of psychiatric disorders and other health-related problems such as depression, bipolar disorder, schizophrenia, panic disorders and other anxiety disorders, substance use disorder, some personality disorders (eg, borderline personality disorder), and serious medical disorders
- Imminence, intent, and the method chosen and its accessibility are the three determinants that indicate the level of lethality and the levels of interventions that are necessary for safety
- Suicidal behavior is treatable
- Outcome criteria for the suicidal client include indications that the client is no longer imminently suicidal and that the client's environment is safe for his or her return home (ie, weapons [eg, guns] are removed); follow-up includes outpatient psychotherapy, the possibility of antidepressant medications, and a support system in place for the client to access
- The plan of care emphasizes a reduction in the risk of self-destructive behaviors by monitoring the client's behaviors, providing a safe environment, promoting feelings of self-worth and hope, improving coping skills, limiting social isolation, and building self-esteem
- The client is encouraged to follow the discharge plan of psychotherapy and medications, if ordered

Etiology

- Three kinds of factors: Biologic, psychologic, and sociologic (Box 6.2)
- Biologic factors
  - Irregularities in the serotonin systems of suicidal clients: Changes in the brain's ability to manufacture and use serotonin
  - Dysregulation of impulse control
  - Great degree of glucocorticoid receptor subsensitivity

BOX 6.2 Etiologic Factors Related to Suicide

Biologic Factors
- The neurotransmitters—principally serotonin, dopamine, norepinephrine, and γ-aminobutyric acid—are linked to emotional responses.
- Serotonin plays a major role in the regulation of mood, and it influences the occurrence of depression and suicidality.
- Genetic influences are evident; researchers believe that they have found a specific gene that predisposes a person to suicide.
- Others have found that dimensions of depression (eg, mood, affect, motivation, cognitive content) are correlated with alterations in specific brain structure.

Psychologic Factors
- Self-directed aggression
- Hopelessness and helplessness
- Unresolved interpersonal conflicts
- Negativistic thinking patterns
- A reduction in positive reinforcement
- Difficulty with problem-solving

Sociologic Factors
- Isolation and alienation from social groups
- Biopsychosocial influences

Modified from Fortinash, K. M., & Holoday, P. A. (2012). *Psychiatric mental health nursing* (5th ed.). St. Louis, MO: Mosby.

- Alterations in the hypothalamic-pituitary-adrenal axis with an increased risk for suicidal thoughts and behaviors
- Psychologic factors
  - Suicide most frequently occurs when and individual is depressed
  - Depression follows the loss of a significant love object and leads to feelings of helplessness, hopelessness, guilt, and diminished self-esteem; suicide serves as a way to end those painful feeling states
  - An experience of intense psychologic pain (eg, social isolation, hopelessness) felt by the individual with suicidal ideation and attempts
  - Particular thought patterns such as negativism, self-worthlessness, and a bleak view of the future
  - Cognitive rigidity, which is the inability to identify problems and solutions, may be a factor in suicide when it is accompanied by stress
  - Abandonment and abandonment anxiety, especially among those individuals with borderline personality disorder
- Sociologic factors
  - Alienation from social groups after the disruption of family, community, or social relationships leads some individuals to attempt or commit suicide

Epidemiology

- Suicide was the tenth leading cause of death for all ages in 2013; it was second leading cause of death among teenagers; it is the seventh leading cause of death for males and the fourteenth leading cause for females
- In 2013 in the United States, there were 12.6 suicides per 100,000 persons, which equals 113 suicides each day or one every 13 minutes
- Older adults, aged 85 and older, have a suicide rate that is approximately 36% higher than all other reported suicidal statistics nationally
- Based on data about suicides in the National Violent Death Reporting System of 16 states, in 2010, 33.4% of suicide decedents tested positive for alcohol, 23.8% for antidepressants, and 20.0% for opiates, including heroin and prescription pain killers
- Almost 4% of US adults had suicide ideation in 2013; among students in grades 9 to 12 in the United States during 2013, 17% of students seriously considered attempting suicide in the previous 12 months
- Males take their own lives at nearly four times the rate of females and represent 77.9% of all suicides
- Firearms are the most commonly used method of suicide among males; poisoning is the most common method of suicide for females
- Suicide crosses all socioeconomic levels
- There are increases in the number of suicide attempts and deaths of soldiers who have returned from the war front in Iraq and Afghanistan
- Firearms are the most used of all methods for the completion of suicide; of the individuals who completed suicide in 2010, 49.5% died by using a firearm
- Protective factors against suicide include marriage, sense of responsibility to family, religious beliefs, satisfaction with life and positive social support, access to health care, effective coping and problem-solving skills, intact reality testing

Predisposing Factors

- Early interpersonal trauma and unresolved anxiety
  - Children or teens who lost a parent to suicide are three times more likely to commit suicide; family history of suicide, especially on anniversary date

- Childhood physical, emotional, or sexual abuse
- Problematic family relations
- History of bullying and victimization
- Socioeconomic problems
- Parental psychopathology
- Peer problems
- Legal and/or discipline problems

Risk Factors

- Nurses need to use their knowledge of risk factors to assist them with the assessment of intent and lethality (Box 6.3)
- *Physical and emotional symptoms:* High-risk indicators are serious depression, significant changes in weight, serious sleep disturbances, extreme fatigue and loss of energy, self-deprecation, anger, feelings of hopelessness, and preoccupation with themes of death and dying; serious depression can lead to suicide ideation and suicidal behaviors.
- *Suicide plan:* The presence and nature of the suicide plan are the most critical factors to consider when assigning suicide risk; a plan clearly signals forethought and intent and often helps to determine the level of lethality; plans that are more precise, detailed, and explicit about the method indicate high risk; if the method described is highly lethal (eg, a gunshot to the head

---

BOX 6.3 Risk Factors for Suicide

- A psychiatric diagnosis: 90% of persons who complete a suicide have a psychiatric diagnosis (including substance use disorder), with affective disorders involved in 50% of completed suicides
- Suicidal ideation with intent
- Lethal suicide plan
- History of suicide attempt
- Cooccurring psychiatric illness
- Cooccurring medical illness
- History of childhood abuse
- Family history of suicide
- Recent lack of social support (isolation)
- Unemployment
- Recent stressful life event (eg, death, other loss, such as job loss; impending incarceration); unresolved grief reactions lead to depression and suicidal behavior
- Hopelessness; pessimism
- Anxiety, panic attacks
- Feeling of shame or humiliation
- Impulsivity
- Aggressiveness
- Loss of cognitive function (eg, loss of impulse control)
- Access to firearms and other highly lethal means
- Substance use (without formal disorder)
- Low frustration tolerance
- Sexual orientation issues and gender dysphoria
- Insomnia
- Inability to communicate needs
- Head injury or neurologic disorder

compared with an overdose of pills) and if the method is readily available, the risk is elevated even more; addition of alcohol and other drugs, poor impulse control, and limited time for rescue attempts, and the risk reaches a critical level; plans often include giving away possessions and sometimes mention of the intent to join a deceased loved one in the afterlife, especially if the loved one had committed suicide

- *History of previous attempts:* The majority of persons who complete suicides have made previous suicide attempts
- *Social supports and resources:* The availability of a support system for a suicidal person often determines the outcome of an emotional crisis; this "lifeline" of caring, support, confrontation, and limit setting—as appropriate from family, friends, and community resources—assists suicidal persons with choosing other alternatives when solving their problems; a real or perceived lack of support systems or the failure to use the support system that is available significantly increases the risk for suicide
- *Recent losses:* One of the major emotional determinants of suicidal behavior is real or perceived losses, separations, or abandonment; unresolved grief reactions lead to depression and suicidal behavior
- *Medical problems:* Persons who suffer painful and debilitating acute or chronic conditions or who have terminal illness are of special concern for suicide risk
- *Alcohol and other drugs:* These substances are often lethal companions to suicidal acts; drugs lower inhibition, heighten depression, and quicken impulsivity; according to estimates, at least 50% of adolescents are legally drunk at the time of their death by suicide and an even higher percentage has a history of recent alcohol or other drug abuse
- *Cognition and problem-solving ability:* The inability to adequately identify problems and corresponding solutions greatly contributes to the choice of suicide as a solution to problems
- Recent release from inpatient psychiatric hospitalization
- Significant changes (eg, divorce, death of a loved one, social isolation, and incarceration) contribute to high suicide rates
- Cooccurrence with related health issues: There is a relationship between suicidal behavior and the occurrence of psychiatric disorders and other health-related problems; psychiatric illness, alcohol and other drug use and abuse, and medical illnesses are important indicators of suicidal events
- The presence of a diagnosable mental disorder increases the risk for suicide, regardless of age; the cooccurrence of mood disorder and substance use disorder increases the probability of suicide; the risk for completed suicide secondary to a mental disorder is higher among men than women; women attempt suicide three times more often than men do, but men complete suicide more often than women do
  - Approximately 90% of individuals who complete suicide have a psychiatric disorder that fits the criteria of the DSM-5
  - Individuals diagnosed with bipolar disorder in a hypomanic or manic state are often impulsive, thus increasing the risk for suicide
  - Suicide is the leading cause of premature death among individuals diagnosed with schizophrenia
  - Panic disorder in conjunction with phobias and obsessive-compulsive disorders is a risk factor
  - Often the individual diagnosed with borderline personality disorder experiences suicidal behavior when there is a loss or a perceived loss
  - Alcoholism increases the rate of suicide completion by six times compared with that seen in the general population

- Drugs contribute to poor and impulsive decisions that lead to high-risk, self-injurious behaviors
- When depression and a medical condition (eg, advanced coronary artery disease) coexist, the client suffer nearly twice the loss of social function that occurs when either condition exists by itself; suicide risk also increased in the presence of such coexisting conditions

Nursing Assessment

- Nursing assessment is critical to ensuring the client's safety; determining an individual's risk for suicide requires evaluation of factors that contribute to suicidality
- Suicide attempts can occur before, during, or after hospitalization; hangings, medication overdoses, and jumping from high places are frequent methods of suicide in hospitals
  - Assess for suicidality
  - Assess for major depressive symptoms, recent losses, substance use disorder, and psychosis (especially command hallucinations)
- The initial assessment helps determine the presence of specific risk factors; symptoms do not necessarily mean that a client is suicidal; however, recognizing a cluster of certain symptoms allows accurate assessment of suicidal intent
- When assessing the client's risk for suicide, the nurse will use these methods:
  - *The observable behavior of the client:* A calm client may be highly suicidal, whereas an agitated client is not always in danger; although appearances can be deceiving, increased irritation often signals an imminent suicide attempt as evidenced by impulsivity, restlessness, excessive motor agitation, and a brightening of affect
    - Some individuals manifest withdrawal, apathy, irritability, and immobility that intensify with suicidality
    - Consistently monitor a suicidal client's behavior, affect, and interactions with others; lethality levels increase during hospitalization, particularly as depression lifts and discharge is about to occur
  - The history from the client: Careful scrutiny sometimes reveals events that contributed to current self-destructive thoughts; it is important to determine why the client is feeling suicidal at this time; when gathering the client's history, the nurse will identify self-defeating, coping patterns and past experiences that negatively affect the client's self-esteem; making a note of significant anniversary dates will help to predict a future suicide attempt
    - Screen adolescents for psychiatric disorders such as substance use disorders, depression, and conduct disorders; individuals are at high risk if they are experiencing difficulty interacting with their peers such as bullying, breakup of a significant relationship, pregnancy, obesity, issues related to sexual orientation or gender dysphoria, or feelings of isolation; adolescents are at a higher risk if the individual feels alienated from the family
    - Monitor adolescents who have experienced a peer who has been suicidal or completed suicide; this increases the possibility of a suicidal attempt
  - *Information from friends or relatives:* Nurses obtain useful information about the client's history from friends or relatives; it is often helpful to interview the client and family both together and separately in case the friend or relative is hesitant to speak openly in front of the client; the nurse assesses how family members and friends feel about the client's suicidal behavior;
  - *History of suicidal gestures or attempts:* The suicide attempt is often a way of coping with painful feelings; people who have used this coping style in the past are at greater risk for using it again
  - *The mental status examination:* Disturbances in concentration, orientation, and memory suggest possible organic brain syndromes or severe major depressive disorders, which reduce the client's impulse control and increase the potential for self-harm; disturbance in

thought processing that is evidenced by command hallucinations places the client at greater risk for acting destructively

- *The physical examination:* Always conduct a physical examination when there are obvious signs and symptoms of substance use disorder (eg, impaired attention, irritability, euphoria, slurred speech, unsteady gait, flushed face, psychomotor agitation, needle tracks), previous suicide attempts (eg, scars on the wrists), or debilitating medical conditions (eg, chronic pain)
- *The nurse's intuition:* The nurse's own feelings of uneasiness, anxiety, or unexplained sadness are sometimes the only clues that a seemingly calm client will act on suicidal impulses; although these feelings seem like intuition, research suggests that "intuitive feelings" tend to be based on previous experiences in similar client care situations; nevertheless, if the nurse does not "feel right" about a client, do not ignore this important source of information

- In addition to suicide risk factors, nurses need to consider the assessment of
  - Lethality or the potential for causing death related to the level of danger associated with the suicide plan
  - Imminence (ie, the likelihood that an event will occur within a specific time period)
  - Intent (ie, the method chosen and its accessibility versus ideation)
  - The client's level of hopelessness often helps to determine the level of lethality and the extent of interventions required for safety
  - Access to means

Nursing Diagnosis

- An accurate nursing diagnosis made on the basis of a thorough and ongoing assessment is necessary when identifying and prioritizing the client's needs for nursing interventions
- If clients deny suicidal intent or the need for extra precautions, a diagnosis related to the possibility of suicide or self-directed violence should be used cautiously

Outcome Identification and Planning

- State outcomes in clear behavioral or measurable terms and prioritize them according to client needs, from most urgent to least urgent
- The client will do the following:
  - Remain safe and free from acting on suicidal thoughts
  - Verbalize an absence of suicidal ideation, planning, or intent
  - Verbalize a desire to live and list several reasons for wanting to live
  - Agree to inform staff immediately if suicidal feelings or thoughts recur
  - Display a brightened affect with a broad range of expression, spontaneity, and speech that reflects a hopeful and optimistic attitude
  - Initiate social interactions with peers and staff, both individually and in groups
  - Use effective coping methods to counteract feelings of hopelessness
  - Express a sense of self-worth
  - Meet the client's own needs with the use of clear and direct methods of communication
  - Verbalize realistic role expectations and goals for meeting them
  - Demonstrate the absence of psychotic thinking (eg, delusions, command hallucinations that instruct the client to self-harm)
  - Make plans for the future that include follow-up psychotherapy and adherence to the prescribed medication regimen
  - List several friends or supportive individuals or use a suicide hotline (eg, 1-800-273-TALK) to prevent a possible suicide attempt when experiencing an increase in suicidal thought

- A plan of care aims to save lives and restore biopsychosocial stability
- The plan of care for the suicidal individual emphasizes a reduction in the risk of self-destructive behaviors by monitoring client behaviors and providing a safe environment; promoting the client's feelings of self-worth and hope; improving coping skills; limiting social isolation; and building self-esteem

Immediate Nursing Interventions

- Primary nursing responsibilities involve the prevention of suicide
- The nurse needs to recognize and effectively intervene in the potentially lethal behaviors of clients who are at risk
- This process involves a continuing assessment of lethality factors to determine the client's risk level while working with the client to restore hope, to connect with support resources, and to develop positive alternatives to assist him or her with improved coping
- Nurses need to implement these interventions consistently with hospitalized suicidal clients:
  - Develop the nurse-client relationship, communicating acceptance of the client's feelings and encouraging expression of suicidal feelings
  - Assess potential suicidality
  - Assess if the patient feels able to resist acting on suicidal impulses
  - If positive, ask client about the lethality of the planIf the client mentions a gun, family members should be told to remove firearms from the home
  - If the client mentions overdosing on medications, restricting access to lethal prescriptions, alcohol, and over-the-counter medications is essential
  - If the client has previously attempted suicide, the nurse asks about the method used, how the client was rescued, and any responses to treatment and follow-up care
  - Nursing interventions are prioritized according to the client's needs for safety
  - Levels of observation include frequent observation and continuous observation; to provide safety and to prevent violence, precautions for preventing suicide should be strictly enforced; this includes maintaining a safe environment by doing the following:
    - Routinely count silverware and all other sharp objects before and after the client's use of them
    - Have an awareness of the client's whereabouts at all times
    - Provide one-to-one observation for the client as necessary on the basis of the assessment of the client's current lethality level
    - Plan the staffing pattern so that the unit always has experienced staff on the floor, especially during staff meal times, breaks, vacations, changes of shift, or unit staff meetings (ie, the times during which most suicides occur in hospitals)
    - Provide a roommate for the suicidal client
    - Request that visitors clear all personal items for the client or any gifts with staff
    - Search the suicidal individual for drugs, sharp objects, cords, shoelaces, and other potential weapons after a return from being off of the unit
    - Thoroughly assess the client before any reason to leave the unit is granted to determine the client's current risk level

Ongoing Nursing Interventions

- Assist with the development of improved coping skills:
  - Nurses use specific techniques that include nonjudgmental and empathic listening, encouragement, the tolerance of expressions of pain, and flexible responses to client needs

- The nurse encourages the client to focus on strengths rather than weaknesses so that the client becomes aware of positive qualities and capabilities that have helped with coping in the past
- Nurses provide learning opportunities for improved coping by introducing the client to therapeutic modalities that assist with more positive thinking; by replacing or substituting irrational and self-deprecating thoughts, beliefs, and images, the client becomes more capable of viewing life realistically and rationally
- Nurses need to explain that clients may still have "bad" days because recovery is not usually consistent
- Nurses help clients to prioritize their concerns:
  - Encourage the client to prioritize problems from most to least significant
  - Support the client in finding immediate solutions for the most urgent problems
  - Postpone seeking solutions to those problems that do not require immediate solutions
  - Encourage the client to delegate problem-solving to others when appropriate
  - Help the individual to acknowledge problems that are beyond his or her control
  - Identify, define, and promote healthy adaptive behaviors in clients
  - Encourage the continuance of healthy behaviors when improved coping strategies are demonstrated (ie, positive reinforcement)
  - Encourage the individual to discuss the feelings that are generated by ineffective coping (eg, frustration, anger, inadequacy)
  - Affirm the client's rational decisions that have been made on the basis of accurate judgment
  - Reinforce the client's attempts to make independent decisions
  - Acknowledge the client's demonstrated willingness to implement improved coping behaviors
  - Respond to delusional statements by stating the reality of the situation without arguing with the client's perceived reality
- To enhance family and social support systems:
  - Enlist the family as partners in the client's treatment; family attendance at psychoeducation groups can help the family learn strategies to support the patient's recovery. For example, family therapy can improve the relationships and functioning of all members of the family unit.
  - Determine the degree of available family support that contributes to overall risk management; inform family members about critical signs that the client will exhibit as the depression lifts and as discharge from the hospital occurs
  - Encourage the removal of any lethal weapons from the client's home environment
  - Provide understanding and encouragement when family members express feelings (eg, frustration, helplessness, guilt) and intense affect
  - Contact social services to assist with any needed vocational or financial support
  - Refer the client to aftercare groups, support groups, and 12-step groups, as needed
  - Refer the client to a suicide hotline (eg, 1-800-273-TALK) to use when the client is feeling overwhelmed and suicidal in the future
- Additional treatment modalities
  - Depending on the client's diagnosis, pharmacologic intervention is often a primary consideration for the treatment of the suicidal client; antidepressants, anxiolytics, and antipsychotic medications are frequently used, depending on the individual's needs, history, and previous responses to medication intervention
  - Psychotherapeutic interventions vary and include insight-oriented techniques, cognitive reframing, and brief solution-focused crisis interventions
  - Electroconvulsive therapy is sometimes used with adults whose response patterns reflect a lack of positive response to medication (ie, intractable or refractory depression); these

adults usually present with long-standing histories of severe depression and express imminent intent to die

Evaluation and Discharge Criteria

- Evaluation helps the nurse target areas of outcomes that are critical to the client's continued survival
  - A client's lack of positive response to nursing interventions indicates the need to change the interventions, to implement other treatment modalities, or to reexamine the target dates for the completion of outcomes
  - The deliberate and conscientious evaluation of a suicidal client's response to nursing interventions helps ensure the client's continued safety and readiness for discharge
- Discharge criteria help both the client and the nursing staff to a completion of treatment goals
- The admission assessment establishes the groundwork for discharge criteria
- Discharge criteria help establish time frames for the achievement of goals; designate areas of responsibility and accountability through documentation; and meet specific institutional, professional, certifying, legal, or funding requirements
- Discharge criteria for the suicidal client include:
  - Indications that the client is no longer imminently suicidal
  - Determination that the client's living environment is safe for his or her return
  - A consistent and available support system for the client that will help the client deal with self-destructive feelings
  - A commitment from the client to use psychotherapy to understand the crises that led to the suicidal ideation or attempt
  - An agreement by the client to use a suicide hotline (eg, 1-800-273-TALK) or to call a supportive friend or family member if suicidal ideation happens again
- Because most suicides occur within 90 days after hospitalization, the nurse needs to reinforce with families, guardians, social services, and legal authorities the necessity of removing any possible weapons (eg, guns, drugs) from the person's home environment to a safe location before the client returns home

Nursing Self-Care

- Because working with suicidal clients is emotionally draining and anxiety producing, nurses must help create a supportive environment for themselves and for other staff, which includes clinical supervision and informal discussions regarding feelings about suicide, death, hostility, anger, depression, and other painful feelings
- Developing an ongoing relationship with a suicidal client is an intense experience during which the client and nurse both examine their feelings about the meaning of life and death
- Receiving support and supervision enables the nurse to develop this kind of intense and caring relationship so that both the nurse and the client experience less anxiety and have increased energy to work toward hope and health

Prognosis

- Suicidal behavior is a treatable mental health problem
- Prognosis is related to the severity of their accompanying mental disorders
- Because most suicidal behavior is connected closely with major depressive disorders, the effective treatment of depression reduces the risk of suicide
- Clients with schizophrenia and panic disorder who maintain therapeutic blood levels of the prescribed psychotropic medications also have a favorable response and a positive outcome related to a reduction in suicide risk

APPLICATION AND REVIEW

16. A client who attempted suicide by slashing the wrists is transferred from the emergency department to a mental health unit. What are the important nursing interventions when the client arrives on the unit? **Select all that apply.**
    1. Obtain vital signs
    2. Assess for suicidal thoughts
    3. Institute continuous monitoring
    4. Initiate a therapeutic relationship
    5. Inspect the bandages for bleeding

17. A nurse plans to evaluate a newly admitted depressed client's potential for suicide. What is the **best** approach to obtain this information?
    1. Question the client about plans for the future
    2. Inquire whether the client is now considering suicide
    3. Discuss suicide with other clients when the client is in the group
    4. Ask family members whether the client has ever attempted suicide

18. A client is admitted to the mental health unit after attempting suicide. When a nurse approaches, the client is tearful and silent. What is the nurse's **best** initial intervention?
    1. Observe the behavior, record it, and notify the health care provider
    2. Sit quietly next to the client and wait for the client to start speaking
    3. Say, "You are crying; that means you feel badly about attempting suicide and really want to live"
    4. Say, "I see you are tearful; tell me about what is going on in your life, and we can work on helping you"

19. A teenager recently committed suicide, and grief counselors have been working with students. What behaviors indicate to the school nurse that a student may be considering suicide? **Select all that apply.**
    1. Withdrawing from friends
    2. Giving away prized possessions
    3. Memorializing the dead teenager
    4. Talking excessively about the event
    5. Becoming involved in student activities

20. A nurse is in the working phase of a therapeutic relationship with a depressed client who has a history of suicide attempts. What question should the nurse ask the client when exploring alternative coping strategies?
    1. "How have you managed your problems in the past"
    2. "What do you feel you have learned from this suicide attempt"
    3. "How will you manage the next time your problems start piling up"
    4. "Were there other things going on in your life that made you want to die"

See Answers on pages 104–107.

ANSWER KEY: REVIEW QUESTIONS

1. **1 Developmental level is essential to understanding a child's response to a crisis situation; the variety of coping abilities usually increases as the child progresses through the stages of growth and development** 2 Although the quality of the child's peer relationships is important and eventually should be done, it is not an initial assessment. 3 The child's perception of the crisis situation should be assessed after the child's developmental level is identified. 4 Although the child's communication patterns with family members are important and eventually should be reviewed, it is not an initial assessment
   Client Need: Psychosocial Integrity; **Cognitive Level:** Application; **Nursing Process:** Assessment/Analysis

2. **4 An adventitious crisis is a crisis or disaster that is unplanned and accidental; its subcategories include natural disasters, national disasters, and crimes of violence**

   1 Recurring crisis is not considered a category in crisis theory. 2 A situational crisis results from an external source and involves the loss of self-concept or self-esteem of an individual or family group. 3 A maturational crisis occurs as an individual moves into a new stage of development and prior coping styles are no longer effective; these crises usually are predictable

   Client Needs: Psychosocial Integrity; **Cognitive Level:** Comprehension; **Nursing Process:** Assessment/Analysis

   > 🔑 **Memory Aid:** Adventitious is *not* the same as advantageous. **A**ssociate Adventitious with **A**ccidental, because most people associate accidents with negative experiences.

3. **2 Situational crises involve an unanticipated loss, such as a divorce, that is threatening to the client**

   1 Social crises involve multiple losses such as those occurring during major disasters. 3 Maturational crises occur in response to stress experienced as one struggles with developmental tasks. 4 Developmental (maturational) crises are associated with developmental tasks; divorce is not a developmental task

   Client Need: Psychosocial Integrity; **Cognitive Level:** Comprehension; **Nursing Process:** Assessment/Analysis

4. **Answers: 1, 5**

   1 The nurse should assume an active role in assessing the current situation and facilitate the interview with authority. 5 During crisis intervention the nurse should be goal-directed to assist the client with coping with the crisis

   2 A passive approach is not appropriate; the client usually needs direction to move forward. 3 A reflective approach might be more appropriate for long-term therapy. 4 An interpretive approach is an analytical approach that is not appropriate for crisis intervention

   Client Need: Psychosocial Integrity; **Cognitive Level:** Comprehension; **Integrated Process:** Caring; **Nursing Process:** Planning/Implementation

5. **3 In a crisis situation, the individual frequently just needs support to regroup strengths and reestablish the ability to cope**

   1 Socialization is part of recovery; this is not done during the initial stage of a crisis. 2 Meeting dependency needs is not possible or realistic. 4 Involving them in a therapy group may have the effect of increasing anxiety, thereby making the crisis situation worse

   Client Needs: Psychosocial Integrity; **Cognitive Level:** Application; **Nursing Process:** Planning/Implementation

6. **Answers: 3, 5**

   3 Healthier coping provides a repertoire of skills to draw upon in future crisis situations. 5 Being able to be objective and review the situation realistically demonstrates progress as the client moves toward resolution of the crisis

   1 Although crying reflects that the client is expressing her feelings, usually it indicates the presence of anxiety and is probably not a resolution of the crisis. 2 Sleeping excessively is a maladaptive strategy. 4 Refusing a referral to support services may indicate denial; one of the goals of crisis intervention is to develop a stronger support system

   Client Needs: Psychosocial Integrity; **Cognitive Level:** Analysis; **Nursing Process:** Evaluation/Outcomes

7. **1 Identification of support networks and relationships is a priority if the victim is to be helped after the immediate crisis is over**

   2 Sexual background eventually may be of value, but at this time, it is irrelevant to assessing the client's present condition or needs. 3 The ability to relate the facts eventually may be of value, but at this time, it is irrelevant to assessing the client's present condition or needs. 4 Knowledge of sexual assault terminology is not necessary for providing care

   Client Needs: Psychosocial Integrity; **Cognitive Level:** Application; **Nursing Process:** Assessment/Analysis

8. **4 A crisis is defined as a situation in which the client's previous methods of adaptation are inadequate to meet present needs**

   1 A crisis is not necessarily related to degree of stress; it occurs when past coping mechanisms are ineffective. 2 The challenge of raising her child alone is not the immediate stress for which the client has no coping

mechanism. **3** That the client's boyfriend left her when she was pregnant is not causing the crisis; the client's lack of coping mechanisms is

Client Needs: Psychosocial Integrity; **Cognitive Level:** Application; **Nursing Process:** Assessment/Analysis

9. **4 After the client has made a decision, the nurse's main responsibility is to assist the client in using the problem-solving process to explore other agencies, facilities, and services**

1 It is not appropriate to question the decision after it has been made. **2** Exploring other problems that the client may be experiencing is not part of the immediate goal during the crisis; the client may be encouraged to seek help later for other problems. **3** The client must take primary responsibility for this intervention

Client Needs: Management of Care; **Cognitive Level:** Application; **Nursing Process:** Planning/Implementation; **Integrated Process:** Communication/Documentation

10. **4 Assessment of the client's present status and ability to perform ADLs is the priority because it will influence the choice of an appropriate therapeutic regimen**

1 Although significant, the nature of the precipitating factor is not the priority at this time; it should have already been addressed. **2** Concern now is for the client, not for how the client's behavior affects others. **3** The present crisis must be dealt with first before coping with successive crises

Client Needs: Psychosocial Integrity; **Cognitive Level:** Application; **Nursing Process:** Assessment/Analysis

11. **1 Crisis intervention deals with the here and now; the past is not important except in building on client strengths**

2 The client is anxious and uncomfortable because of the current situation; the focus is on the present, not the past or stressors in the past. **3** Psychotherapy is not appropriate for crisis intervention; psychotherapy focuses on the causes of current feelings and behavior and may be provided long term. **4** Exploring the past history of mental health problems is not significant to crisis intervention

Client Needs: Psychosocial Integrity; **Cognitive Level:** Application; **Nursing Process:** Planning/Implementation; **Integrated Process:** Caring

12. **3 The client needs continued assistance, including additional information and referral regarding other community resources, to facilitate resolution of unresolved conflicts and problems**

1 Discharging the client on time whether or not the crisis is fully resolved is unethical; referral for ongoing therapy is warranted in this situation. **2** If immediate issues have not been resolved during crisis intervention, then further therapy is an appropriate option; thus referral to other services is appropriate. **4** Underlying personality conflicts in preparation for referral to long-term therapy are not the focus of crisis intervention and should be left to the therapist who undertakes long-term therapy with the client

Client Needs: Management of Care; **Cognitive Level:** Application; **Nursing Process:** Planning/Implementation; **Integrated Process:** Communication/Documentation

13. **1 The most significant factor in either precipitating or avoiding a crisis is not the events but how the individual perceives them**

2 Changes in role may occur, but again, the individual's perception of these changes is most influential. **3** Anticipation of negative changes associated with old age may be a factor, but perception is most important. **4** Lack of support from family members is not a significant factor; the family may provide support and a crisis can still occur

Client Need: Psychosocial Integrity; **Cognitive Level:** Comprehension; **Nursing Process:** Planning/Implementation

---

Memory Aid: **I**ndividual **p**erception or "IP" is the key to crisis resolution; think of it as the psychological **I**nternet **p**rovider for connecting to new coping skills and resources.

---

14. **2 Crisis intervention is short-term therapy with the major goal of restoring clients to their precrisis state of psychologic equilibrium**

1 Referring the client for occupational therapy is not a goal but an action to help achieve a goal; it is not part of crisis intervention. **3** Scheduling the client for follow-up counseling is not a goal, but rather an intervention that may be necessary if psychologic equilibrium cannot be restored. **4** Having the client gain insight into the problem is not always necessary for clients to be able to function effectively

Client Need: Psychosocial Integrity; **Cognitive Level:** Application; **Nursing Process:** Planning/Implementation

15. **4 This assessment assists the nurse to determine what the situation means to the client**

1 The client's work habits are not the priority but should be included in a later assessment. **2** Any significant physical health data are not the priority but should be included in a later assessment. **3** A history of emotional problems in the family is not the priority but should be included in a later assessment

Client Need: Psychosocial Integrity; **Cognitive Level:** Application; **Integrated Process:** Communication/Documentation; **Nursing Process:** Assessment/Analysis

16. **Answers: 1, 2, 3, 4, 5**

1 Obtaining vital signs is required in this situation; physiologic stability must be maintained; **2** Suicidal impulses take priority, and the client must be stopped from acting on them when treatment is in progress. **3** Suicidal impulses take priority, and the client must be stopped from acting on them when treatment is in progress. **4** A therapeutic relationship must develop so that the client can trust the nurse to provide a safe environment and help emotional recovery. **5** This intervention is required in this situation; physiologic stability must be maintained

Client Need: Safety and Infection Control; **Cognitive Level:** Application; **Nursing Process:** Planning/Implementation

17. **2 Directness is the best approach at the first interview because this sets the focus and concern and lets the nurse know what the client is feeling now**

1 At this point the client is most likely unable to think past the present, much less deal with future plans; **3** Discussing suicide with other clients when the client is in the group is an indirect approach, but initially the direct approach is best. **4** Asking family members whether the client has ever attempted suicide is one resource for input; but regarding suicide, it is best to approach the client directly

Client Need: Safety and Infection Control; **Cognitive Level:** Application; **Integrated Process:** Communication/Documentation; **Nursing Process:** Planning/Implementation

18. **4 Saying, "I see you are tearful; tell me about what is going on in your life, and we can work on helping you" is a response that recognizes feelings and behavior and encourages the client to share feelings; it also promotes trust, which is essential to a therapeutic relationship**

1 Although it is important to observe and record behavior and notify the health care provider, it is not enough and does not meet the client's needs. **2** Sitting quietly next to the client and waiting for the client to start speaking will not meet the depressed client's needs. **3** Saying "You are crying; that means you feel badly about attempting suicide and really want to live" is a response that assumes too much and may be inaccurate

Client Need: Psychosocial Integrity; **Cognitive Level:** Analysis; **Integrated Process:** Caring; Communication/Documentation; **Nursing Process:** Planning/Implementation

19. **Answers: 1, 2**

1, 2 Giving away prized possessions indicates that the student expects no future

3 It is typical to pay tribute to dead friends. **4** Talking about the event helps to resolve the conflict involved. **5** Becoming involved in school activities demonstrates a return to usual life patterns.

Client Need: Psychosocial Integrity; **Cognitive Level:** Application; **Nursing Process:** Assessment/Analysis

20. **3 The question "How will you manage the next time your problems start piling up" focuses the interaction toward the future and invites the client to explore alternative coping strategies**

1 The question "How have you managed your problems in the past" explores past coping strategies and should have been asked as a part of the initial assessment. **2** The question "What do you feel you have learned from this suicide attempt" attempts to explore the client's insight into present coping strategies, which should have been done before discussing the alternatives. **4** The question "Were there other things going on in your life that made you want to die" asks the client once more to ensure that all the precipitating stressors have been identified; this should have been done in the initial assessment

Client Need: Psychosocial Integrity; **Cognitive Level:** Application; **Integrated Process:** Communication/Documentation; **Nursing Process:** Planning/Implementation

7 Mental Health and Mental Illness

MENTAL HEALTH

Overview

- The World Health Organization (WHO) defines mental health as "a state of well-being in which each individual is able to realize his or her own potential, cope with the normal stresses of life, work productively and fruitfully, and make a contribution to his or her community" (WHO, 2014)
- Quality of life, effective daily functioning, and overall perception of well-being are linked to mental health
- Healthy individuals live productive, creative, and satisfying lives; experience relatively low internal and external stress; are cognitively, emotionally, physically, and behaviorally stable; have realistic perceptions, ordered thought patterns, and feelings of overall well-being; are able to function autonomously and in harmonious relationships with others; and maintain the capacity, abilities, and motivation to meet life's daily needs, demands, inevitable changes, and challenges
- Mentally healthy people are prone to recover relatively quickly from illnesses, thus making it important for nurses to identify, reinforce, support, and promote health when interacting and working with clients
- Life is a continually changing process, and when these changes occur in areas of significance, they often produce distinct emotional responses:
  - Resistance to change: The individual hesitates to accept or adapt to the change and may attempt to deny its occurrence or reject its outcome
  - Regression: The individual returns to an earlier type of behavior that, at the time, provided some satisfaction and gratification and now provides an escape from the unacceptable or anxiety-producing situation
  - Acceptance and progression: The individual adapts to the change and expends energy on outside objects rather than self-centered aims
- Attempts to define mental health and mental health disorder in simple terms fall short of the depth and breadth of the meanings of both terms; various definitions and descriptions are available from multiple reliable sources, but no single definition of either term is considered to be official
- Mental health is more than the absence of mental illness

Factors of Mental Health

- Some of the factors and indicators of mental health in Box 7.1 and Figure 7.1 are considered to be intrinsic (internal or intrapersonal; or occurring within the individual), whereas other factors and indicators are extrinsic (external or interpersonal) and refer to influences that exist or occur outside of the individual
- Interpersonal factors are said to be relational, which refers to a person's relationships with others and the environment; identifying these internal and external factors and influences is a helpful step as nurses assess and treat their clients
- *Resiliency* means a person returns to previous level of functioning after life crisis

| BOX 7.1 | Indicators of Mental Health |

- Intact anatomy and physiology of the brain and central nervous system
- Absence of signs and symptoms of mental health disorder
- Freedom from excessive mental and emotional disability and pain
- Demonstrates mental and physical competence and skills
- Perceives self, others, and events correctly and realistically
- Recognizes own strengths, weaknesses, capabilities, and limitations
- Separates fantasy from reality
- Thinks clearly
  - Solves problems
  - Uses good judgment
  - Reasons logically
  - Reaches insightful conclusions
- Negotiates each developmental stage
- Attains and maintains a positive self-system
  - Self-concept
  - Self-image
  - Self-esteem
- Accepts self and others as uniquely different but humanly similar
- Appreciates life
- Finds beauty, joy, and goodness in self, others, and the environment
- Is creative
- Is optimistic but realistic
- Is resilient
- Is autonomous
- Uses talents to the fullest
- Involves self in purposeful and meaningful life work
- Engages in play
- Develops and demonstrates an appropriate sense of humor
- Expresses emotions
- Exhibits congruent thoughts, feelings, and behaviors
- Accepts responsibility for actions
- Controls impulses and behavior
- Is accountable for own behaviors
- Respects societal rules and sanctions
- Learns from experiences
- Maintains wholesome values and belief system
- Copes with internal and external stressors in constructive and adaptive ways
- Returns to usual or higher function after crises
- Delays gratification
- Functions independently
- Maintains reasonable expectations of self and others
- Adapts to social environment
- Relates to others
  - Forms relationships
  - Maintains close, meaningful, loving, and adaptive relationships
  - Works and plays well with others
  - Is appropriately and selectively intimate
  - Responds to others in need
  - Feels and exhibits compassion and empathy toward others
  - Demonstrates culturally and socially acceptable interpersonal interactions
  - Manages interpersonal conflict constructively
  - Gives and receives gracefully
  - Learns from and teaches others
  - Functions interdependently
  - Considers their own safety and the safety of others in decisions/thinking
- Seeks self-actualization
- Attains self-defined spirituality

Modified from Fortinash, K. M., & Holoday, P. A. (2012). *Psychiatric mental health nursing* (5th ed.). St. Louis, MO: Mosby.

- *Autonomy* includes an internal locus of control and self-efficacy
- *Positive attitude toward self* is evident in how a person views himself or herself
- *Sense of self-actualization* means a person is accomplishing what they think they need to accomplish
- *Formation of relationships with individuals and groups* describes a social component to mental health
- *Adaptation to life changes* refers to Erikson's stages as well as other changes
- *Ability to function in prescribed settings,* including work, home, and social settings
- *Comfort with one's sexuality* forms another dimension of mental health

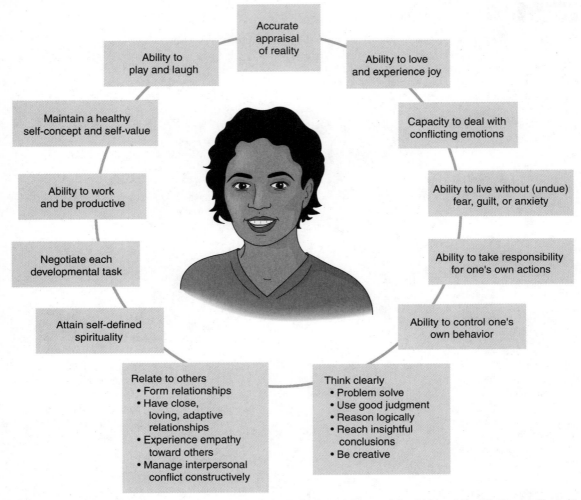

FIG. 7.1 Attributes of mental health. (From Varcarolis, E. M. [2014]. *Essentials of Mental Health Nursing* [2nd ed., revised reprint]. St. Louis, MO: Saunders/Elsevier.)

APPLICATION AND REVIEW

1. Which of these terms describes a person's ability to return to previous level of functioning after life crisis?
   1. Sense of self-actualization
   2. Resiliency
   3. Formation of relationships with individuals and groups
   4. Positive attitude toward self
2. Which of these terms means the individual adapts to the change and expends energy on outside objects rather than self-centered aims?
   1. Regression
   2. Resistance
   3. Intolerance
   4. Acceptance and progression

See Answers on page 117.

MENTAL ILLNESS

Definition and Description

- The American Psychiatric Association (APA) defines mental illness as "health conditions involving changes in thinking, emotion, or behavior (or a combination of these). Mental illnesses are associated with distress and/or problems functioning in social, work or family activities" (APA, 2015)
- Not all mental, emotional, or behavioral disturbances are mental health disorders
  - People who experience great losses (eg, the death or disappearance of a loved one, divorce), traumatic crises, and other events (eg, war, hurricane, earthquake, rape) may demonstrate dramatic withdrawal or explosive acting out behaviors that are determined to be normal responses
  - Nurses and other health professionals recognize these distinctions and respond with certain principles in mind
  - The continuum of mental health to mental health disorders is recognized by nursing; nursing practice addresses a broader scope than just mental health disorders
- The term *mental health disorder* defies simple definitions
  - A mental health disorder is identified by the client's responses to the disorder, and manifestations are specific for each disorder; one symptom or trait alone is not considered a disorder; rather, a syndrome (a cluster of symptoms) that express impaired perception, cognition, mood, affect, behavior, or a combination of these must be present
  - The syndrome may cause distress to the individual in some cases, and this distress varies with the type of disorder
  - The person's ability to function and their relationships are usually impaired at some level; symptoms vary depending on the type of disorder, and more than one disorder may occur at the same time (comorbid)
- Acute episodes that signal the emergence or recurrence of a mental health disorder usually occur rapidly, are intense, and have a relatively brief course (eg, brief reactive psychosis)
  - There also may be acute episodes of a long-term, persistent disorder (eg, an acute psychotic episode in an individual diagnosed with schizophrenia)
- Long-term, persistent mental health disorders are marked by symptoms that remain more constant, and the course is longer in duration (eg, autism spectrum disorder, schizophrenia, Alzheimer's disease)
- Symptoms of both acute episodes and long-term, persistent conditions are also considered on a continuum from mild to moderate to severe
- Mental health disorders are sometimes referred to as "mental illness"
  - There were times when that term was strongly contested as a result of theoretic and conceptual differences regarding the etiology (the source or origin) of mental health disorders
  - Clients, families, students of psychiatric nursing, and others want to know what causes the symptoms that they witness during disruptive episodes of mental health disorders
- Early recognition of symptoms and early treatment of mental health disorders is a primary objective
- It is necessary for psychiatric nurses as well as the nurses who work with clients in any area to be skilled at discerning healthy responses from disordered ones
  - Symptoms that are associated with mental health disorders may manifest and be demonstrated in any type of setting, including homes, schools, workplaces, neighborhoods, public places, hospitals (all units), clinics, places of worship, organizational meetings, battlefields, and correctional facilities

- Nurses must be prepared by being able to identify symptoms of mental health disorders when they occur and then to intervene; such skills begin with a knowledge base related to mental health and illness

Dysfunctional Patterns of Behavior

- Various theories (psychoanalytic, developmental, neurobiologic, sociocultural, behavioral, cognitive) identify factors that lead to patterns of behavior that are dysfunctional
  - Psychoanalytic theories focus on interpersonal relationships and communication patterns that are especially influenced by childhood experiences
  - Developmental theories focus on the ability to accomplish age-related tasks
  - Neurobiologic theories focus on brain structure and/or neurochemistry
  - Sociocultural theories focus on learned values, beliefs, norms, and rituals that reinforce behavior
  - Behavioral theories focus on behaviors as learned patterns that have been reinforced
  - Cognitive theories focus on the relationship among beliefs, mindsets, and behavior
- Most dysfunctional behavior result from multiple stressors
- It is the frequency, extent, and effect these behaviors have on overall functioning that will determine whether they are dysfunctional
- Dysfunctional behavior is precipitated by stressors that become overwhelming; influencing factors include the severity, multiplicity, and duration of stressors
- Dysfunctional patterns of behavior usually reflect problems in ability to cope with stressors; continued use of these patterns impairs the individual's ability to grow and change and therefore creates further stress
- Dysfunctional patterns of behavior and specific psychiatric diagnoses that can be correlated to certain patterns of dysfunctional behavior include:
  - Withdrawn behavior
    - Pathologic retreat from, or an avoidance of, people and reality; withdrawn behavior can range from poor socialization to retreat into a private world of delusion, hallucination, and fantasy
    - Associated with autism spectrum disorders, major depressive disorder, anxiety, dementia, and schizophrenia and other psychotic disorders
  - Projective behavior
    - Denial of one's own feelings, faults, and failures and attributing them to other people or objects; projective behavior can range from displacing anger onto a less threatening person to blaming others for one's own addiction or aggressive behavior
    - Associated with substance use disorder, antisocial personality disorder, paranoid personality disorder, phobias
  - Aggressive behavior
    - Physical, symbolic, or verbal behavior that is forceful or hostile and enacted to intimidate others or as a result of fear; aggression occurs on a continuum ranging from angry body language to physical violence
    - Associated with substance use disorder, conduct disorders, mania, delirium, dementia, domestic violence, sexual assault; for some of these the aggressive behavior is purposeful
  - Self-destructive behavior
    - Indulging in actions that could lead to self-harm (eg, nonadherence to medical regimens, substance use disorder, engaging in high-risk activities) or violence against self (eg, cutting, overdose); self-destructive behaviors can range from a client with a cardiac problem who fails to follow dietary restrictions to a client who attempts suicide
    - Associated with depression, manic episode of bipolar disorder, borderline personality disorder

- Addictive behavior
  - Repeated or chronic use of a substance (eg, alcohol, drugs, cigarettes); continued use of the substance despite the occurrence of related problems; the use of a substance may be a form of self-medication for an underlying mental illness; behaviors such as gambling addiction and compulsive overeating that continue despite occurrence of related problems are viewed as addictive disorders
  - Associated with substance use disorder, personality disorders, bipolar disorder, schizophrenia, attention deficit hyperactivity disorder (ADHD)

Risk Factors

- Risk factors are internal predisposing characteristics and external influences that increase a person's vulnerability and potential for developing mental health disorders; types of risk factors and some examples include:
  - Biologic (ie, genetic predisposition for a specific disorder; person's age; gender; blood relative with mental illness; long-term medical disorder, brain damage)
  - Psychologic (ie, influence of a mentally disordered family member in the home; difficult temperament; pessimistic or suspicious worldview; negative attitudes; lower level of intelligence)
  - Sociocultural (ie, absence of parents; being orphaned; abusive or neglectful home; poverty; inadequate social skills; rejection by ethnic or religious group; punitive gangs; school bullies, trauma)
  - Environmental (ie, exposure to toxins, illegal drugs, or pollution)
- Some risk factors are fixed and unchanging, whereas others may change over time to positively or negatively influence mental health
  - Genetic predisposition
  - Mentally disturbed family member in the household
  - Suspicious worldview
  - Negative attitudes
  - Impaired functioning
  - Threatening belief systems
  - Abusive relationships
  - Rejection
  - Ineffective coping
  - Significant life event at vulnerable age

Protective Factors

- Protective factors are characteristics that guard against risks and that may decrease an individual's potential for developing the risk for mental health disorders; factors are either internal or external (Fig. 7.2)
- Some examples of a person's internal protective factors are resilience; good overall health; high stress tolerance; average or higher intelligence; optimism; high strong motivation; competence in several areas; flexibility; healthy curiosity and interest in life; and useful skills
- Examples of external protective factors include healthy, skilled, and caring parents, family, and friends; supportive teachers, bosses, cultures, and subcultures; sufficient income; and available and appropriate resources, recreation, and hobbies
- Altered factors may influence client responses and affect the outcome toward mental health or mental health disorder; lives of individuals, their families, and their communities are all affected by the emergence or recurrence of mental health disorders

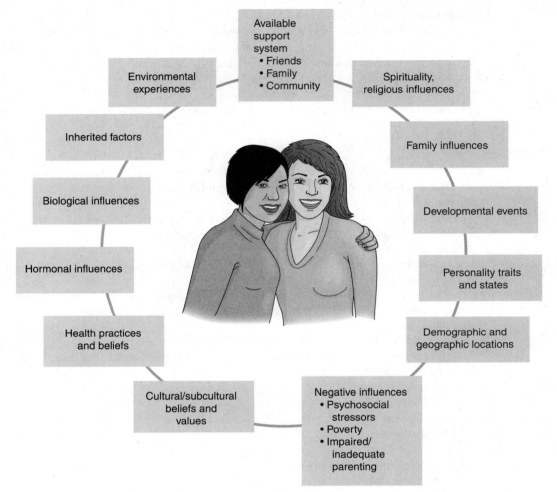

FIG. 7.2 Influences that can have an effect on an individual's mental health. (From Varcarolis, E. M. [2014]. *Essentials of Mental Health Nursing* [2nd ed., revised reprint]. St. Louis, MO: Saunders/Elsevier.)

CLASSIFICATION OF MENTAL HEALTH DISORDERS

Overview

- Mental health disorders continue to occur in all areas of the world and require identification and diagnosis before treatment begins
  - To facilitate this process, standardized diagnostic classifications have been developed and are widely used by mental health practitioners of all disciplines in the United States and beyond
  - The diagnostic manuals describe specific symptoms to identify each mental health disorder, and they are valuable tools for that reason
- Two published diagnostic classification manuals currently dominate the health care industry: *The Diagnostic and Statistical Manual of Mental Disorders* (DSM-5 APA, 2013) and *The International Classification of Diseases* (ICD-10; WHO, 2014)
  - Both are currently utilized in psychiatric facilities and other settings and both list categories for each mental health disorder and the symptoms that identify the disorders

- Nurses familiarize themselves with the DSM for practical and collaborative purposes but are reminded that the primary emphasis in their profession remains unchanged
  - That emphasis focuses on the care and treatment of the whole client and the clients' *responses* to their disorders versus a focus on treating clients' disorders
- General purposes of diagnoses include communication, treatment, prognosis, and funding
  - Communication: Diagnoses define disorders and the manifestations that accompany them; naming a diagnosis facilitates communication and avoids unnecessary repetitive explanations of diagnosis-specific symptoms
  - Treatment: Diagnoses direct treatment approaches and guide the staff to interact and intervene accordingly; for example, the treatment plan and approach for a depressed, withdrawn client who is threatening suicide will be different from that for a client who is admitted for drug-induced hallucinations
  - Prognosis: A diagnosis often carries an initial prognosis; for example, schizophrenia has a long-term persistent prognosis, whereas adjustment disorders have a more favorable prognosis; the outcome from any diagnosis may change or vary with time and circumstances, but prognoses are guides that direct the delivery of care
  - Funding: Diagnostic criteria dictate payment for treatments and services in the health care setting; in addition, the allocation of research funds in both the public and private sectors is designated for specifically named diagnoses

Diagnostic and Statistical Manual of Mental Disorders 5 (DSM-5)

- "The diagnostic classification is the official list of mental disorders recognized in DSM. Each diagnosis includes a diagnostic code, which is typically used by individual providers, institutions, and agencies for data collection and billing purposes. These diagnostic codes are derived from the coding system used by all U.S. health-care professionals" (APA, 2017)
- DMS-5's prime purpose is to provide a classification of types of mental health disorders and guidelines to aid in making a diagnosis
- The DSM-5 does not contain nursing diagnoses

DSM Format

- Standardized language is used to provide a classification of types of mental health disorders
  - "Specifiers" help the clinician describe the precise character of the illness such as frequency, intensity (mild, moderate, severe), number of episodes, and duration (eg, brief, less than 1 month, 1–6 months, more than 6 months)
- Defining characteristics and symptoms give specific guidelines to aid in making a diagnosis
  - For instance, specific codes identify schizophrenia with hallucinations or with delusions
- Factors related to diagnosis, such as with or without stressors, onset, and accompanying diagnoses, help further clarify the diagnosis
- DSM-5 divides diagnostic criteria into these categories:
  - Neurodevelopmental disorders: Includes autism spectrum disorder, attention-deficit/hyperactivity disorder, specific learning disorder, motor disorders, tic disorders, and other neurodevelopmental disorders
  - Schizophrenia spectrum and other psychotic disorders
  - Bipolar and related disorders
  - Depressive disorders
  - Anxiety disorders
  - Obsessive-compulsive and related disorders
  - Trauma-related and stressor-related disorders

- Dissociative disorders
- Somatic symptom and related disorders
- Feeding and eating disorders
- Elimination disorders
- Sleep-wake disorders: Includes breathing-related sleep disorders and parasomnias
- Sexual dysfunctions
- Gender dysphoria
- Disruptive, impulse-control, and conduct disorders
- Substance-related and addictive disorders: Includes alcohol-, caffeine-, cannabis-, hallucinogen-, inhalant-, and opioid-related disorders; sedative-, hypnotic- or anxiolytic-related disorders; stimulant-related disorders (includes tobacco-related disorders); other substance-related disorders; and nonsubstance-related disorders (such as gambling disorders)
- Neurocognitive disorders: Major and mild neurocognitive disorders, including those due to Alzheimer's disease and others
- Personality disorders, including clusters A, B, and C, and other
- Paraphilic disorders
- Other mental health disorders
- Medication-induced movement disorders
- Other adverse effects of medication; other conditions that may be a focus of clinical attention such as abuse and neglect and others

APPLICATION AND REVIEW

3. Risk factors for the development of physical and mental health disorders include which of the following? **Select all that apply.**
   1. A parent who gets drunk every night after work and says that it is relaxing
   2. A school in which students either ignore or bully the new students
   3. A higher-than-average intelligence level and many satisfying hobbies
   4. A large circle of friends who play sports together
   5. A lack of difficulty with relationships at school or work
4. Which of these is a protective factor against the development of mental illness?
   1. Abusive relationships
   2. High stress tolerance
   3. Negative attitudes
   4. Ineffective coping
5. What is the prime purpose of the *Diagnostic and Statistical Manual of Mental Disorders*, 5th edition (DSM-5)?
   1. Facilitate communication between researchers and clinicians
   2. Aid in teaching psychopathology to mental health professionals
   3. Assist in collecting accurate public health statistics through the use of diagnostic codes
   4. Provide a classification of types of mental health disorders and guidelines to aid in making a diagnosis
6. Which of these are classifications of diagnosis in DSM-5. **Select all that apply.**
   1. Anxiety disorders
   2. Obsessive-compulsive and related disorders
   3. Trauma-related and stressor-related disorders
   4. Dissociative disorders
   5. Breathing disorders

See Answers on page 117.

ANSWER KEY: REVIEW QUESTIONS

1. **2 Resiliency is a person's ability to restore to previous level of functioning after life crisis**
   1 A sense of self-actualization means a person is accomplishing what they think they need to accomplish. **3** *Formation of relationships with individuals and groups* describes a social component to mental health. **4** Positive attitude toward self is evident in how a person views himself or herself
   Client Need: Management of Care; **Cognitive Level:** Knowledge; **Nursing Process:** Assessment/Analysis

2. **4 Acceptance and progression means the individual adapts to the change and expends energy on outside objects rather than self-centered aims**
   1 Regression means that the individual returns to an earlier type of behavior that, at the time, provided some satisfaction and gratification and now provides an escape from the unacceptable or anxiety-producing situation. **2** Resistance to change means that the individual hesitates to accept or adapt to the change and may attempt to deny its **occurrence** or reject its outcome. **3** Intolerance means a person is not accepting of another
   Client Need: Management of Care; **Cognitive Level:** Knowledge; **Nursing Process:** Assessment/Analysis

3. **Answers: 1, 2**
   1 Absence of a caring parent, dysfunctional family functions, and abusive behavior place the person at risk for anxiety or depression. 2 Stressful environmental and sociocultural factors, such as bullying, can affect a person's feeling of self-worth
   3 A higher-than-average intelligence level and many satisfying hobbies are not risk factors for the development of physical and mental health disorders. **4** A large circle of friends who play sports together is not a risk factor for the development of physical and mental health disorders. **5** A lack of difficulty with relationships at school or work is not a risk factor for the development of physical and mental health disorders
   Client Needs: Management of Care; **Cognitive Level:** Knowledge; **Nursing Process:** Assessment/Analysis

4. **2 High stress tolerance is a protective factor against the development of physical and mental health disorders**
   1 Abusive relationships are a risk factor for the development of mental illness. **3** Negative attitudes are a risk factor for the development of mental illness. **4** Ineffective coping is a risk factor for the development of mental illness
   Client Needs: Management of Care; **Cognitive Level:** Knowledge; **Nursing Process:** Assessment/Analysis

5. **4 The prime purpose of the DSM-5 is to serve the clinician as a guide in determining a client's mental health/psychiatric diagnosis**
   1 Although facilitating communication between researchers and clinicians is a benefit of the DSM-5, it is not the prime purpose of this publication. **2** Although to aid in teaching psychopathology to mental health professionals is a benefit of the DSM-5, it is not the prime purpose of this publication. **3** Although assistance in collecting accurate public health statistics through the use of diagnostic codes is a benefit of the DSM-5, it is not the prime purpose of this publication
   Client Needs: Management of Care; **Cognitive Level:** Knowledge; **Nursing Process:** Assessment/Analysis

6. **Answers: 1, 2, 3, 4**
   1 Anxiety disorders is a classification in DSM-5. **2** Obsessive-compulsive and related disorders is a classification in DSM-5. **3** Trauma-related and stressor-related disorders is a classification in DSM-5. **4** Dissociative disorders is a classification in DSM-5
   5 Breathing disorders is not a classification in DSM-5
   Client Needs: Management of Care; **Cognitive Level:** Knowledge; **Nursing Process:** Assessment/Analysis

8 Psychotherapy

NONPHARMACOLOGIC THERAPEUTIC MODALITIES

Overview

- Many therapists use a variety of therapeutic approaches to mental health based on client need

Cognitive Theory

- Cognitive theorists believe that
  - Patterns of thinking, mindsets, and belief systems influence feelings and behavior
  - Dysfunctional cognitive patterns and cognitive distortions (eg, pessimism, overgeneralizing, unrealistic expectations) lead to alterations in mood and behavior
- Cognitive therapy is evidence-based, and most effective in treating clients diagnosed with anxiety and mood disorders
- Interventions focus on identification of dysfunctional thought patterns or "cognitive distortions" and replacement with healthier, more reality-based thinking
- Examples of cognitive therapy include
  - Thought journals: Client records situations in which cognitive distortions occur and the thoughts and feelings that follow
  - Cognitive restructuring (cognitive reframing) whereby the client is helped to look at cognitive distortions (unrealistic thoughts) in a more realistic light and to restructure these thoughts in a healthier way.
  - Cognitive rehearsal: Client prepares mental script to address situations that usually trigger cognitive distortions

Behavioral Theory

- Behavioral theorists believe that
  - All behavior is motivated and learned
  - Automatic or habitual behavior patterns develop over time through reinforcement but can be unlearned
- Behavioral therapy is effective in developing skills in individuals with limited cognitive skills (eg, children, developmentally disabled) and for individuals diagnosed with disorders that include significant behavioral components (eg, phobias, compulsions)
- Consistent nursing responses are essential for behavioral interventions
- Examples of behavioral therapy include
  - Behavioral Contracting: Client agrees, orally or in writing, to change dysfunctional behavior; contracts include specific behavior to be modified, the positive reinforcers, and the consequences if contract is broken
  - Token/reward system: Desired behavior receives concrete positive reinforcement (eg, colorful stickers during toilet training for child)
  - Desensitization (exposure therapy): Client is exposed to slowly increasing experiences with an anxiety-producing stimulus when practicing behavioral techniques such as relaxation or deep breathing

- Flooding: Client is exposed to anxiety-producing stimulus continuously in a supportive environment until intensity of response diminishes

Maslow's Humanistic Theory

- Maslow's humanistic theory, a nondevelopmental theory, postulates that people are guided by a variety of needs, from basic physiologic ones to self-actualization, the need to achieve one's full potential
- The existence of unmet needs and the desire to achieve optimum self-potential are fundamental sources of human motivation; Maslow's Hierarchy of Needs is:
  - Physiologic—satisfying needs for oxygen, water, food, shelter, sleep, and relief of sexual tension
  - Safety—avoiding harm and achieving security and safety
  - Love and belonging—giving and receiving affection, developing companionship, group acceptance
  - Esteem—achieving recognition from others leads to self-esteem, prestige, and work success
  - Self-actualization—achieving one's own unique potential
- With the gratification of basic needs, other higher needs emerge, moving one toward self-potential
- People may simultaneously be working to achieve needs on more than one level
- Maslow's Hierarchy can help nurses determine priority of nursing interventions. In mental health, safety may be the priority need.

Group Therapy

- Group therapy uses the dynamics of the group to achieve results less likely to occur in a one-to-one nurse-client relationship (eg, decreasing sense of isolation, instilling hope through example of others, providing opportunities to help others)
- Group process describes how the group is functioning, including all the verbal and nonverbal behaviors that occur within the group; group content describes what topics or tasks are addressed
- Groups can be effective or ineffective (Table 8.1)
  - Universality, a perception of sharing, can enhance bonding
- Nursing care associated with group therapy
  - Select clients suitable for the group (level of attention and communication skills)
  - Orient group members to the group process; explain confidentiality
  - Maintain individual member's psychologic and physical safety
  - Facilitate healthy group process when necessary
  - Assist the group to achieve therapeutic goals by encouraging member participation; all communication has value
  - Note that leading group therapy is an advanced practice skill

Therapeutic Milieu

- Therapeutic milieu is the provision of an environment that consistently encourages the highest level of functioning of clients
- The environment supports client independence and responsibility, as well as improves social interactions (eg, daily schedule of activities, communal dining, wearing street clothes) while maintaining safety
- Clients and health team members interact and work together to improve clients' function

TABLE 8.1	Comparison of Group Effectiveness	
Factor	**Effective Group**	**Ineffective Group**
Atmosphere	Relaxed and interested	Tense and bored
Goal setting	Clearly defined and accepted Modified as needed	Vague and not supported
Goal emphasis	Process and task functions balanced	Tasks and process needs are not balanced
Cohesiveness	Built through trust and mutual support	Too close and overcontrolling or limited connection among members
Conflict	Accept differences Work to resolve conflicts	Avoid facing conflicts or unresolved ongoing conflicts
Power	Shared Determined by ability	Based on position only
Leadership	Based on needs and ability Delegates appropriately	Overcontrolling or weak
Communication	Open and two-way	Closed and one-way Dominated by a few members
Decision making	Consensus when appropriate	From leader down with little input from members
Problem-solving	Encourage constructive criticism	Limited by inflexibility
Creativity	Open to new ideas	New ideas discouraged
Self-evaluation	Open to all members Frequently performed	Performed by only a few members infrequently

From Nugent, P. M., Green, J. S., Hellmer Saul, M. A., & Pelikan, P. K. (2012). *Mosby's comprehensive review of nursing for the NCLEX-RN examination* (20th ed.). St. Louis, MO: Mosby.

- Milieu varies with treatment settings, both inpatient and outpatient
- The nurse is responsible for structuring and /or implementing many aspects of the therapeutic milieu, including establishing a supportive and emotionally safe environment
- Nursing care associated with maintaining a therapeutic milieu
  - Prioritize safety; maintain client safety by increasing supervision and removing dangerous objects
  - Structure
    - Develop and maintain a schedule of unit activities and routine, which may include formal and informal group activities with periods of time to be alone
    - Safe physical environment
    - Formal and informal rules
  - Have clear expectations of behavior
  - Encourage client independence in daily activities gradually, as appropriate
  - Provide opportunities for healthy socialization

Relaxation Therapy

- Promotion of relaxation through meditation, progressive relaxation, deep breathing, guided imagery, and biofeedback

- Integration of many types of treatment for clients who need to develop healthier methods for coping with stress
- Nursing care associated with relaxation therapy
  - Teach and reinforce relaxation techniques
  - Lead relaxation groups

Family Therapy

- Derived from systems theory and group therapy
- The guiding principle is that treating the individual in isolation from the family allows dysfunctional interpersonal patterns to continue once the client returns to the family environment, which often undermines progress made in individual therapy
- The focus of family therapy is on the family as a system and improving family functioning. Nurses work with families by helping them identify resources and improve family communication and understanding of illnesses through psychoeducation. The National Alliance on Mental Illness has Family Support Groups for family members of clients diagnosed with mental illnesses.

Additional Nonpharmacologic Therapies

- *Occupational Therapy*
  - The occupational therapist assesses a patient's abilities and disabilities and helps the patient increase his or her functioning and independent living skills in areas such as self-care, work, and leisure activities
  - Therapists teach adaptive skills for home, school, and job functioning
  - They plan and lead groups that focus on areas such as stress management, enhancing parenting skills, conflict resolution, time management, money management, budgeting, feeling, and self-awareness
- *Art Therapy*
  - Art therapists use art as a means of helping the patient express thoughts and feelings that he or she is not able to verbalize
  - This intervention helps the patient understand problem areas from a symbolic standpoint
  - Therapists also teach the patient an alternative means of expression and self-soothing
- *Music Therapy*
  - Music therapists use music to help the patient express feelings and thoughts that are not easy to verbalize
  - Music helps the patient relax and learn alternative self-soothing strategies
- *Movement Therapy*
  - Teaches patients how to move their bodies when they are stressed, and it helps them learn about methods of relaxation
  - Movement therapy is helpful for patients who become numb when experiencing intense feelings (e.g., abandonment, anger) to teach them to use methods of self-touching to reestablish a feeling state rather than self-mutilating
- *Recreational Therapy*
  - Helps patients with personality disorders explore ways to enjoy themselves without the use of self-destructive behaviors, such as abusing alcohol or drugs
  - Helpful for patients who have difficulty socializing, because recreation strengthens social skills

APPLICATION AND REVIEW

1. A nurse encourages a client to join a self-help group after being discharged from a mental health facility. What is the purpose of having people work in a group?
   1. Support
   2. Confrontation
   3. Psychotherapy
   4. Criticism

2. During a group meeting a client tells everyone, "I am afraid of my impending discharge from the hospital." What is the **most** appropriate response by the nurse facilitator?
   1. "You ought to be happy that you're leaving"
   2. "Maybe you're not ready to be discharged yet"
   3. "Maybe others in the group have similar feelings that they would share"
   4. "How many in the group feel that this member is ready to be discharged"

3. At a group therapy session a client tearfully tells the other members, "I just lost my job this week." What is the nurse leader's **most** appropriate response?
   1. Ask the client to consider the reasons this may have occurred
   2. Quietly observe how the group responds to the client's statement
   3. Gently suggest that the client check the help-wanted advertisements in the local paper
   4. Request that the group help the client reflect on how the dismissal may have been prevented

4. A nurse is assigned to lead a relaxation group. Which techniques should the nurse incorporate? **Select all that apply.**
   1. Meditation
   2. Mental imagery
   3. Token economy
   4. Operant conditioning
   5. Deep-breathing exercises

See Answers on pages 138-142.

PSYCHOPHARMACOLOGY

Overview

- Chemicals produce profound effects on the mind, emotions, and body
- Within one decade (the 1950s), three major classes of psychotropic drugs—antimanic, antipsychotic, and antidepressant—were developed; the decrease in state hospital census has been attributed to the introduction of psychotropic drugs
- These compounds significantly advanced the treatment of bipolar illness, psychoses, and depression
- Psychotropic drugs include antianxiety or anxiolytic agents and sedative and hypnotic agents; antipsychotic agents; antidepressants, antimanic, and mood-stabilizing agents; stimulant agents; and antidementia agents
- The safety of psychotropic drugs during pregnancy is of concern; consultations with a health care provider and a pharmacist before administration is advised
- Response to psychotropic medications, both therapeutic and side effects, varies greatly from person to person
- The goal of psychopharmacology is to administer the medication and dosage that will maximize therapeutic effects and minimize side effects
- Medication is only one component of treatment; it is used to increase clients' abilities to engage in other forms of therapy
- Relapse in clients diagnosed with psychiatric problems most often is related to failure to adhere to the medication regimen
- Psychotropic drugs affect major neurotransmitters (Fig. 8.1)

NEUROTRANSMITTERS

ACETYLCHOLINE (ACh)
DOPAMINE (DA)
GABA
NOREPINEPHRINE (NE)
SEROTONIN (5-HT)

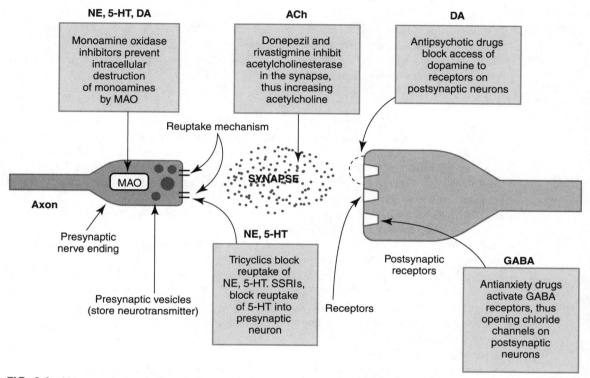

FIG. 8.1   How psychotropic drugs affect five major neurotransmitters. (Modified from Stuart, G., & Sundeen, S. [1995]. *Principles and practice of psychiatric nursing* [5th ed.]. St. Louis, MO: Mosby.)

ANTIANXIETY/ANXIOLYTIC MEDICATIONS

Description

- Used in the treatment of acute anxiety, for alcohol withdrawal, and in the induction of sleep
- Potentiates brain chemicals that help decrease anxiety
- Available in PO, IM, IV, rectal preparations
- Exert a general depressing effect on the central nervous system (CNS); many also exert skeletal muscle-relaxant and anticonvulsant effects
- Available in oral and parenteral (intramuscular [IM], IV) preparations
- Intended for short-term use when the individual has difficulty in coping with environmental stresses and accomplishing daily activities
- Benzodiazepines: Enhance the gamma-aminobutyric acid (GABA) activity (the primary inhibitory neurotransmitter in the brain), resulting in further opening of the chloride ion

channel and a further inhibition of neuronal activity; a decrease in the firing rate of neurons results in lowering of anxiety

Types

- Benzodiazepines
  - Short-acting: Alprazolam, midazolam, oxazepam, triazolam
  - Medium-acting: Lorazepam, temazepam
  - Long-acting: Chlordiazepoxide, clonazepam, clorazepate, diazepam, flurazepam
- Nonbenzodiazepines: Buspirone, diphenhydramine, hydroxyzine, eszopiclone, ramelteon, zaleplon, zolpidem; some are used to treat anxiety, others for insomnia
- Antidepressants indicated for anxiety disorders: Clomipramine, fluoxetine, fluvoxamine, paroxetine, sertraline, venlafaxine, duloxetine

Precautions

- Drug interactions: These drugs potentiate depressant effects of alcohol or sedatives
- Adverse effects: Related to diminished mental alertness; caution about driving or operating hazardous machinery until tolerance develops; Asians and Eskimos at greater risk for toxic levels
- Tolerance to the sedative and hypnotic effects develop eventually with all these drugs, although they develop more slowly with the benzodiazepines than other drugs; tolerance can contribute to self-medication and dosage escalation
- Anxiolytics/sedative hypnotic (not antidepressants) can lead to physical and emotional addiction if taken in large enough doses or for extended time periods
- A drop in blood pressure (BP) of 20 mm Hg (systolic) on standing warrants withholding the drug and notifying the health care provider
- Physical withdrawal symptoms can occur any time these drugs (anxiolytics/sedative hypnotics) are stopped after being taken continuously for more than 2 weeks; signs and symptoms closely resemble the original sleep or anxiety problems
- Caffeine can worsen symptoms of anxiety; it is thought to interfere with medications used to treat these disorders
- Benzodiazepines
  - Should not be discontinued abruptly to avoid a withdrawal syndrome
  - Should be discontinued if the client is receiving electroconvulsive therapy (ECT)
  - Because tolerance and addiction may develop with long-term use, chronic anxiety disorders are usually treated with antidepressant medications
  - Overdose necessitates administration of flumazenil to counter adverse effects
- Buspirone
  - Potent antianxiety agent with no identified addictive potential
  - Not effective in the management of drug or alcohol abuse
  - Therapeutic effects are not apparent for 3 to 6 weeks; this is a much longer lag time than other drugs in this category
  - Can be taken long-term

Nursing Care of Clients Receiving Antianxiety/Anxiolytic Medications

- Safety is the first priority with the use of these medications
- Assess the client's medication history, knowledge level, and use of current medications (eg, prescribed, over-the-counter [OTC], and illicit drugs), medication allergies, and pattern of alcohol, tobacco, and herbal use because all may interfere with the action of anxiolytics

- Explore the client's perceptions and feelings about medications; clarify misinformation and concerns
- Monitor for suicidal ideation, mental status, CNS changes
- Monitor the effects of medication (eg, effects on target symptoms, side effects, and adverse reactions)
- Monitor BP, blood studies (including renal/hepatic status), and for infection
- Administer medications exactly as prescribed and in accordance with schedule restrictions
- Teach the client about the medication: desired effect; side effects; food, herbal, and activity restrictions; and lag period between onset of treatment and symptom remission for antidepressants and buspirone
- Teach client to take exactly as prescribed and not to use anxiolytics/sedative-hypnotics for more than 4 months unless prescriber approves
- Provide education regarding benzodiazepines
  - OTC drugs such as antihistamines may increase potency
  - Driving or working with machinery should be avoided when sedative side effects are present
  - CNS depressants and alcohol potentiate effects
  - Drugs should not be discontinued abruptly
  - If prior assessment reveals use of herbal or related products (St. John's wort, kava, ginseng, etc.), consult with health care provider and pharmacist
  - Teach that drug may be addicting and affect CNS function
  - Teach to avoid OTC products unless prescriber approves
  - Teach to avoid alcohol and other psychotropic medications
  - Teach client to change positions slowly
  - Teach client to report signs and symptoms of infection
- Monitor for addiction/withdrawal/toxicity with anxiolytics/sedative hypnotics
- Supplement verbal teaching with appropriate written or audiovisual materials
- Evaluate client's response to medications and understanding of teaching
- Encourage client involvement in therapy to decrease stressors and improve coping to limit long-term need for antianxiety medication

Antipsychotic Agents

- Used to treat agitated and aggressive behavior and psychotic symptoms (eg, out of touch with reality); makes client better able to participate in therapy
- Act by blocking a subtype of dopamine receptors in the CNS; they also block the muscarinic receptors for acetylcholine and the alpha receptors for norepinephrine
  - Positive (type I) symptoms of schizophrenia (eg, hallucinations, delusions) respond to traditional and newer antipsychotic drugs
  - Negative (type II) symptoms (eg, apathy, flat affect) are more responsive to the newer atypical antipsychotic drugs
- Available in oral (PO) and parenteral (IM, IV) preparations
- Effective in treating symptoms of psychosis noted in schizophrenia, schizoaffective disorder, and delusional disorder
- May be prescribed in conjunction with benzodiazepines
- May be prescribed at the onset of mania for sedative effects until therapeutic levels of antimanic medication is achieved
- Antipsychotic effects usually occur within 1 to 2 weeks after initiating treatment, but sedative effect can be immediate

- Ethnic/racial differences in response to antipsychotic medications have been reported and may be due to genetics, kinetic variations, dietary or environmental factors, or variations in the prescribing practices of clinicians

Types

- Traditional drugs (first-generation drugs)—phenothiazines (depresses limbic system to decrease aggression): Chlorpromazine, thioridazine, fluphenazine, piperazine, piperidine, prochlorperazine, triflupromazine
- Traditional drugs (first-generation drugs)—nonphenothiazines (depress cerebral cortex, hypothalamus, limbic system to decrease aggression): Haloperidol, thiothixene, loxapine, pimozide, molindone
- Atypical drugs (second-generation drugs; block dopamine and serotonin receptor activity): Aripiprazole, clozapine, olanzapine, quetiapine, risperidone, ziprasidone

Precautions

- Drug interactions
  - Potentiate the action of alcohol, barbiturates, antihypertensives, and anticholinergics; concomitant use should be avoided if possible
  - Should be temporarily discontinued when spinal or epidural anesthesia is necessary
- Adverse effects
  - Agranulocytosis (may be manifested by signs and symptoms of a cold or sore throat, chills or fever; highest risk is with clozapine)
  - Jaundice (hepatotoxicity)
  - Drowsiness (highest incidence in initial days of therapy because of CNS depression)
  - Orthostatic hypotension (autonomic nervous system [ANS] depression)
  - Anticholinergic side effects: Dry mouth, blurred vision, tachycardia, constipation and urinary retention
  - Hypersensitivity reactions: Tissue fluid accumulation, visual changes, impotence, cessation of menses or ovulation
  - Cardiac toxicity (direct toxic effect)
  - Weight gain and metabolic syndrome (abdominal obesity, dyslipidemia, hypertension, and insulin resistance leading to diabetes)
  - Photosensitivity
  - Extrapyramidal side effects (EPS)
    - Dystonia: Occurs early in treatment, possibly after initial dose; involves grimacing, torticollis, intermittent muscle spasms
    - Pseudoparkinsonism: Resembles true parkinsonism (tremor, masklike facies, drooling, restlessness, shuffling stooped gait, rigidity)
    - Akathisia: Motor agitation (restless legs, "jitters," nervous energy); *most common of all EPS*
    - Akinesia: Fatigue, weakness (hypotonia), painful muscles, lack of energy (anergia)
    - Tardive dyskinesia: Late-appearing after prolonged use of antipsychotic drugs; not related to dopamine-acetylcholine imbalance; most severe effect characterized by involuntary movements of face, jaw, and tongue or by lip smacking, grinding of teeth, rolling or protrusion of tongue, tics, and diaphragmatic movements that may impair breathing; condition disappears during sleep; antiparkinsonian drugs ineffective and condition is usually irreversible; all antipsychotics should be discontinued to determine whether symptoms subside

BOX 8.1   Summary of Major Adverse Responses to Antipsychotic Drugs

Anticholinergic Side Effects
- *Cause:* Blockade of cholinergic receptors (muscarinic receptors)
- *Offending agents:* Anticholinergic drugs, such as low-potency antipsychotics and anticholinergic-antiparkinsonian drugs
- *Signs and symptoms: Constipation,* decreased sweating, dilated pupils, dry mouth, slowed bowels and bladder

Extrapyramidal Side Effects
- *Cause:* Blockade of D2 receptors
- *Offending agents:* Typically high-potency antipsychotics
- *Signs and symptoms:* Akathisia, akinesia, dystonia, parkinsonism, tardive dyskinesia

Neuroleptic Malignant Syndrome
- *Cause:* Blockade of D2 receptors
- *Offending agents:* Typically high-potency antipsychotics
- *Signs and symptoms:* High fever and rigidity—can be fatal

(From Keltner, N. L., & Steele, D. (2015). *Psychiatric nursing* [7th ed.]. St. Louis, MO: Mosby/Elsevier.)

- Neuroleptic malignant syndrome: Infrequent yet extreme life-threatening condition occurring in severely ill clients and thought to be the result of dopamine blockage in the hypothalamus; associated with high-potency antipsychotic drugs, especially when given in a large loading dose; symptoms are hyperthermia (cardinal symptom), muscular rigidity, tremors, impaired ventilation, muteness, altered consciousness, unstable BP, and autonomic hyperactivity (Box 8.1)
  - Used for treatment of symptoms of neuroleptic malignant syndrome: dantrolene, bromocriptine, amantadine, antipyretics
- Antiparkinsonian drugs are given to block the EPS that are related to dopamine and acetylcholine imbalance, but may mask symptoms of tardive dyskinesia
- Anticholinergics are most used for EPS: Benztropine, biperiden, trihexyphenidyl; a missed dose should be taken up to 2 hours before next dose; has an additive anticholinergic effect with that of the antipsychotics
- Antihistamine: Diphenhydramine
- Other treatments for side effects
  - Used for neuroleptic malignant syndrome: Dantrolene, bromocriptine, amantadine, antipyretics
  - Used for akinesia and akathisia: Lorazepam, diazepam, clonazepam, propranolol, amantadine

Nursing Care of Clients Receiving Antipsychotic Agents
- Monitor BP
  - Assess in both supine and standing position
  - Assess before each dose is administered
  - Assess for tachycardia, which usually is a response to hypotension
  - Consult health care provider as to safe systolic/diastolic parameters for each client
  - Maintain safety if hypotension occurs (eg, assist with ambulation, assist client to rise from bed slowly and sit on bed before ambulating, keep side rails up when nonambulatory)
- Monitor geriatric clients closely for serious reactions

- Monitor mental status, CNS/neurologic/mood/personality changes
- Monitor for neuroleptic malignant syndrome
- Assess for EPS, antiparkinsonism agent may be prescribed to decrease symptoms
- Monitor laboratory results during long-term therapy (eg, periodic complete blood counts [CBCs], liver function tests, lipid profiles, glucose tolerance, blood glucose levels, and chemistry analysis); monitor weekly white blood cell (WBC) count if administering clozapine
- Monitor for signs of hepatic toxicity (eg, jaundice) and renal toxicity
- Monitor for signs of agranulocytosis such as infection (eg, sore throat)
- Monitor for weight gain associated with metabolic syndrome
- Monitor intake and output
- For nonphenothiazines, monitor ECG in clients with cardiovascular disease
- Instruct client to
  - Take medication as prescribed; do not discontinue abruptly
  - Take with food, milk, or full glass of water to prevent GI distress; some of the newer atypical antipsychotics require a full meal to facilitate absorption
  - Report suicide ideation or behavior
  - Avoid OTC products without prescriber permission
  - Avoid administration with other CNS depressants, including concurrent use of alcohol
  - Avoid engaging in potentially hazardous activities
  - Avoid exposure to direct sunlight; wear protective clothing and sunglasses outdoors
  - Recognize signs and symptoms of EPS and report their occurrence immediately
  - Avoid changing positions rapidly
  - Notify health care provider if sore throat, fever, or weakness occur; avoid crowded, potentially infectious places
  - Use sugar-free chewing gum or hard candy to increase salivation and relieve dry mouth
  - Increase water intake and eat high-fiber diet to avoid constipation
  - Expect weight gain; control weight with appropriate diet
  - Avoid mixing with certain juices or liquids (eg, coffee, tea, or cola beverages), which may decrease effectiveness of drug
  - Avoid antacids or take them 1 to 2 hours after antipsychotic drug is taken because antacids decrease absorption of antipsychotics
  - Eliminate or minimize smoking because it decreases serum levels of antipsychotics
- Recognize that nonadherence to drug regimen is common; monitor clients during administration to ensure medication is taken to prevent "cheeking" (client may discard tablet or save tablets to attempt overdose); consult health care provider about use of longer-acting drugs such as fluphenazine, haloperidol, or risperidone, about liquid forms of medications, or about rapidly dissolving tablets such as olanzapine
- Evaluate client's response to medication and understanding of teaching
- Consider long-acting forms of some antipsychotic agents for noncompliant patients

APPLICATION AND REVIEW

5. What is the **most** important information a nurse should teach to prevent relapse in a client diagnosed with a serious and persistent psychiatric illness?
   1. Develop close support systems
   2. Create a stress-free environment
   3. Refrain from activities that cause anxiety
   4. Follow the prescribed medication regimen

6. A client diagnosed with a psychosis is receiving olanzapine. What is important for a nurse to consider when administering this drug?
   1. It can be given rectally
   2. A special tyramine-free diet is required
   3. It dissolves instantly after oral administration
   4. An empty stomach increases its effectiveness

7. A nurse administers an antipsychotic medication to a client. For which **common** manageable side effect should the nurse assess the client?
   1. Jaundice
   2. Melanocytosis
   3. Drooping eyelids
   4. Unintentional tremors

8. What medication should the nurse expect to administer to actively reverse the overdose sedative effects of benzodiazepines?
   1. Lithium
   2. Flumazenil
   3. Methadone
   4. Chlorpromazine

9. A client with a diagnosis of schizophrenia is discharged from the hospital. At home the client forgets to take the medication, is unable to function, and must be hospitalized again. What medication may be prescribed that can be administered on an outpatient basis every 2 to 3 weeks?
   1. Lithium
   2. Diazepam
   3. Fluvoxamine
   4. Fluphenazine

10. A health care provider prescribes haloperidol for a client. What should the nurse teach the client to avoid when taking this medication?
    1. Driving at night
    2. Staying in the sun
    3. Ingesting aged cheeses
    4. Taking medications containing aspirin

11. A client diagnosed with anxiety is to receive fluoxetine. What precaution should the nurse consider when initiating treatment with this drug?
    1. It must be given with milk and crackers to avoid hyperacidity and discomfort
    2. Eating cheese or pickled herring or drinking wine may cause a hypertensive crisis
    3. Blood levels may not be sufficient to cause noticeable improvement for 2 to 4 weeks
    4. Blood levels should be obtained weekly for 3 months to monitor for appropriate levels

12. In conjunction with which classification of medication are trihexyphenidyl, biperiden, or benztropine often prescribed?
    1. Anxiolytics
    2. Barbiturates
    3. Antipsychotics
    4. Antidepressants

13. A nurse is educating a client who is taking clozapine for a diagnosis of schizophrenia. What should the nurse emphasize about the side effects of clozapine as a priority concern?
    1. Risk for falls
    2. Inability to sit still
    3. Increase in temperature
    4. Dizziness upon standing

14. A primary nurse observes that a client has become jaundiced after 2 weeks of antipsychotic drug therapy. The primary nurse continues to administer the antipsychotic until the health care provider can be consulted. What does the nurse manager conclude concerning this situation?
    1. Development of jaundice is sufficient reason to withhold the antipsychotic
    2. The blood level of antipsychotics must be maintained once established
    3. Jaundice is a benign side effect of antipsychotics that has little significance
    4. The prescribed dose for the antipsychotic should have been reduced by the nurse

15. A client diagnosed with schizophrenia is receiving an antipsychotic medication. For which potentially irreversible extrapyramidal side effect should a nurse monitor the client?
    1. Torticollis
    2. Oculogyriccrisis
    3. Tardivedyskinesia
    4. Pseudoparkinsonism

    See Answers on pages 138-142.

ANTIDEPRESSANTS

Description

- Primarily used for major depressive illness; also used in the treatment of panic disorder, other anxiety disorders, posttraumatic stress disorder, narcolepsy, attention deficit disorders, and enuresis in children
- Treatment is based on the restoration of acceptable levels of neurotransmitter systems by blocking the uptake in the presynaptic nerve ending, inhibiting breakdown, stimulating the release, and reducing stimulation at the site of the postsynaptic beta receptors (ie, down-regulation)
- Affect the neurotransmitters norepinephrine and/or serotonin by partially blocking their reuptake; roles for other neurotransmitters are unclear and under study
- Available mainly in oral preparations
- May need to be taken for 1 to 4 weeks before therapeutic response occurs; side effects may occur with initial doses
- Bupropion, an atypical antidepressant, also is used as an adjunctive treatment for smoking cessation
- Selective serotonin reuptake inhibitors, with their low side effect profile, are being used to treat eating disorders and obsessive-compulsive disorder
- Monoamine oxidase inhibitors (MAOIs) elevate norepinephrine levels in brain tissues by interfering with the enzyme MAO; act as psychic energizers; rarely used because of serious drug and food interactions that cause hypertensive crisis

Types

- Tricyclic drugs (TCAs; increase amount of norepinephrine and serotonin in nerve cells by preventing their reuptake): Amitriptyline, clomipramine, desipramine, doxepin, imipramine, nortriptyline, protriptyline, trimipramine
- Monoamine oxidase inhibitors (MAOIs; inhibit monoamine oxidase, thus increasing norepinephrine, dopamine, serotonin at receptor sites): Isocarboxazid, phenelzine, selegiline, tranylcypromine
- Selective serotonin reuptake inhibitors (SSRIs; inhibit neuronal reuptake of serotonin): Citalopram, fluoxetine, fluvoxamine, escitalopram, paroxetine, sertraline
- Atypical or second-generation antidepressants (affect one or two of the three neurotransmitters: Serotonin, norepinephrine, dopamine): bupropion, mirtazapine, trazodone
- Serotonin-norepinephrine reuptake inhibitors (SNRIs; Inhibits neuronal reuptake of serotonin and norepinephrine): Desvenlafaxine, duloxetine, venlafaxine

Precautions

- Tricyclic antidepressants (TCAs)
    - Drug interactions: Potentiate effects of anticholinergic drugs and CNS depressants (eg, alcohol and sedatives)

- Adverse effects
  - Orthostatic hypotension, skin rash, drowsiness, dry mouth, blurred vision, constipation, urine retention, tachycardia, mydriasis
  - CNS stimulation in older adults (eg, excitement, restlessness, incoordination, fine tremor, nightmares, delusions, disorientation, insomnia)
- Should not be prescribed for clients with narrow-angle glaucoma or benign prostatic hyperplasia
- Contraindicated during recovery phase of myocardial infarction or when client's history indicates cardiac dysrhythmias and cardiac conduction defects
- Should not be administered concurrently with MAOIs to prevent hypertensive crisis; there should be a minimum of 14 days between switching the TCA-resistant client to an MAOI
- Abrupt discontinuation of TCAs can cause nausea, headache, and malaise
- Highly lethal in overdose
- Low doses used as adjunctive treatment of chronic pain
- MAOIs
  - Drug interactions: MAOIs potentiate the effects of alcohol, barbiturates, anesthetic agents, cocaine, antihistamines, narcotics, corticoids, anticholinergics, and sympathomimetic drugs; can cause hypertensive crisis
  - Drug-food interactions: Hypertensive crisis with vascular rupture, occipital headache, palpitations, stiffness of neck muscles, emesis, sweating, photophobia, and cardiac dysrhythmias may occur when neurohormonal levels are elevated by ingestion of foods with high tyramine content (eg, pickled herring, beer, wine, chicken livers, aged or natural cheese, chocolate, caffeine, cola, licorice, avocados, bananas, and bologna); processed cheeses and fresh cheese (eg, cottage cheese) are low in tyramine
  - Adverse effects
    - Orthostatic hypotension (CNS effect)
    - Skin rash (hypersensitivity)
    - Drowsiness (CNS depression)
    - Dry mouth, blurred vision, urinary retention, tachycardia (anticholinergic effect)
    - Sexual dysfunction (autonomic effect)
    - Nightmares, delusions, disorientation, insomnia (CNS stimulation)
- Selective serotonin reuptake inhibitors (SSRIs) and serotonin-norepinephrine reuptake inhibitors (SNRIs)
  - Drug interactions: May interact with tryptophan, diazepam, warfarin, and digoxin; should be discontinued 4 to 6 weeks before switching to an MAOI
  - Adverse effects: Insomnia, headache, dry mouth, sexual dysfunction, anxiety, diarrhea, and other GI complaints
  - Serotonin syndrome: Confusion, coma, agitation, tachycardia, BP changes, nausea, myoclonus, hyperreflexia, tremors, ataxia, hyperpyrexia; usually resolves with elimination of SSRIs and supportive care
  - Hyponatremia, especially in the elderly
  - Usually these drugs are administered before noon to avoid insomnia or sleep disturbances
- Atypical second-generation antidepressants
  - Adverse effects: Increased appetite, weight gain, and sleep disturbances; mild anticholinergic side effects noted
  - Bupropion is thought to affect dopamine reuptake and agitation is sometimes produced

Nursing Care of Clients Receiving Antidepressants

- Monitor CNS/mood/personality changes and for self-destructive behavior, particularly during the second week of drug therapy when suicidal ideation remains and energy increases; maintain suicide precautions
- Monitor serum glucose levels in clients diagnosed with diabetes
- Monitor blood studies: Renal/hepatic function and cardiac status
- Monitor weight regularly for clients taking SSRIs, SNRIs, and atypical antidepressants
- Monitor for serotonin syndrome
- Instruct client to
  - Report suicide ideation, behavior; signs/ symptoms of serotonin syndrome
  - Change positions slowly
  - Avoid engaging in hazardous activities
  - Take medication as prescribed; NOT to abruptly discontinue medication
  - Use sugar-free chewing gum or hard candy to stimulate salivation
  - Check with the health care provider before taking all OTC preparations, alcohol, and cough or herbal medicines (eg, St. John's wort)
  - Expect therapeutic effect to be delayed; may take up to 3 weeks with MAOIs and 2 to 4 weeks with other antidepressants
  - Avoid alcohol, CNS depressants, other antidepressants and antipsychotics unless prescriber approves
- Avoid concurrent administration of adrenergic drugs; limit or eliminate caffeine use to prevent exacerbation of depression
- MAOIs
  - Maintain dietary restrictions; avoid foods containing tyramine (aged cheese, sauerkraut, cured meats, draft beer, fermented soy products; provide for nutritional education
  - Monitor client for signs and symptoms of hypertensive crisis (eg, occipital headache, palpitations, and stiff neck); treat with nifedipine and phentolamine
  - Administer during the day to prevent insomnia
  - Teach client to report signs/symptoms of hypertensive crisis
- TCAs
  - Monitor ECG in clients with history of cardiovascular disease
  - Monitor for withdrawal, chronic pain
  - Teach client to wear sunscreen, protective clothing, sunglasses
- SSRIs
  - Monitor cardiac status and heart rhythm
  - Do not administer within 14 days of MAOIs
  - Administer with food or milk to prevent GI distress
  - Use of concurrent herbal medication can cause serotonin syndrome
- SNRIs
  - Monitor cardiac status and heart rhythm
  - Teach client to report urinary retention
- Atypical antidepressants
  - Teach client to report auditory, visual, CNS changes
  - Teach client to notify prescriber if urinary retention occurs
- Fluoxetine, weekly capsule (90 mg), may be recommended if client responds to a daily maintenance dose of 20 mg without serious effects, for clients who have trouble adhering to daily regime
- Evaluate client's response to medication and understanding of teaching

ANTIMANIC AND MOOD-STABILIZING DRUGS

Description

- Used for maintenance in clients with a history of mania to decrease severity and frequency of manic episodes
- Improves productivity by decreasing psychomotor activity or response to environmental stimuli
- Available in oral capsules and tablets (both regular and sustained-release forms) and in concentrates
- Lithium affects the neurotransmitters of multiple systems including dopamine, norepinephrine, serotonin, acetylcholine, and GABA

Types

- Antimanic agents and mood stabilizers (increase norepinephrine and serotonin uptake): Lithium (extended release), lithium (regular release)
- Alternative antimanic agents and mood stabilizers: carbamazepine, lamotrigine, valproic acid, divalproex, topiramate, tiagabine, gabapentin
- Antipsychotics approved to treat mania and bipolar disorders: Olanzapine, ziprasidone, aripiprazole (see Antipsychotic section); some antipsychotic agents such as aripiprazole and ziprasidone may be used during the acute manic phase of bipolar illness to assist with symptom control until therapeutic levels of other antimanic medications are achieved

Precautions

- Drug interactions: Diuretics increase the reabsorption of lithium, resulting in possible toxic effects; when given with haloperidol, encephalopathic syndrome can occur; sodium bicarbonate or sodium chloride increases the excretion of lithium
- Drug-food interaction: Restriction of sodium intake increases drug substitution for sodium ions, which causes signs of hyponatremia (eg, nausea, vomiting, diarrhea, muscle fasciculations, stupor, seizures); daily intake of more than 250 mg of caffeine with lithium decreases effect of antianxiety drugs
- Adverse effects: Headache, drowsiness, dizziness, dry mouth, anorexia, nausea, hypotension, edema, fine hand tremor
- Toxic effects: Vomiting, diarrhea, tremors, weakness, lassitude, severe thirst, tinnitus, dilute urine; drug blood levels higher than 1.5 mEq/L indicate toxicity; toxicity easily occurs because the difference between the therapeutic level and toxic level is slight
- One to 2 weeks of treatment is necessary to achieve a clinical response; antipsychotic agents or benzodiazepines may be used in combination with lithium to control manic symptoms initially until antimanic clinical response occurs

Nursing Care of Clients Receiving Antimanic and Mood-Stabilizing Agents

- Recognize that therapeutic effects will be delayed for several weeks
- Check concurrent medications for potential interactions
- Administer with meals to reduce gastrointestinal (GI) irritation; ensure that drug is not crushed or chewed; liquid forms are available
- Encourage avoidance of hazardous activities
- Monitor mental status/CNS changes
- Teach that medication should not be discontinued abruptly and that if it is discontinued, it should be done with medical supervision

- Teach not to use OTC products unless prescriber approves
- Provide nursing care specific to lithium
  - Assess therapeutic blood levels (0.5–1.5 mEq/L) weekly for 1 month and then at 2-month to 3-month intervals; monitor for lithium toxicity
  - Maintain and encourage sodium and adequate fluid intake because dehydration and hypo- natremia predispose to lithium toxicity; monitor intake and output
  - Monitor weight and for signs of dependent edema; assess skin turgor daily
  - Monitor electrolyte status
  - Teach to report signs and symptoms of side effects and toxicity; teach that it takes 1 to 3 weeks to reach therapeutic levels
  - Refer pregnant woman to health care provider; cessation of lithium during pregnancy is recommended to avoid teratogenic effects during first trimester
  - Monitor ECG in clients with history of CV disease
- Provide nursing care specific to valproic acid
  - Administer with food or increase dose slowly to avoid GI distress
  - Teach about side effects: Sedation, drowsiness, nausea, vomiting, diarrhea, constipation, heartburn, ataxia, asthenia, insomnia, suicide ideation, thrombocytopenia
  - Teach about signs of toxicity: Visual disturbances, diplopia, rash, diarrhea, light-colored stools, jaundice, protracted vomiting
- Evaluate client's response to medication, including CBC results and liver function studies
- Evaluate client's understanding of self-care related to the medication regimen

SEDATIVE AND HYPNOTIC AGENTS

Description

- Benzodiazepines have almost entirely replaced barbiturates in the treatment of anxiety and sleep disorders; sedative and hypnotic agents are primarily used in general medicine rather than psychiatry
- Sedative-hypnotic preparations are generally intended for either occasional or short-term use
- Insomnia, hypersomnia, narcolepsy, parasomnias, periodic leg movements (nocturnal myoclonus), and sleep apnea are among the disorders that are responsive to these agents; specific psychiatric conditions predispose clients to insomnia (mood disorders, anxiety, and dementias)
- CNS depressants have antianxiety effects in low dosages, produce sleep in high dosages, and have general anesthetic-like states in very high dosages
- Sedatives reduce nervousness, excitability, and irritability without inducing sleep, but a sedative can become a hypnotic in large doses
- All hypnotic drugs probably alter either the character or the duration of rapid eye movement (REM) sleep
- Hypnotics cause sleep and have a more potent effect on the CNS than sedatives
- Sedative-hypnotics are classified chemically into three groups: barbiturates, benzodiazepines, and nonbenzodiazepines

Types

- Barbiturates: Pentobarbital
- Benzodiazepines: See Antianxiety/Anxiolytic Medications
- Nonbenzodiazepine hypnotics: See Antianxiety/Anxiolytic Medications

- Antidepressant: Trazodone (see previous mention)
- Antihistamines: Diphenhydramine; hydroxyzine
- Beta-adrenergic blocker: Propranolol

Precautions

- The sedative-hypnotics are CNS depressants
- Adverse effects:
  - Hypnotic drugs have undesirable effects (eg, physiologic addiction, fatal overdose potential, and dangerous interactions with other drugs and alcohol)
  - Barbiturate sedatives increase the metabolism of anticoagulants because they induce liver enzyme synthesis
- Tolerance develops to sedative and hypnotic agents; therefore the client in the outpatient setting may resort to increasing doses to produce the desired effect
- Physical and emotional addiction occurs if taken in large dosages or for a long time period; once physical dependence develops, abrupt discontinuation of sedative-hypnotics leads to withdrawal
- Once physical dependence develops, abrupt discontinuation of sedative-hypnotics leads to withdrawal
  - Withdrawal characteristics: Insomnia, weakness, muscle tremors, anxiety, irritability, sweating, anorexia, fever, nausea and vomiting, headache, incoordination, and restlessness
  - After several days, severe symptoms of withdrawal may develop: Postural hypotension, tinnitus, incoherence, delirium, psychosis, seizures, status epilepticus, cardiovascular collapse, loss of temperature regulation, and/or death
- To avoid severe withdrawal that could result in death, it is important to slowly and gradually taper the dose with the same drug or one that is cross-tolerant
- Treatment for overdose: Removal of the drug from the stomach by aspiration, resuscitative measures (eg, assisted ventilation, cardiac massage); hemodialysis of diffusible drug; vasopressor administration to counteract vascular collapse; and correction of acidosis
- Follow-up drug supervision is needed to avoid repetition of the problem
- Psychotherapy may be required for depressed clients
- Refer to Antianxiety/Anxiolytic Medications for additional information

Nursing Care of Clients Receiving Sedative and Hypnotic Agents

- Assess for history of drug or alcohol abuse or suicide attempts by overdose because of the increased risk for abuse
- Assess for pregnancy and breastfeeding because safe use has not been established
- Explore the client's perceptions and feelings about medications; clarify any misinformation and concerns
- Plan for client teaching about specific sedative-hypnotic agents; institute safety precautions
- Supplement verbal teaching with appropriate written or audiovisual materials
- Administer controlled substances according to schedule restrictions
- Evaluate client's response to medication and understanding of teaching
- Assess for undesired effects (eg, respiratory depression, increased sedation, and hypotension)
- Review methods to improve sleep (eg, minimizing daytime napping, increasing physical activity except just before bedtime, eliminating caffeine intake after dinner, establishing bedtime routines, maintaining a regular sleep schedule)
- Refer to Nursing Care of Clients Receiving Antianxiety/Anxiolytic Medications

STIMULANTS

Description and Types

- For attention-deficit disorder: Methylphenidate (possible mechanism—changes to serotonergic pathways occurs by affecting changes in dopamine transport); also used for narcolepsy
  - Some nonstimulants are also available for treatment of ADHD
- Amphetamines (central nervous system stimulants): Amphetamine sulfate, dextroamphetamine sulfate, lisdexamfetamine dimesylate

Precautions

- Can cause anorexia; give after breakfast or meal to ensure dietary intake
- Any second dose should be administered before 6 PM to limit insomnia
- Contraindicated in hyperthyroidism, Tourette syndrome, cardiac disease

Nursing Care of Clients Receiving Stimulants

- Involve family in parenting education training
- Provide parents with list of available community resources
- Support attendance at school or special education program
- Monitor weight, sleep patterns, mental status, as well as height and growth in children
- Monitor for hepatotoxicity, exfoliative dermatitis, thrombocytopenia, stroke
- Monitor children for onset of Tourette syndrome
- Instruct parents and clients to:
  - Administer medication as prescribed; do **not** abruptly discontinue; consult prescriber before modifying dose
  - Avoid foods/beverages and OTC products containing caffeine
  - Avoid alcohol and hazardous activities
  - Report adverse effects: Tachycardia, hypertension, growth suppression, palpitations, seizures, transient weight loss in children
  - Monitor side effects: Anorexia, dry mouth, nausea, vomiting, dizziness, insomnia, irritability, tremors, euphoria, blurred vision, headache, abdominal pain, anemia
- Evaluation/outcomes:
  - Participates in work, home, and school activities
  - Hyperactivity decreased, attention span increased (completes tasks and follows directions)
  - Blood pressure and heart rate within normal limits

ANTI-ALZHEIMER DRUGS

Description

- Temporary improvement in cognitive function but progression of disease continues
- Cholinesterase inhibitors: Impedes cholinesterase in the CNS thereby increasing acetylcholine
  - Used to treat mild to moderate Alzheimer disease
  - Unlabeled use includes vascular dementia
- N-methyl-d-aspartate (NMDA) receptor antagonist: Impedes action of CNS NMDA receptors, thereby lowering the glutamate level in the brain; protects CNS neurons
  - Used to treat moderate to severe Alzheimer disease
  - Unlabeled use includes vascular dementia

Types

- Acetylcholinesterase inhibitors: Donepezil, rivastigmine, galantamine
- NMDA receptor antagonist: Memantine

Precautions

- Acetylcholinesterase inhibitors
  - Drug interactions: Synergistic effect with other cholinesterase inhibitors; donepezil should not be administered within 2 weeks of MAOIs because hypertensive crisis may occur
  - Adverse effects: GI disturbances (eg, nausea, vomiting, diarrhea), headache, insomnia, dizziness
- NMDA receptor antagonist
  - Drug interactions: Alter effects of both NMDA and other medication; hydrochlorothiazide (HCTZ), H_2-histamine antagonists (eg, cimetidine), ranitidine
  - Adverse effects: Dizziness, confusion, headache, vomiting, constipation

Nursing Care of Clients Receiving Anti-Alzheimer Agents

- Administer rivastigmine and galantamine with meals; administer donepezil and memantine without regard to meals
- Provide assistance with ambulation and activity because dizziness may occur
- Assess GI and urinary status and for behavioral changes, less confusion, increase in mood
- Assess ability to swallow medication; some are supplied in oral solution, oral disintegrating tablets, transdermal route, extended release product that can be sprinkled on food
- Monitor vital signs for bradycardia or hypotension
- Monitory for adverse effects

APPLICATION AND REVIEW

16. A depressed client has been prescribed a tricyclic antidepressant. How long should the nurse inform the client it will take before noticing a significant change in the depression?
    1. 4 to 6 days
    2. 2 to 4 weeks
    3. 5 to 6 weeks
    4. 12 to 16 hours

17. A nurse is teaching clients about dietary restrictions when taking an MAOI. What response does the nurse tell them to anticipate if they do not follow these restrictions?
    1. Occipital headaches
    2. Generalized urticaria
    3. Severe muscle spasms
    4. Sudden drop in blood pressure

18. An MAOI is prescribed. What should the nurse include in the teaching plan about what to avoid when taking this drug?
    1. Ingesting aged cheeses
    2. Prolonged exposure to the sun
    3. Engaging in active physical exercise
    4. Over-the-counter antihistamine drugs

19. A client has been receiving escitalopram for treatment of a major depressive episode. On the fifth day of therapy the client refuses the medication stating, "It doesn't help, so what's the use of taking it?" What is the nurse's **best** response?
    1. "Sometimes it takes 1 to 4 weeks to see an improvement"
    2. "It takes 6 to 8 weeks for this medication to have an effect"
    3. "I'll talk to your health care provider about increasing the dose; that may help"
    4. "You should have felt a response by now; I'll notify your health care provider immediately"

20. A client is receiving doxepin. For which **most** dangerous side effect of tricyclic antidepressants should a nurse monitor the client?
    1. Mydriasis
    2. Dry mouth
    3. Constipation
    4. Polyuria

21. Imipramine, 75 mg three times per day, is prescribed for a client. What nursing action is appropriate when administering this medication?
    1. Tell the client that barbiturates and steroids will not be prescribed
    2. Warn the client not to eat cheese, fermenting products, and chicken liver
    3. Monitor the client for increased tolerance and report if the dosage is no longer effective
    4. Have the client checked for increased intraocular pressure and teach about symptoms of glaucoma

22. A client diagnosed with bipolar disorder is receiving lithium. What is an important nursing intervention when this medication is being administered?
    1. Restrict the client's daily sodium intake
    2. Test the client's urine specific gravity weekly
    3. Check the lab report about the client's drug blood level regularly
    4. Withhold the client's other medications for several days

23. A client in the hyperactive phase of a mood disorder, bipolar type, is receiving lithium. A nurse identifies that the client's lithium blood level is 1.8 mEq/L. What is the **most** appropriate nursing action?
    1. Continue the usual dose of lithium and note any adverse reactions
    2. Discontinue the drug until the lithium serum level drops to 0.5 mEq/L
    3. Ask the health care provider to increase the dose of lithium because the blood lithium level is too low
    4. Hold the drug and notify the health care provider immediately because the blood lithium level may be toxic

24. A nurse is caring for a client who abruptly discontinued use of a barbiturate medication. What should the nurse anticipate that the client may experience?
    1. Ataxia
    2. Seizures
    3. Diarrhea
    4. Urticaria

25. A client is to receive donepezil for treatment of dementia of the Alzheimer's type. The nurse teaches the primary caretaker and client about the purpose of the drug, its dosage, and the usual side effects. What side effect identified by the caretaker leads the nurse to conclude that further teaching is needed?
    1. Nausea
    2. Dizziness
    3. Headache
    4. Constipation

See Answers on pages 138-142.

ANSWER KEY: REVIEW QUESTIONS

1. **1 Self-help group members share similar experiences and can provide valuable understanding and support to each other**

   2 Although confrontation may occur, it is not the primary purpose of self-help groups; **3** Self-help groups provide an opportunity for people to interact, not engage in professional psychotherapy; **4** Criticism is not the primary purpose of self-help groups

   Client Need: Psychosocial Integrity; **Cognitive Level:** Comprehension; **Integrated Process:** Caring; **Nursing Process:** Planning/Implementation

2. **3 Stating, "Maybe others in the group have similar feelings that they would share" permits the client to see that personal feelings are not unique but are shared by others**
   1 The statement "You ought to be happy that you're leaving" makes the client worry about not feeling happy; **2** The statement "Maybe you're not ready to be discharged yet" is a nonsupportive response to a realistic fear of leaving the safe hospital and going back to where problems must be confronted; **4** How the others feel about whether the client is ready to be discharged is irrelevant
   Client Need: Psychosocial Integrity; **Cognitive Level:** Application; **Integrated Process:** Caring; Communication/Documentation; **Nursing Process:** Planning/Implementation

3. **2 The leader should not intervene at this point; the client addressed the statement to the group, and the group response should be fostered**
   1 Asking the client to consider the reasons this may have occurred may be viewed as aggressive and may make other members fearful of contributing because they might be confronted; **3** Gently suggesting that the client check the help-wanted advertisements in the local paper denies the client's feelings; **4** Requesting that the group help the client reflect on how the dismissal may have been prevented may be viewed as aggressive and may make other members fearful
   Client Need: Psychosocial Integrity; **Cognitive Level:** Application; **Integrated Process:** Communication/Documentation; **Nursing Process:** Planning/Implementation

4. **Answers: 1, 2, 5**
   1 Meditation lowers heart and blood pressure rates, decreases levels of adrenal corticosteroids, improves mental alertness, and increases a sense of calmness and peace; **2** Imagery is the internal experience of memories, dreams, fantasies, and visions that serves as a bridge connecting the body, mind, and spirit; its distractive ability decreases adrenal corticosteroids, promotes muscle relaxation, and increases a sense of calmness and peace; **5** Deep breathing increases oxygenation and releases tension in the muscles of the neck, shoulders, and torso
   3 Token economy is a behavioral theory that acknowledges acceptable behavior with a reward (token) that can be redeemed for something that has a perceived value (eg, a desirable activity); **4** Operant conditioning, a behavioral therapy, is the learning of a particular type of behavior followed by a reward
   Client Needs: Psychosocial Integrity; **Cognitive Level:** Application; **Nursing Process:** Planning/Implementation; **Integrated Process:** Communication/Documentation

5. **4 Following the prescribed medication regimen is important because side effects and denial of illness may cause clients to stop taking their medications; this is a common cause of relapse**
   1 Although developing close support systems is beneficial, this may not always be possible to achieve; **2** It is impossible to create a stress-free environment; clients need to learn better ways to cope with stress; **3** Refraining from any activity that may cause anxiety is too restrictive
   Client Need: Psychosocial Integrity; **Cognitive Level:** Analysis; **Integrated Process:** Teaching/Learning; **Nursing Process:** Planning/Implementation

6. **3 Olanzapine is an oral disintegrating tablet, which will instantly dissolve on contact with moisture. It is also available for IM injection.**
   1 Olanzapine can be given orally or via IM injection; **2** Tyramine-free diets are necessary with MAOIs, not antipsychotics; **4** An empty stomach is not necessary with olanzapine
   Client Need: Pharmacological and Parenteral Therapies; **Cognitive Level:** Knowledge; **Nursing Process:** Planning/Implementation

Memory Aid: To recall that olanzapine is available as an oral disintegrating ("disappearing") tablet, use the o's: *O*lanzapine is *o*ral; then imagine a magician doing a disappearing act, but instead of saying, "Prest*o*!" the magician says "*O*lanzapine!"

7. **4 Unintentional tremors are one of the extrapyramidal side effects of the antipsychotics and are considered common and manageable**
   1 Jaundice is a severe but not a common occurrence; periodic liver function tests should be performed; **2** An excessive number of melanocytes is not a side effect of antipsychotics; **3** Drooping eyelids is not a common side effect
   Client Need: Pharmacological and Parenteral Therapies; **Cognitive Level:** Application; **Nursing Process:** Assessment
8. **2 Flumazenil is the drug of choice in the management of overdose when a benzodiazepine is the only agent ingested by a client not at risk for seizure activity; this medication competitively inhibits activity at benzodiazepine recognition sites on GABA/benzodiazepine receptor complexes**
   1 Lithium is used in the treatment of mood disorders; **3** Methadone is used for narcotic addiction withdrawal; **4** Chlorpromazine is contraindicated in the presence of central nervous system depressants
   Client Need: Pharmacological and Parenteral Therapies; **Cognitive Level:** Knowledge; **Nursing Process:** Planning/Implementation
9. **4 Fluphenazine can be given IM every 2 to 3 weeks for clients who are unreliable in taking oral medications; it allows them to live in the community while keeping the disorder under control**
   1 Lithium is a mood stabilizing medication that is given to clients with bipolar disorder; this drug is not given for schizophrenia; **2** Diazepam is an antianxiety/anticonvulsant/skeletal muscle relaxant that is not given for schizophrenia; **3** Fluvoxamine is a selective serotonin reuptake inhibitor (SSRI); it is administered for depression, not schizophrenia
   Client Need: Pharmacological and Parenteral Therapies; **Cognitive Level:** Comprehension; **Nursing Process:** Planning/Implementation
10. **2 Haloperidol causes photosensitivity; severe sunburn can occur on exposure to the sun**
    1 There is no known side effect that affects night driving; **3** "Ingesting aged cheeses" would be true if the client were taking an MAO inhibitor; however, people taking psychotropic medications should avoid alcohol; **4** Aspirin is not contraindicated
    Client Need: Pharmacological and Parenteral Therapies; **Cognitive Level:** Comprehension; **Integrated Process:** Teaching/Learning; **Nursing Process:** Planning/Implementation
11. **3 Fluoxetine does not produce an immediate effect; nursing measures must be continued to decrease the risk for suicide**
    1 Giving fluoxetine with food as a precaution is not necessary; **2** The food precautions of avoiding cheese and pickled herring or drinking wine are appropriate with the MAOI medications; **4** Checking blood levels weekly for 3 months is not necessary with fluoxetine
    Client Need: Pharmacological and Parenteral Therapies; **Cognitive Level:** Comprehension; **Nursing Process:** Planning/Implementation
12. **3 These medications are used to** control **the extrapyramidal (parkinsonism-like) symptoms that often develop as a side effect of antipsychotic therapy**
    1 There is no documented use of trihexyphenidyl, biperiden, or benztropine with antianxiety agents because they do not have extrapyramidal side effects; **2** Barbiturates do not have extrapyramidal side effects that respond to these drugs; **4** Antiparkinsonian drugs usually are not prescribed in conjunction with antidepressants because antidepressants do not cause parkinsonism-like symptoms
    Client Need: Pharmacological and Parenteral Therapies; **Cognitive Level:** Analysis; **Nursing Process:** Planning/Implementation
13. **3 Clozapine, an atypical antipsychotic medication, may cause agranulocytosis, which can result in acquiring an infection**
    1 Risk for falls is more common with typical antipsychotic medications because they may cause orthostatic hypotension and extrapyramidal side effects; **2** An inability to sit still (akathisia) is more common with typical antipsychotics because they may cause extrapyramidal side effects; **4** Dizziness upon

standing (orthostatic hypotension) is more common with typical antipsychotics because they may cause extrapyramidal side effects

Client Need: Pharmacological and Parenteral Therapies; **Cognitive Level:** Analysis; **Integrated Process:** Teaching/Learning; **Nursing Process:** Planning/Implementation

14. **1 Liver damage is a well-documented toxic side effect of antipsychotics; by continuing to administer the drug, the nurse failed to use professional knowledge in the performance of responsibilities as outlined in the Nurse Practice Act**

    2 Blood levels must be reduced when signs of liver damage are present; **3** Liver damage, indicated by jaundice, is a well-documented side effect; **4** The antipsychotic should be stopped, not reduced; liver damage is a well-documented toxic side effect

    Client Need: Management of Care; **Cognitive Level:** Analysis; **Nursing Process:** Evaluation/Outcomes

15. **3 Tardive dyskinesia occurs as a late and persistent extrapyramidal complication of long-term antipsychotic therapy; it is most often manifested by abnormal movements of the lips, tongue, and mouth**

    1 Torticollis is reversible with administration of an anticholinergic (eg, benztropine) or an antihistamine (eg, diphenhydramine) or by stopping the medication; **2** Oculogyric crisis is reversible with administration of an anticholinergic (eg, benztropine) or an antihistamine (eg, diphenhydramine) or by stopping the medication; **4** Pseudoparkinsonism is reversible with administration of an anticholinergic (eg, benztropine) or an antihistamine (eg, diphenhydramine) or by stopping the medication

    Client Need: Pharmacological and Parenteral Therapies; **Cognitive Level:** Comprehension; **Nursing Process:** Assessment

16. **2 It takes 2 to 4 weeks for the drug to reach a therapeutic blood level**

    1 Four to six days is too short a time for a therapeutic blood level of the drug to be achieved; **3** Improvement in depression should be demonstrated earlier than 5 to 6 weeks; **4** Twelve to 16 hours is too short a time for a therapeutic blood level of the drug to be achieved

    Client Need: Pharmacological and Parenteral Therapies; **Cognitive Level:** Comprehension; **Integrated Process:** Teaching/Learning; **Nursing Process:** Planning/Implementation

17. **1 Occipital headaches are the beginning of a hypertensive crisis that results from excessive tyramine**

    2 Generalized urticaria is unrelated to the ingestion of tyramine; **3** Severe muscle spasms are unrelated to the ingestion of tyramine; **4** Excessive tyramine causes an increase, not a decrease, in blood pressure

    Client Need: Pharmacological and Parenteral Therapies; **Cognitive Level:** Application; **Integrated Process:** Teaching/Learning; **Nursing Process:** Evaluation/Outcomes

18. **1 The monoamine oxidase inhibitors can cause a hypertensive crisis if food or beverages that are high in tyramine are ingested**

    2 Prolonged sun exposure is important for clients taking one of the phenothiazines; **3** Active physical exercise is not contraindicated; **4** Antihistamines are not prohibited with MAOI medications

    Client Need: Pharmacological and Parenteral Therapies; **Cognitive Level:** Comprehension; **Integrated Process:** Teaching/Learning; **Nursing Process:** Planning/Implementation

19. **1 It usually takes 1 to 4 weeks to attain a therapeutic blood level of this MAOI**

    2 Escitalopram works within 1 to 4 weeks; **3** Escitalopram works within 1 to 4 weeks; **4** The client needs a longer time to see an effect from this medication

    Client Need: Pharmacological and Parenteral Therapies; **Cognitive Level:** Application; **Integrated Process:** Teaching/Learning; **Nursing Process:** Planning/Implementation

20. **1 Mydriatic action causes dilated pupils, which can precipitate an acute attack of glaucoma, resulting in blindness**

    2 Although dry mouth is a side effect, it is not serious and can be resolved; **3** Although constipation is a side effect, it is not serious and can be resolved; **4** Urinary retention is a side effect, and can be serious; polyuria is not a side effect.

Client Need: Pharmacological and Parenteral Therapies; **Cognitive Level:** Comprehension; **Nursing Process:** Evaluation/Outcomes

21. **4 The development of glaucoma is one of the side effects of imipramine, and the client should be taught the symptoms**

    1 That barbiturates and steroids will not be prescribed is true of MAOIs; imipramine is not an MAOI; **2** Avoidance of cheese, fermenting products, and chicken liver is important with MAOIs; imipramine is not an MAOI; **3** Tolerance is not an issue with tricyclic antidepressants such as imipramine

    Client Need: Pharmacological and Parenteral Therapies; **Cognitive Level:** Application; **Nursing Process:** Planning/Implementation

22. **3 Lithium alters sodium transport in nerve and muscle cells and causes a shift toward intraneuronal metabolism of catecholamines; because the range between therapeutic and toxic levels is very small, the client's serum lithium level should be monitored closely**

    1 Sodium restriction may cause electrolyte imbalance and lithium toxicity; **2** Testing the client's urine specific gravity is not necessary or useful; **4** Withholding the client's other medications for several days may or may not be necessary; it depends on what the client is receiving; also, it requires a health care provider's order

    Client Need: Pharmacological and Parenteral Therapies; **Cognitive Level:** Application; **Nursing Process:** Planning/Implementation

23. **4 The lithium level should be maintained between 0.5 and 1.5 mEq/L**

    1 Continuing the usual dose of lithium and noting any adverse reactions is unsafe; **2** The lithium level is currently unsafe, but it does not need to drop to 0.5 mEq/L before being resumed; **3** Asking the health care provider to increase the dose of lithium because the blood lithium level is too low is unsafe

    Client Need: Pharmacological and Parenteral Therapies; **Cognitive Level:** Analysis; **Nursing Process:** Planning/Implementation

24. **2 Seizures are a serious side effect that may occur with abrupt withdrawal from barbiturates**

    1 Ataxia is not associated with barbiturate withdrawal; **3** Diarrhea is not associated with barbiturate withdrawal; **4** Urticaria is not associated with barbiturate withdrawal

    Client Need: Pharmacological and Parenteral Therapies; **Cognitive Level:** Comprehension; **Nursing Process:** Assessment

25. **4 Donepezil, a cholinesterase inhibitor, may cause nausea, vomiting, increased salivation, diarrhea, and involuntary defecation related to the increase in gastrointestinal secretions and activity caused by parasympathetic nervous stimulation; it does not cause constipation**

    1 Common side effects of donepezil include anorexia, nausea, and vomiting that result from stimulation of the parasympathetic nervous system; **2** Dizziness is a common side effect of donepezil that results from central nervous system cholinergic effects; **3** Headache is a common side effect of donepezil that results from central nervous system cholinergic effects

    Client Needs: Pharmacological and Parenteral Therapies; **Cognitive Level:** Application; **Nursing Process:** Evaluation/Outcomes; **Integrated Process:** Teaching/Learning

---

Memory Aid: Connect the d's of *d*onepezil, *d*efecation, and *d*iarrhea to recall that donepezil does not cause constipation.

Neurocognitive Disorders 9

OVERVIEW

- Neurocognitive disorders (NCD) can be divided into delirium, dementia, and amnestic disorders
- The primary initial deficit occurs in cognition (ability to think, perceive, and reason), although there may be changes in mood and behavior
- NCD includes disorders associated with
  - Temporary or permanent changes in brain tissue that were formerly classified as organic brain syndrome or organic mental disorders (eg, delirium, dementia)
  - Persistent disturbances in memory resulting from a medical condition or substance use
  - Psychosis that may be acute and short-term or chronic and debilitating; brief psychotic disorders; and psychotic disorders caused by medical conditions or substance use
- Cognitive disorders range from mild memory loss to full (pervasive) dementia
- Major disorders of alterations in cognition and perception include delirium and dementia

Nondementia Cognitive Disorders

- Mild cognitive impairment (memory loss that does not interfere with activities of daily life)
- Delirium

Types of Dementia

- Potentially reversible dementias: Dementias caused by normal-pressure hydrocephalus, Vitamin B_{12} deficiency, brain tumor, subdural hematoma
- Irreversible dementias
  - Alzheimer disease (most common; 60%–80% of dementias)
  - Vascular dementia (second most common; 10%–20% of dementias)
  - Other irreversible dementias: Frontotemporal lobe dementia, dementia related to Parkinson's disease, dementia with Lewy bodies, Creutzfeldt-Jakob Disease (prion disease), AIDS dementia complex, dementia associated with alcoholism, dementia related to Huntington's disease

Classification of Dementias as Primary or Secondary

- Primary: These dementias are not caused by another disease; examples include Alzheimer's disease and vascular dementia
- Secondary: These dementias are secondary to another disease process, such as B12 deficiency, AIDs, alcoholism, Parkinson's disease, or Huntington disease: note that very few secondary dementias are reversible (see **Irreversible Dementias**)

General Nursing Care of Clients with Disorders Related to Alterations in Cognition and Perception

- Provide a safe, familiar environment–including cultural considerations, direct supervision as necessary (direct supervision reduces fear because constant reassurance is needed), and a consistent caregiver to foster trust; have all caregivers use a *consistent* approach; these clients need structure and routines; they resist change

- Have all caregivers use a consistent schedule and consistent approach
- Reorient to time, place, person, and situation (eg, clocks, calendar, incorporation of statements into ordinary conversation that reorient the client); reorientation usually reduced anxiety; however, avoid excessive use of reorientation because it may cause anxiety; keep statements short, simple, and concrete and use nonverbal cues
- Keep involved in reality-based activities and in the home situation as long as possible
- Allow to assume as much responsibility for self-care as possible; respect the individual
- Provide a quiet environment but do not understimulate; reduce unfamiliar stimuli; promote relationships
- Plan care so that the client can be approached when receptive
- Attempt to follow familiar routines; keep schedule of activities flexible to make use of the client's labile mood and easy distractibility
- Provide prompting for completion of activities of daily living (ADLs); the goal is to maintain the highest level of safe, independent functioning
- Encourage adequate nutritional intake; set limits on hyperorality; monitor intake and output (I&O)
- Provide diversional activities including exercises that are enjoyable and realistic
- Observe for changing physiologic and neurologic signs and symptoms
- Protect from physical harm to self or others related to confusion, aggression, or fluid and electrolyte imbalance
- Support and educate family caregivers; maintain nonjudgmental attitude
- Encourage the responsible others to obtain periodic relief from total care; refer to community agencies that provide home care helpers or respite care if appropriate
- Support family's decision to place client in a long-term facility when appropriate (culturally as well as for the client), or recommend family's acceptance of help from outside resources

APPLICATION AND REVIEW

1. Nurses working with clients who have a diagnosis of dementia should adopt a common approach of care because these clients need to:
   1. Relate to staff in a consistent manner
   2. Learn that the staff cannot be manipulated
   3. Accept controls that are concrete and fairly applied
   4. Have sameness and consistency in their environment
2. What is the priority nursing objective of the therapeutic psychiatric environment for a confused client?
   1. Assist the client to relate to others
   2. Make the hospital atmosphere more home-like
   3. Help the client become accepted in a controlled setting
   4. Maintain the highest level of safe, independent functioning
3. What is the **most** appropriate nursing intervention for clients who exhibit mild cognitive impairment?
   1. Reality orientation
   2. Behavioral confrontation
   3. Reflective communication
   4. Reminiscence group therapy
4. An older adult is brought to the clinic by a family member because of increasing confusion over the past week. Which technique can the nurse use to assess the client's orientation to place?
   1. Explain a proverb
   2. State where they were born
   3. Identify the name of the town
   4. Recall what they had eaten for breakfast

5. A nurse is admitting a client with the diagnosis of dementia. What should the nurse ask the client to **best** assess orientation to place?
   1. "Where are you"
   2. "Who brought you here"
   3. "Do you know where you are"
   4. "Do you know the day you arrived"

See Answers on pages 154-157.

DELIRIUM

Definition

- An acute state of confusion, altered attention, and altered perception

ETIOLOGIC AND PREDISPOSING FACTORS

- Mortality rates increase in accordance with the severity of delirium symptoms; therefore the cause of the delirium must be quickly identified and corrected
- *Temporary,* usually *reversible,* syndrome from which the client usually recovers after treatment
- Cognitive changes usually the result of a medical condition, substance use, or both
- Clinical manifestations develop over a short period (hours or days), and cognitive impairment fluctuates during a 24-hour period
- Stressors
  - Infection
    - Intracranial or nervous system (eg, meningitis or encephalitis)
    - Systemic (eg, infection, acute or chronic respiratory disorders)
  - Head trauma
  - Circulatory disturbances resulting in impairment of blood flow to the brain
  - Metabolic disorders: Electrolyte imbalances resulting from dehydration, diarrhea, or vomiting; fever; endocrine imbalances
  - Ingestion of substances, accumulative central nervous system (CNS) effect of prescribed medications (including some anticholinergics, cardiac medications, sedative-hypnotics, narcotics, and others) or street drugs, or withdrawal syndromes (eg, alcohol withdrawal delirium)
  - Multiple etiologies (eg, combination of medical condition and substance interaction)

Behavioral/Clinical Findings

- Acute onset and rapid progression
- Confusion, hallucinations (perception in absence of an external stimulus; visual and tactile hallucinations are the most common hallucinations associated with metabolic disease), illusions (misinterpretation of an actual stimulus), and delusions (fixed false belief)
- Disorientation and confusion as to time, place, person, and situation
- Memory defects for both recent and remote events and facts
- Slurring or rapid speech that may occur concurrently with an indistinct pronunciation or use of words
- Tremors, incoordination, imbalance, and incontinence
- Physical signs and symptoms such as hyperthermia, tachycardia, and gastrointestinal (GI) changes (eg, anorexia, nausea, vomiting, diarrhea)
- Agitation and irritability
- Insomnia
- Fluctuating level of consciousness

Distinguishing Delirium from Dementia (Table 9.1)

- Distinguishing delirium from dementia is critical **before** beginning care
- Note that an acute state of delirium can occur in a person with dementia

Therapeutic Interventions

- Reduction of causative agent such as fever or toxins
- Prevention of further damage
- Diet high in calories, protein, and vitamins and an adequate fluid intake if not contraindicated by physical status; elimination of caffeine
- Mild sedatives if necessary

NURSING CARE OF CLIENTS WITH DELIRIUM

Assessment/Analysis

- History of onset and progression of symptoms from family members
- Potential causative factors (eg, illness, medications, substance abuse)
- Orientation to time, place, person, and situation
- Occurrence of memory defects
- Mood swings or behavior associated with delirium

TABLE 9.1 Comparison of Clinical Findings of Delirium and Dementia

Delirium	Dementia
Acute onset (hours/days)	Chronic
Rapidly progressive	Insidious
Intense anxiety and irritability	Short attention span Blunted or labile affect
Tremors/hyperreflexia	Motor disturbance
Insomnia	Sundowning Possible day-night confusion
Hyperactivity and purposeless movement	Lack of initiative/apathy Wandering
Fever and tachycardia	Vital sign stability
Hypertension and other vital sign changes	Vital sign stability
Visual and tactile hallucinations, illusions, and delusions	Impaired new learning Loss of judgment Recent memory loss; later long-term loss
Seizures	Exaggeration of traits
Death	Memory problems that progress to loss of ADLs and immobility in late stages Lower personal care standards Progressive to death

Modified from Nugent, P. M., Green, J. S., Hellmer Saul, M. A., & Pelikan, P. K. (2012). *Mosby's comprehensive review of nursing for the NCLEX-RN examination* (20th ed.). St. Louis, MO: Mosby.

- Level of consciousness
- Vital signs and physical symptoms
- Assessment of labs (for example, mild elevations of BUN can cause confusion in the elderly)
- Assessment of polypharmacology or drug-drug interactions as potential cause

Planning/Implementation

- See General Nursing Care of Clients with Disorders Related to Alterations in Cognition and Perception, Nursing Care of Clients with Dementia, and Nursing Care of Clients with Amnestic Disorders
- Implement prescribed measures to reduce causative factors
- Reassure family members that symptoms associated with delirium may subside with treatment
- Assign a one-to-one caregiver during restless or agitated periods
- Provide a safe (proper lighting, no fall risk hazards), quiet environment with increased supervision
- Reorient to time, place, person, and situation
- Communicate with simple direct statements in calm voice; use nonverbal cues
- Channel agitation into safe activities

Evaluation/Outcomes

- Remains free from injury
- Remains oriented ×4 (time, place, person, and situation) to time, place, person, and situation
- Assumes increased responsibility for self-care
- Maintains a diet high in calories, protein, and vitamins
- Avoids intake of pharmacologic substance associated with delirium
- Continues to visit health care provider for treatment and amelioration of underlying cause

APPLICATION AND REVIEW

6. When distinguishing between dementia and delirium, which factors are unique to delirium? **Select all that apply.**
   1. Slurred speech
   2. Lability of mood
   3. Long-term memory loss
   4. Visual or tactile hallucinations
   5. Insidious deterioration in cognition
   6. Fluctuating levels of consciousness

See Answers on pages 154-157.

ALZHEIMER'S DISEASE/DEMENTIA

Database

- Death occurs after years of mental and physical decline; Alzheimer's disease is the sixth leading cause of death in the United States
- Etiologic and predisposing factors
  - Not associated with expected aging processes, although increased age does increase risk
  - Anatomic changes in the brain from trauma, tumors, and degeneration of tissue (eg, atrophy, widening ventricles, senile plaques caused by deposits of amyloid protein, neurofibrillary tangles) (Figs. 9.1, 9.2)
  - Infections such as tertiary syphilis and acquired immunodeficiency syndrome (AIDS)
  - Circulatory disturbances causing anoxia and permanent brain damage (eg, cerebral arteriosclerosis, stroke)

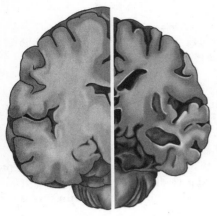

FIG. 9.1 Drawing of effects of Alzheimer's disease on the brain. Left shows a coronal view of a normal brain; right shows a brain with Alzheimer's disease. Note the diffuse atrophy and increased sulci in the brain with Alzheimer's disease. (From Lewis, S. L., Bucher, L., Heitkemper, M. M., & Harding, M. M. [2017]. *Medical-surgical nursing* [10th ed.]. St. Louis, MO: Elsevier.)

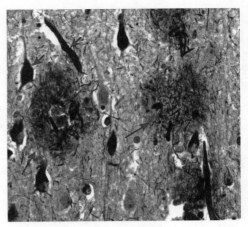

FIG. 9.2 Histopathologic changes in Alzheimer's disease. Beta-amyloid protein deposits (plaques) in the neutrophil *(long arrows)* and neurofibrillary tangles *(short arrows)*. (From Kumar, V., Abbas, A. K., & Aster, J. [2013]. *Robbins basic pathology* [9th ed.]. Philadelphia: Saunders.)

- Vascular dementia may develop after a stroke, although strokes don't always cause vascular dementia; it may result from other conditions that damage blood vessels and reduce circulation, depriving the brain of vital oxygen and nutrients; risk factors for heart disease and stroke (eg, high blood pressure, high cholesterol, smoking) also raise the risk for vascular dementia
  - Nutritional deprivation of brain cells (eg, pellagra)
  - Toxins (eg, chronic alcohol use)
  - Decreased level of neurotransmitters, especially acetylcholine
  - Chromosomal defects (eg, Huntington disease)
  - Immunologic defects creating prolonged inflammatory response in brain tissue
- Behavioral/clinical findings (Table 9.1)
  - Progressive: Dementia has an insidious onset with symptoms after a progressively downhill course
  - Early recognition of cognitive deficits may lead to anger, anxiety, and depression; as cognitive deficits progress and self-awareness declines, symptoms may be replaced by apathy and social withdrawal; anxiety may occur when cognitive abilities are overwhelmed and confusion increases
  - May repeat old defense mechanisms to defend against their memory and cognitive deficits, but they are not capable of learning new ones
  - May use confabulation (making up stories in place of actual memories) to help their self-esteem, or perseveration (repeated phrases or behaviors) especially under stress; may not answer questions in order to preserve self-esteem
  - Two important symptoms that tend to be hard to control include wandering and catastrophic reactions

- Neurologic Deficits
  - Progression moves from mild forgetfulness for recent events and mild expressive aphasia to inability to perform ADLs and mutism
  - "4 As" of dementia of the Alzheimer's type:
    - Amnesia (loss of memory)
    - Apraxia (impaired motor activities)
    - Agnosia (inability to recognize familiar objects)
    - Aphasia (language disturbance)
  - Ataxia (impaired coordination)
  - Disturbance in planning, organizing, sequencing, and abstracting (executive function)
  - Emotional lability or flat affect
  - Hallucinations, illusions, and delusions
  - Sundowning phenomenon: Agitated behaviors of physical aggression and increased confusion between 2 PM and 9 PM; nighttime sleeplessness and wandering between midnight and 6 AM
  - People with recent memory loss have difficulty shifting to the present and at advanced stages may seem to live in or dwell on the past

Nursing Diagnosis

- Nursing diagnoses are varied and may be related to safety or health risks, the client's cognitive state, or the role of the caregiver

Nursing Interventions and Medications

- The same as those for delirium with greater emphasis on preventing further damage (see Delirium—Therapeutic Interventions)
- Medications for depression, agitation, and cognitive decline
  - Antidepressants: May improve overall level of functioning (see Chapter 8, Psychopharmacology—Antidepressants)
  - Antipsychotics: May decrease agitation and aggressive behavior (see Chapter 8, Psychopharmacology—Antipsychotic Agents); be alert for black box warnings because some are not approved for dementia-related psychosis
  - Antidementia agents: Provide a temporary improvement in cognitive function but progression of disease continues (see Chapter 8, Psychopharmacology—Anti-Alzheimer's Drugs)
  - Avoid use of benzodiazepines because of safety issues

NURSING CARE OF CLIENTS WITH DEMENTIA

Assessment/Analysis

- History of onset and progression of symptoms
- Physical and emotional status in relation to needs associated with nutrition, fluid and electrolyte status, hygiene and toileting capabilities, and safety
- History of premorbid personality, abilities, and level of functioning
- History of impaired memory
- History of hallucinations (often visual) and delusions (often persecution)
- Identification of caregivers and their ability to provide adequate care
- Existence of advance directives
- Screening with the Mini-Mental State Examination (MMSE); assesses orientation (eg, identifying year, date, location), registration (eg, repeating names of objects), attention and calculation

(eg, identifying serial numbers, spelling a word backward), recall (eg, restating words previously said by examiner), language (eg, naming objects, obeying a three-stage command, reading and obeying a command); maximum score is 30; score less than 23 is indicative of cognitive impairment
  - Used to determine the stage of Alzheimer's disease (Table 9.2)
  - Distinguish between dementia and depression because some symptoms overlap

Planning/Implementation

- See Nursing Care of Clients with Delirium and Nursing Care of Clients with Amnestic Disorders
- Toilet frequently
- Provide skin care
- Assist with feeding, especially if swallowing difficulty is present; be alert for respiratory issues; ensure adequate fluid and nutrient intake
- Protect from self and environment; modify and simplify environment to prevent injury and wandering; increase supervision
- Support attempts at independence when appropriate
- Support family's decisions regarding present and future care; encourage completion of advance directives while client has capacity
- Assess effectiveness of medication to delay progression of cognitive symptoms
- Support caregivers as necessary (eg, respite care, home health aides, long-term residence, support groups)
- Identify stressors for undesirable behavior and remove the stressor when possible
- Give simple directions one at a time
- Prevent arguments from escalating into acting out by giving the client directions in a firm, low-pitched voice; explain any actions, such as separating the client from others, in an adult manner helps maintain self-esteem

TABLE 9.2 Stages of Alzheimer's Disease

Stage	MMSE* Score	Duration (yr)	Changes
Mild	20–30	2–3	Decreased short-term memory Word-finding and name-finding difficulties Decision making, concentration, reasoning, and judgment problems Difficulty performing usual activities Denial Getting lost Repetitive questioning
Moderate	10–19	3–4	Apraxia, agnosia, aphasia with poor comprehension, disorientation, blunting of affect, misidentification, sleep disturbance, delusions, needs assistance with activities of daily living Redirectable, extreme emotional lability, self-absorption, supervision with meals, wandering, urinary incontinence, requires supervision
Severe	0–9	5–10	Gait disturbance, unable to feed self, double incontinence, bowel impaction, bed bound, difficulty swallowing, fetal position; requires 24-hour supervision, close observation, or both

*MMSE: Mini-Mental state examination
Modified from: Folstein, M. F. (1997). Differential diagnosis of dementia: The clinical process. *Psychiatric Clinics of North America, 20(1)*, 45.

Evaluation/Outcomes

- Remains free from injury
- Maintains maximal potential for as long as possible
- Family uses community resources as necessary

AMNESTIC DISORDERS

Database

- Condition in which a person has difficulty learning new information or with remembering previously learned information that does not occur during delirium or dementia
- Categorized as a major NCD due to another medical condition, substance use, or an unknown etiology

Etiologic Factors

- Disturbance in memory related to medical condition (eg, head trauma, brain attack) or psychological trauma
- Disturbance in memory related to persistent effects of substance (eg, substance use disorders, medication, or toxin exposure)

Behavioral/Clinical Findings

- Impaired ability to learn new information
- Difficulty recalling previously learned information or past events
- Absence of anxiety related to a traumatic event
- Impaired social and occupational abilities
- Therapeutic Interventions: See Dementia

NURSING CARE OF CLIENTS WITH AMNESTIC DISORDERS

Assessment/Analysis

- History of onset and progression of symptoms
- History of previous level of functioning
- Causative agent
- Physical and emotional status

Planning/Implementation

- See Nursing Care of Clients with Substance-Induced Amnestic Disorders, Nursing Care of Clients with Delirium, and Nursing Care of Clients with Dementia
- Maintain a safe environment
- Support attempts at independence when appropriate
- Support client and family regarding present and future care decisions
- Support interventions regarding memory

Evaluation/Outcomes

- Demonstrates remission of amnesia
- Returns to previous level of functioning
- Family utilizes community resources

APPLICATION AND REVIEW

7. A nurse is teaching a client and family about the characteristics of dementia of the Alzheimer's type. What characteristic should the nurse include?
   1. Periodic exacerbations
   2. Aggressive acting-out behavior
   3. Hypoxia of selected areas of brain tissue
   4. Areas of brain destruction called senile plaques

8. A client diagnosed with dementia has been cared for by the spouse for 5 years. During the last month the client has become agitated and aggressive and is incontinent of urine and feces. The possibility of delirium in addition to the dementia has been ruled out. What is the **priority** nursing objective when this client is in an inpatient mental health facility?
   1. Managing the behavior
   2. Preventing further deterioration
   3. Focusing on the needs of the spouse
   4. Establishing an elimination retraining program

9. Which nursing intervention is **most** helpful in meeting the needs of an older adult with the diagnosis of dementia of the Alzheimer type? Select all that apply.
   1. Providing nutritious foods high in carbohydrates and proteins
   2. Offering opportunities for choices in the daily schedule to stimulate interest
   3. Developing a consistent plan with fixed time schedules to provide for emotional needs
   4. Simplifying the environment as much as possible
   5. Eliminating the need for decisions and choices

10. When attempting to assess the behavior of an older adult diagnosed with dementia, a nurse considers that the client probably is:
    1. not capable of using any defense mechanisms.
    2. using one method of defense for every situation.
    3. making exaggerated use of old, familiar mechanisms.
    4. attempting to develop new defense mechanisms to meet the current situation.

11. Which intervention should a nurse include in the plan of care for a client diagnosed with vascular dementia?
    1. A reeducation program
    2. Plan for supportive care
    3. An introduction of new leisure-time activities
    4. Plans for involvement in group therapy sessions

12. A nurse's **best** approach when caring for a confused, older client is to provide an environment with
    1. space for privacy.   3. trusting relationships.
    2. group involvement.   4. activities that are varied.

13. An older adult on the mental health unit begins acting out when in the day room. What is a nurse's initial intervention?
    1. Instruct the client to be quiet
    2. Allow the client to act out until fatigue sets in
    3. Give the client directions in a firm, low-pitched voice
    4. Guide the client from the room by gently holding the client's arm

14. A nurse is assessing an older adult with the diagnosis of dementia. Which manifestations are expected in this client? **Select all that apply.**
    1. Resistance to change
    2. Inability to recognize familiar objects
    3. Preoccupation with personal appearance
    4. Inability to concentrate on new activities or interests
    5. Tendency to dwell on the past and ignore the present

15. When answering questions from the family of a client diagnosed with Alzheimer disease, the nurse explains, "This disease is:
    1. One that emerges in the fourth decade of life"
    2. A slow and progressive deterioration of the mind"
    3. Functional in origin that occurs in the later years"
    4. Diagnosed through laboratory and psychologic tests"

16. A client in the early dementia stage of Alzheimer disease is admitted to a long-term care facility. Which interventions should the nurse initiate? **Select all that apply.**
    1. Weigh the client once a week
    2. Have specialized rehabilitation equipment available
    3. Keep the client in pajamas and robe most of the day
    4. Establish a schedule with periods of rest after activities
    5. Review the client's weekly budget and use of community resources
    6. Set up a plan for weekly entertainment through a senior citizens group

17. A nurse is assessing a client diagnosed with dementia. Which clinical manifestations are expected? **Select all that apply.**
    1. Agitation
    2. Pessimism
    3. Short attention span
    4. Disordered reasoning
    5. Impaired motor activities

18. What are the four "As" for which nurses should assess clients suspected of having Alzheimer's disease?
    1. Amnesia, apraxia, agnosia, aphasia
    2. Avoidance, aloofness, asocial, asexual
    3. Autism, loose association, apathy, affect
    4. Aggressive, amoral, ambivalent, attractive

19. A nursing home resident diagnosed with dementia of the Alzheimer's type is engaging in numerous acting-out behaviors. On what should the nurse base the **initial** plan of care?
    1. Assessing the client's level of consciousness
    2. Identifying the stressors that precipitated the client's behavior
    3. Observing the client's performance of activities of daily living
    4. Monitoring any side effects associated with the client's medications

20. A 54-year-old client has demonstrated increasing forgetfulness, irritability, and antisocial behavior. After being found walking down a street, disoriented and seminaked, the client is admitted to the hospital and is diagnosed with dementia of the Alzheimer's type. The client expresses fear and anxiety. What is the **best** approach for the nurse to take?
    1. Explore the reasons for the client's concerns
    2. Reassure the client by the frequent presence of staff
    3. Initiate the program of planned interaction and activity
    4. Explain the purpose of the unit and why admission was necessary

See Answers on pages 154-157.

ANSWER KEY: REVIEW QUESTIONS

1. **4 A consistent approach and consistent communication from all members of the health team help the client who has dementia remain more reality-oriented**

   1 It is the staff members who need to be consistent; **2** Clients who have this disorder do not attempt to manipulate the staff; **3** Concrete and fair application is not needed when working with clients who have this disorder; consistency is most important

   Client Need: Psychosocial Integrity; **Cognitive Level:** Comprehension; **Nursing Process:** Planning/Implementation

2. **4 The therapeutic milieu is directed toward helping the client develop effective ways of functioning safely and independently**

   1 Assisting the client to relate to others is one small part of the overall objectives; **2** The therapeutic milieu allows some items from home to make the client less anxious; however, the objective is not to duplicate a home situation; **3** Helping the client become accepted in a controlled setting is a worthwhile objective but not as important as maximizing safe, independent functioning

   Client Need: Psychosocial Integrity; **Cognitive Level:** Application; **Nursing Process:** Planning/Implementation

3. **1 Reality orientation generally is helpful to clients exhibiting mild cognitive impairment; these clients are aware of their impairment, and orientation then reduces anxiety**

   2 Behavioral confrontation is not therapeutic because it may cause frustration and increase psychomotor agitation in a client with cognitive impairment; **3** Reflective communication is a technique in which the nurse restates or repeats the client's statements; it can be used to clarify thoughts but can also lead to frustration when the approach is overdone; **4** Reminiscence group therapy is helpful with severely confused, disorganized clients because it reinforces identity, acknowledges what was significant, and often compensates for the dullness of the present

   Client Need: Psychosocial Integrity; **Cognitive Level:** Application; **Nursing Process:** Planning/Implementation

4. **3 Orientation to place refers to an individual's awareness of the objective world in its relation to the self; orientation to time, place, and person is part of the assessment of cerebral functioning**

   1 Explaining a proverb requires abstract thinking, which involves a higher integrative function than orientation to place; **2** Stating where they were born assesses remote memory, not orientation; **4** Recalling what they ate for breakfast assesses recent memory, not orientation

   Client Need: Psychosocial Integrity; **Cognitive Level:** Application; **Nursing Process:** Assessment/Analysis

5. **1 "Where are you" is the best question that can be asked to elicit information about the client's orientation to place because it encourages a response that can be assessed**

   2 "Who brought you here" focuses on recent memory; it does not assess orientation to place; **3** "Do you know where you are" probably will be answered with a "Yes" or "No"; this will not reveal the client's orientation objectively; **4** "Do you know the day you arrived" focuses on orientation to time, not place

   Client Need: Psychosocial Integrity; **Cognitive Level:** Application; **Nursing Process:** Assessment/Analysis; **Integrated Process:** Communication/Documentation

6. **Answers: 1, 4, 6**

   1 Delirium, a transient cognitive disorder caused by global dysfunction in cerebral metabolism, causes sparse or rapid speech that may be slurred and incoherent; **4** Visual or tactile hallucinations and illusions may occur with delirium because of altered cerebral functioning; hallucinations are not prominent with dementia; **6** Clients with delirium fluctuate from hyperalert to difficult to arouse; they may lose orientation to time and place; clients with dementia do not have fluctuating levels of consciousness, but they may be confused and disoriented

   2 Clients with delirium consistently are irritable, anxious, and fearful; lability of mood is associated with dementia; **3** Short-term memory loss is associated with both delirium and dementia; eventually, long-term memory loss is associated with dementia; **5** The onset of delirium is abrupt (hours to days) and has an organic basis; it is often precipitated by drugs such as anesthesia, analgesics, and antibiotics or by conditions such as infections, end-stage kidney disease, and substance abuse or withdrawal; the onset of dementia is slow and insidious (years)

Client Need: Psychosocial Integrity; **Cognitive Level:** Comprehension; **Nursing Process:** Assessment/Analysis

---

Memory Aid: Whether you are waiting for a pizza deli*very* or a baby deli*very*, you want *rapid* delivery! *Deli*rium has *acute onset and rapid progression.* Because it can progress to seizures and death, your rapid recognition of delirium is crucial!

---

7. **4 When an older person's brain atrophies, some unusual deposits of iron are scattered on nerve cells; throughout the brain, areas of deeply staining amyloid, called senile plaques, can be found; these plaques are end stages in the destruction of brain tissue**

    1 Dementia is associated with a chronic deterioration, not with remissions and exacerbations; **2** Aggressive acting-out behavior may or may not be part of the disorder; **3** Hypoxia of areas of brain tissue is typical of vascular dementia, not dementia of the Alzheimer's type

    Client Need: Psychosocial Integrity; **Cognitive Level:** Comprehension; **Nursing Process:** Planning/Implementation

8. **1 The client must be kept from harming self or others; the client needs a calm, supportive environment that meets needs and maintains dignity**

    2 Alzheimer's dementia is characterized by progressive deterioration that is not preventable; however, some drugs such as donepezil (Aricept) may slow mild to moderate dementia; **3** Although addressing the needs of family members is important, the focus of care primarily is on the client; **4** Establishing an elimination retraining program may be unrealistic and is not the priority

    Client Need: Psychosocial Integrity; **Cognitive Level:** Analysis; **Nursing Process:** Planning/Implementation

9. **Answers: 4, 5**

    Clients with this disorder need a simple environment; because of brain cell destruction, they are unable to make choices

    1 A well-balanced diet is important throughout life, not just during senescence; a diet high in carbohydrates and protein may be lacking other nutrients such as fats; **2** The client may be incapable of making choices; providing alternative choices will increase anxiety; **3** Emotional needs must be met on a continuous basis, not just at fixed times

    Client Need: Psychosocial Integrity; **Cognitive Level:** Application; **Nursing Process:** Planning/Implementation

10. **3 These clients attempt to use defense mechanisms that have worked in the past but use them in an exaggerated manner; because of brain cell destruction, they are unable to develop new defense mechanisms**

    1 Clients with dementia will depend on old, familiar defense mechanisms; **2** The client is not capable of focusing on one defense mechanism; **4** The client is incapable of developing new defense mechanisms at this time

    Client Need: Psychosocial Integrity; **Cognitive Level:** Comprehension; **Nursing Process:** Assessment/Analysis

11. **2 Damaged brain cells do not regenerate; care is therefore directed toward preventing further damage and providing protection and support**

    1 The deterioration of the brain cells makes plans for a reeducation program unrealistic; **3** A client with this disorder may not be able to grasp, understand, or enjoy new leisure activities; **4** It is beyond the scope of the client's ability to function in a group therapy session

    Client Need: Psychosocial Integrity; **Cognitive Level:** Application; **Integrated Process:** Caring; **Nursing Process:** Planning/Implementation

12. **3 A one-to-one trusting relationship is essential to help the client become more involved and interested in interpersonal relationships**

    1 Privacy usually is not an issue for a confused client who requires increased supervision; **2** A confused individual needs to start with a one-to-one relationship before progressing to group involvement; **4** Selected activities, rather than a large variety of activities, are best

    Client Need: Psychosocial Integrity; **Cognitive Level:** Application; **Integrated Process:** Caring; **Nursing Process:** Planning/Implementation

13. **3 Clients who are out of control are seeking control and frequently respond to simple directions stated in a firm voice**

    1 "Be quiet" is an order that is nontherapeutic; furthermore, this is demeaning to the client; **2** Allowing the client to act out until fatigue sets in will not help the client gain control and might be frightening to other clients in the day room; **4** Guiding the client from the room is done only after an attempt at calming the client has failed

    Client Need: Safety and Infection Control; **Cognitive Level:** Application; **Integrated Process:** Communication/ Documentation; **Nursing Process:** Planning/Implementation

14. **Answers: 1, 2, 4, 5**

    1 Resistance to change is a clinical finding associated with dementia; these client need structure and routines; **2** An inability to recognize familiar objects (agnosia) is a typical cognitive dysfunction associated with dementia; **4** A short attention span and little or no interest in new activities are typical of dementia; **5** The past is where these clients feel more comfortable rather than the threatening present

    3 Clients with delirium, dementia, or other cognitive disorders rarely express any concern about personal appearance; the staff must meet most of these clients' personal needs

    Client Need: Psychosocial Integrity; **Cognitive Level:** Comprehension; **Nursing Process:** Assessment/Analysis

15. **2 Explaining that Alzheimer's disease is a slow and progressive deterioration of the mind is a true statement; clients become progressively worse over time**

    1 Alzheimer's disease usually appears in people 60 years of age and older; **3** Alzheimer's disease is an organic, not a functional, disorder; **4** At this time, there are no diagnostic tools other than autopsy that can provide a definite confirmation of Alzheimer's disease

    Client Need: Management of Care; **Cognitive Level:** Comprehension; **Integrated Process:** Communication/ Documentation; **Nursing Process:** Planning/Implementation

16. **Answers: 1, 2, 4**

    1 Monitoring weight is an objective way to assess nutritional status; **2** Specialized equipment can facilitate the client's participation in self-care; **4** Incorporating rest periods into the client's day prevents fatigue and energizes the client for the next period of activity

    3 The client needs to wear clothes to help maintain a positive view of self; **5** It is not appropriate to review budgeting and use of community resources with a client in the early dementia stage of Alzheimer's disease; these activities may produce frustration, withdrawal, and/or self-absorption; **6** A client with early dementia stage of Alzheimer's disease usually is unable to participate in or travel with a local senior citizens group

    Client Need: Physiological Integrity; **Cognitive Level:** Application; **Nursing Process:** Planning/Implementation

17. **Answers: 1, 3, 4, 5**

    1 The behavior of clients with dementia tends to be inappropriate, restless, and agitated; **3** Cognitive abilities are impaired, evidenced by a short attention span, limited ability to focus, and limited judgment and insight; **4** Cognitive abilities are impaired, evidenced by disordered reasoning; speech may be incoherent; memory, particularly short-term memory, is impaired; **5** Impaired motor activity (apraxia) and impaired coordination (ataxia) are associated with dementia

    2 Pessimism is more characteristic of depression, not dementia; the two often occur together and should be identified and treated appropriately

    Client Need: Psychosocial Integrity; **Cognitive Level:** Comprehension; **Nursing Process:** Assessment/Analysis

18. **1 Neurofibrillary tangles in the hippocampus cause recent memory loss (amnesia); temporoparietal deterioration causes cognitive deficiencies in speech (aphasia), purposeful movements (apraxia), and comprehension of visual, auditory, and other sensations (agnosia)**
    2 Avoidance, aloofness, asocial, and asexual are characteristics are related to schizoid personality;
      3 Autism, loose association, apathy, and affect are characteristics are related to schizophrenia;
      4 Aggressive, amoral, ambivalent, and attractive are characteristics are related to antisocial personality
    Client Need: Psychosocial Integrity; **Cognitive Level:** Knowledge; **Nursing Process:** Assessment/Analysis

> **Memory Aid:** To help you recall the "4 A's" of Alzheimer's dementia, say this sentence aloud: **Agn**es (**agn**osia), **Apr**il (**apr**axia), **Am**anda (**am**nesia), and **Aph**rodite (**aph**asia) had Alzheimer's dementia.

19. **2 If the areas that cause stress can be identified and avoided, the client should be better able to control the acting-out behavior**
    1 Clients who have Alzheimer's disease may be confused or disoriented, but they usually do not experience altered levels of consciousness; altered levels of consciousness are associated with delirium, not dementia; 3 Observing the client's performance of activities of daily living this may be done, but it is only one area of functioning that should be assessed; 4 Although monitoring side effects associated with the client's medications is important, it is not the priority
    Client Need: Psychosocial Integrity; **Cognitive Level:** Application; **Nursing Process:** Assessment/Analysis

20. **2 The client needs constant reassurance because forgetfulness blocks previous explanations; frequent presence of staff serves as a continual reminder**
    1 Clients who have Alzheimer's dementia will be unable to explain the reasons for concerns; 3 Too many varied activities will increase anxiety in a confused client; clients with dementia need simple, structured, routine environments and activities; 4 Clients with Alzheimer's dementia will not remember the explanation from one moment to the next
    Client Need: Psychosocial Integrity; **Cognitive Level:** Analysis; **Nursing Process:** Planning/Implementation; **Integrated Process:** Caring

10 Schizophrenia and Other Psychotic Disorders

SCHIZOPHRENIA

Overview

- Occurs in all cultures and socioeconomic groups
- Incidence (approximately 1 person per 100 people) is about equal between men and women (slightly higher in men); 95% of people have it for their lifetime
- Age of onset is late adolescence/early adulthood
  - In men usually between ages 18 and 25 years; men have a more severe course
  - Later onset for women, between 25 and 35 years
- DSM-5 no longer classifies subtypes of schizophrenia

Predisposing Factors

- Foremost etiology is the biologic perspective (eg, neuroanatomy, biochemical, genetics, perinatal; trauma and disease as causation continue to be researched)
- Biologic theories
  - Heredity and genetics (relatives have a greater incidence)
  - Neuroanatomic differences (enlarged ventricles, brain atrophy, decreased cerebral blood flow
  - Neurochemicals (eg, dopamine hyperactivity or overproduction; too little glutamate)
    - Dopamine hypothesis is that persons diagnosed with schizophrenia have an increased level of dopamine in certain areas of the brain such as the nigrostriatal tract, which runs from the substantia nigra to the basal ganglia; excess dopamine causes symptoms of psychosis (eg, hallucinations, delusions) because it disrupts cognition and thought; people diagnosed with schizophrenia smoke more cigarettes than the general population, presumably because nicotine affects dopamine release, producing a therapeutic effect
    - Recent research has indicated that alterations of other neurochemicals, including serotonin, are also involved in the pathology of schizophrenia
  - Estrogen's effect on dopamine function in women may have a protective effect
  - Neurotransmitter function: Abnormal neurotransmitter-endocrine interactions
  - Perinatal risk factors
    - Viral exposure during pregnancy (such as influenza)
    - Prenatal lead exposure
    - Complications during labor and delivery
- Psychodynamic theories
  - Susceptible genes interacting with environmental factors
    - Environmental factors include exposure to pollutants, toxins; and other substances, and stress
  - Developmental theories
    - Events early in life, especially during the trust-or-mistrust stage (neglect or rejection); lack of nurture
  - Family theories: "Blame" theories—when the family is blamed for the offspring's disease—have been discredited

- Stress theory
  - Predispositions + stress = multifactorial etiology
  - Psychosocial considerations are significant; causative models postulate that biologic vulnerability interacts with stressful environmental influences

Manifestation of Symptoms

- Symptoms include changes in perception, thought, consciousness, and affect
  - Symptoms interrupt an individual's ability to distinguish reality from unreality
  - Symptoms can be both acute and chronic; severe, and debilitating; include disruptions in sensory-perceptions, cognition, language, emotions, moods, attention, motivation, and reality testing
- Symptoms may come from different mechanisms; therefore they may respond to a variety of psychosocial and psychopharmacologic treatments
- Signs include changes in relationships, behaviors, and activities
  - Decline in interpersonal relationships and social functioning

Positive and Negative Symptoms

- Characteristic symptoms generally fall into two broad categories (Table 10.1)
- Positive symptoms (additional behaviors)
  - Theoretically related to *excessive* dopamine processes
  - Respond favorably to hospitalization, medication, reduced stimuli, and therapeutic interventions; more responsive than negative symptoms
  - More apparent during acute relapses
  - Disorganized or bizarre alterations in thinking, speech, perception (eg, altered reality testing, hallucinations, delusions), behavior, and mood
    - Disorganized thinking (formal thought disorder) is generally implied from the person's speech patterns
    - The person typically switches from one topic to another (loose associations or *derailment*)
    - Speech is *tangential* (digressive or rambling), and some responses to questions may be somewhat related to the questions, or completely unrelated (*tangentiality*); *clang associations* (selecting words based on sound versus meaning, often rhyming

TABLE 10.1 Schizophrenia: Symptom Categorization

Positive Symptoms	Negative Symptoms
Hallucinations	Apathy
Delusions	Social withdrawal
Loose association and other symptoms of formal though disorder	Flat affect
Concrete thinking	Poor ADLs*
Neologisms	Anhedonia
Bizarre behavior	Poverty of ideas and speech

*ADLs—activities of daily living
Modified from Nugent, P. M., Green, J. S., Hellmer Saul, M. A., & Pelikan, P. K. (2012). *Mosby's comprehensive review of nursing for the NCLEX-RN examination* (20th ed.). St. Louis, MO: Mosby.

- Hallucinations: Perceptions that occur in the absence of an external stimulus
  - They are not under voluntary control and can be quite vivid and clear to the individual
  - They may occur in any of the five senses (auditory, visual, olfactory, gustatory, and tactile), but *auditory hallucinations* are the most common type
  - Auditory hallucinations most often occur as voices that the client hears, which he can distinguish from his own thoughts; the voices may or may not be familiar to him, and if they are command-type hallucinations, they may be instructing the client to harm self or others
  - During acute episodes the voices heard may say derogatory things about the individual
- Delusions: Fixed or erroneous beliefs that typically involve a misinterpretation of understanding and experiences and cannot be corrected by logic
  - Content includes a variety of themes (eg, persecutory, referential, somatic, religious, or grandiose); although delusions occur in schizophrenia, they are also part of a separate disorder. See Delusional Disorder for descriptions of various delusions
  - The difference between a delusion and a strongly held belief is often difficult to discern and may depend on the degree of conviction held by the person in spite of obvious contrary evidence
  - Bizarre delusions are often difficult to judge, especially across different cultures; delusions are considered to be bizarre if they are obviously unlikely, not understandable by persons of the same culture, and do not evolve from ordinary life experiences
- Grossly disorganized or abnormal motor behavior, including agitation and catatonic behavior:
  - *Stereotypic movements* (odd postures, eg, swaying and rocking; and strange hand movements, eg, clapping and flapping)
  - *Catatonic behavior* is a severe decrease in reactions to the environment; this can range from resistance to directions *(negativism);* to exhibiting a sustained, bizarre, rigid posture; to a complete absence of motor and verbal responses *(stupor and mutism);* it can also include excessive and purposeless motor activity without obvious provocation *(catatonic excitement);* although catatonia has typically been associated with schizophrenia, catatonic symptoms are *not* specific to the disorder
- Negative symptoms (deficits of behaviors)
  - Flat/blunted affect, diminished emotional expression
  - Apathy/avolition (lack of motivation)
  - Attention deficit
  - No social engagement; poor rapport
  - Poverty of speech, communication difficulties
  - Poor grooming, hygiene

Course of Illness

- *Premorbid phase* includes features that contribute to the later development of the illness
  - Mild deficits in social, motor, and cognitive functions that occur during childhood and adolescence, such as subtle motor abnormalities during infancy and deficits in social functioning, organizational ability, and intellectual functioning around the ages of 16 to 17 years
- *Prodromal phase* (also known as the *prepsychotic phase*) includes symptoms and behaviors that signal the approaching onset of the illness
- *Psychotic phase* progresses through an *acute phase, a recovery or maintenance phase,* and a *stable phase:*
  - *Acute phase*: Individuals experience florid positive symptoms such as delusions and hallucinations as well as negative symptoms such as apathy, withdrawal, and avolition; they

are unable to perform self-care activities, and they may require brief hospitalization for their own safety and treatment
- *Recovery, maintenance, or stabilizing phase:* Symptoms are present, but they are less severe than during the acute phase; by 5 to 10 years after onset, most clients have a leveling off of their illness and functioning; they are generally able to care for themselves with some supervision
- *Stable phase:* This is the time during which symptoms are in remission, although some symptoms may persist or remain present in milder forms (residual symptoms); some people are able to live independently in the community during this time
- Onset and relapse can be related to stress

Clinical Description (Fig. 10.1)

- Symptom duration of at least 6 months
- Problems in cognitive functioning and thought processing: Attention deficits, abstract concept formation, decision making, and problem-solving
- Perceptual problems (hallucinations, delusions)
- Disturbed reality testing
- Problems in motivation

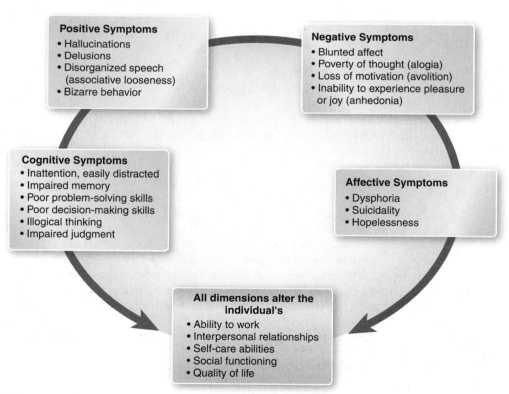

FIG. 10.1 Treatment-relevant symptoms in schizophrenia. (From Varcarolis, E. M. [2015]. *Essentials of mental health nursing* [2nd ed. revised reprint]. St. Louis, MO: Saunders/Elsevier.)

- Flat or inappropriate affect
- Behavioral changes such as social withdrawal and occupational role dysfunction

APPLICATION AND REVIEW

1. A client diagnosed with schizophrenia is admitted to an acute care psychiatric unit. Which clinical findings indicate positive signs and symptoms associated with schizophrenia?
   1. Withdrawal, poverty of speech, inattentiveness
   2. Flat affect, decreased spontaneity, asocial behavior
   3. Hypomania, labile mood swings, episodes of euphoria
   4. Hyperactivity, auditory hallucinations, loose associations
2. As a nurse enters a room and approaches a client diagnosed with schizophrenia, the client states, "Get out of here before I hit you—go away." The nurse concludes that this aggressive behavior is probably related to the fact that the client felt
   1. that voices were directing the behavior.
   2. trapped when the nurse walked into the room.
   3. afraid of doing harm to the nurse if the nurse came closer.
   4. that nurse was similar to someone who was previously frightening
3. What should the nurse identify as the foremost basis for the development of schizophrenia?
   1. Biologic perspective
   2. Seasonal approach
   3. Immunologic basis
   4. Psychoanalytic perspective

See Answers on pages 169-173.

Therapeutic Interventions

- Psychotherapeutic nurse-client relationship (see Nursing Care of Clients Diagnosed with Schizophrenia)
- Pharmacologic therapy (see Chapter 8—Antipsychotic Agents) is essential for schizophrenia
  - Antipsychotic medications reduce or alleviate the signs and symptoms associated with psychoses
  - Positive symptoms: Traditional/conventional/typical antipsychotics block the activity of dopamine
  - Negative symptoms: Unconventional/atypical antipsychotic drugs block serotonin and change levels of dopamine in different parts of the brain
- Psychotherapy (eg, individual, family, group) such as cognitive behavioral therapy
- Clients in the community who are more likely to be a danger to self or others with relapses may require mandatory outpatient treatment programs; mandatory outpatient treatment is court-ordered treatment for those clients diagnosed with mental illness who may not use services or who refuse treatment without a court order; it should be considered a last resort
- Day hospital treatment programs in community settings that foster interpersonal relationships
- Combination of medication, support, and group education decreases relapse rate substantially

NURSING CARE OF CLIENTS DIAGNOSED WITH SCHIZOPHRENIC DISORDERS

Assessment/Analysis

- History of onset of disorder
- Delusional ideation (fixed false belief) and/or hallucinations (perceived stimuli without external stimuli); specific assessment for command hallucinations (demand an action that may hurt self or others)

- Suspiciousness and/or feelings of paranoia; presence and extent of fear of other clients and staff
- Assess risk for violence
- History of work and social functioning
- Precipitating or current stress factors
- Assess responses of significant others, such as family
- Physical status

Planning/Implementation

- Adjust implementation based on the individual client (Box 10.1)
- Respect as a human being with both dignity and worth; establish a therapeutic relationship
- Accept at present level of functioning; meet basic physiologic needs; initially focus interactions on nonthreatening topics

---

BOX 10.1 General Principles to Address the Environment of Clients Diagnosed with Schizophrenia

For Disruptive Clients:
- Set limits on disruptive behavior
- Use affirmative language; state what can be done (instead of what not to do)
- Decrease environmental stimuli; for example, many nurses find that soft or classical music calms an environment, whereas hard rock or rap music creates agitation
- Observe escalating clients frequently to intervene; intervention (eg, medication) before acting out occurs protects clients and others physically and prevents embarrassment for escalating clients
- Modify the environment to minimize objects that can be used as weapons; some units use furniture so heavy that it cannot be lifted by most people
- Be careful in stating what the staff will do if a client acts out; however, follow through once a violation occurs (eg, "We can't allow anyone to hurt themselves or others, so the staff will have to use measures like restraints if you act in a dangerous manner like breaking a window")
- When using restraints, provide for safety by evaluating the client's status of hydration, nutrition, elimination, and circulation

For Withdrawn Clients:
- Arrange nonthreatening activities that involve clients in doing something (eg, a walking tour of a park, painting)
- Arrange furniture in a semicircle or around a table, which forces clients to sit with someone; interactions are permitted in this situation but should not

be demanded; sit in silence with clients who are not ready to respond; some may move the chair away despite the nurse's efforts
- Help clients to participate in decision making as appropriate
- Reinforce appropriate grooming and hygiene
- Provide psychosocial rehabilitation—training in community living, social skills, and health care skills

For Suspicious Clients:
- Be matter-of-fact when interacting with these clients
- Staff members should not laugh or whisper around clients unless the clients can hear what is being said; the nurse should clarify any misperceptions that clients have
- Do not touch suspicious clients without warning; avoid close physical contact
- Be consistent in activities (time, staff, approach)
- Maintain eye contact

For Clients with Impaired Communication:
- Be client and do not pressure clients to make sense
- Do not place clients in group activities that would frustrate them, damage their self-esteem, or overtax their abilities
- Provide opportunities for purposeful psychomotor activity

For Clients with Hallucinations:
- Attempt to provide distracting activities
- Discourage situations in which clients talk to others about their disordered perceptions

Continued

BOX 10.1	General Principles to Address the Environment of Clients Diagnosed with Schizophrenia—cont'd

- Monitor television selections; some programs seem to cause more perceptual problems than others (eg, horror movies)
- Monitor for command hallucinations that might increase the potential for clients to become dangerous
- Have staff members available in the day room so that clients can talk to real people about real people or real events

For Disorganized Clients:
- Remove disorganized clients to a less stimulating environment
- Provide a calm environment; the staff should appear calm
- Provide safe and relatively simple activities for these clients

Modified from Keltner, N. L., & Steele, D. (2015). *Psychiatric nursing* (7th ed.). St. Louis, MO: Mosby/Elsevier.

- Accept that hallucinations and delusions are real to client and possibly frightening; avoid trying to argue out of delusions or hallucinations; stay with client and provide support; focus on feelings, not misperceptions of reality
- Maintain safety, especially during acute phase; safety is the priority because of impaired judgment, paranoia, and/or command hallucinations
- Encourage development of interpersonal relationships; provide consistent interactions to promote development of trust
- Point out reality but do not impose staff's concept of reality; involve in reality-based activities such as activities of daily living (ADLs)
- Monitor nutritional status (although a client's suspiciousness may interfere with eating) and hygiene; reinforce grooming
- Monitor sleep because suspiciousness may make it difficult for client to sleep in strange environment
- Use distraction or set limits on inappropriate or unsafe behavior
- Modify the environment as needed for safety
- Clarify unclear communication; it may be necessary to give the patient extra time to respond verbally due to cognitive processing problems. It is helpful to use clear and concrete techniques when communicating
- Encourage to follow a plan of organized activity and the prescribed drug regimen
- Monitor for adverse reactions to antipsychotic medications
- Teach to recognize and report extrapyramidal side effects (EPS); administer prescribed antiparkinsonian agents to minimize EPS (see Chapter 8)
- Encourage to continue medications even after signs and symptoms abate
- Support families through education and family therapy, including multiple-family format

Evaluation/Outcomes

- Remains free from injury to self and others
- Differentiates between hallucinations and reality
- Demonstrates a reduction in anxiety through verbalization or body language
- Demonstrates improved functioning with ADLs and socialization
- Remains free from adverse side effects of psychotropic drug regimen
- Continues therapeutic/pharmacologic regimen

APPLICATION AND REVIEW

4. A nurse is assigned to care for a regressed college student who has been talking to unseen people and refusing to get out of bed, go to class, or get involved in daily grooming activities. What is the nurse's initial effort toward helping this client?
   1. Providing frequent rest periods
   2. Reducing environmental stimuli
   3. Facilitating the client's social relationships with a peer group
   4. Establishing a meaningful relationship with the client

5. An acutely ill client with the diagnosis of schizophrenia has just been admitted to the mental health unit. What is the **most** therapeutic initial nursing intervention?
   1. Spend time with the client to build trust and demonstrate acceptance
   2. Involve the client in occupational therapy and use diversional activity
   3. Delay one-to-one client interactions until medications reduce the psychotic symptoms
   4. Involve the client in multiple small-group discussions to distract attention from the fantasy world

6. A client diagnosed with schizophrenia plans an activity schedule with the help of the treatment team. A written copy is posted in the client's room. What should the nurse say when it is time for the client to go for a walk?
   1. "It's time for you to go for a walk now"
   2. "Do you want to take your scheduled walk now"
   3. "When would you like to go for your walk today"
   4. "You are supposed to be going for your walk now"

7. During the admission procedure, a client appears to be responding to voices. The client cries out at intervals, "No, no, I didn't kill him. You know the truth; tell that police officer. Please help me!" What is the nurse's **most** appropriate response?
   1. Sit quietly and not respond to the client's statements
   2. Listen attentively and assume a facial expression of disbelief
   3. Respond by saying, "I want to help you; I realize you must be very frightened"
   4. Say, "Do not become so upset; no one is talking to you; those voices are part of your illness"

8. A client with a history of schizophrenia attends the mental health clinic for a regularly scheduled group therapy session. The client arrives agitated and exhibits behaviors that indicates the hearing of voices. When a nurse begins to walk toward the client, the client pulls out a large knife. Which is the nurse's **best** approach?
   1. Firm   3. Empathetic
   2. Passive   4. Confrontational

9. While a nurse is talking with a client, another client comes up and yells, "I hate you! You're talking about me again," and throws a glass of juice at the nurse. What is the nurse's **best** response to this outburst?
   1. Repeat the client's words and ask for clarification
   2. Remove the client from the room because limits must be placed on the behavior
   3. Ignore both the behavior and the client, clean up the juice, and talk with the client later
   4. Verbalize feelings of annoyance as an example to the client that it is more acceptable to verbalize feelings than to act them out

10. A client who experiences auditory hallucinations agrees to discuss alternative coping strategies with a nurse. For the next 3 days, when the nurse attempts to focus on alternative strategies, the client gets up and leaves the interaction. What is the nurse's **most** therapeutic response?
    1. "Come back; you agreed that you would discuss other ways to cope"
    2. "You get up and leave every time I bring up a new way to cope"
    3. "Did you agree to talk about other ways to cope because you thought that was what I wanted"
    4. "You walk out each time I start to discuss the hallucinations; does that mean you've changed your mind"

11. What should the nurse do first to achieve a primary objective of providing a therapeutic environment for a client who is withdrawn and reclusive?
    1. Foster a trusting relationship
    2. Administer medications on time
    3. Involve the client in a group with peers
    4. Remove the client from the family home

12. A client experiencing hallucinations tells a nurse, "The voices are telling me I'm no good." The client asks whether the nurse hears the voices. Which is the nurse's **most** appropriate response?
    1. "No, I do not hear the voices, but I believe you can hear them"
    2. "It is the voice of your conscience, which only you can control"
    3. "Those voices are coming from within you; only you can hear them"
    4. "Hearing the voices are a symptom of your illness; don't pay attention to them"

13. A nurse enters a client's room and notices that the client appears preoccupied. Turning to the nurse, the client states, "They are saying terrible things about me. Can't you hear them?" What is the nurse's **most** therapeutic response?
    1. "It seems you heard them before"
    2. "Try to get control of your feelings"
    3. "There is no one here but me"
    4. "I don't hear anyone else talking, but I can see you are upset"

14. A nurse observes a regressed, emotionally disturbed client using the hands to eat soft foods. What is the **best** nursing intervention?
    1. Give the client a spoon and suggest it be used
    2. Say in a joking way, "Well, I guess fingers were made before forks"
    3. Ignore the behavior and observe several additional meals before intervening
    4. Remove the food and say, "You can't have any more until you use your spoon"

15. What clinical manifestation is the **most** serious indication of impending assaultive behavior by a client on a mental health unit?
    1. Uses profane language
    2. Touches people excessively
    3. Exhibits a sudden withdrawal
    4. Experiences command hallucinations

16. A client is admitted to the psychiatric unit during the first episode of an acute psychotic disorder. The plan of care calls for psychiatric, medical, and neurologic evaluation. What essential intervention should be included by the provider in the plan?
    1. Assessing the symptoms and teaching the client about the disorder
    2. Encouraging participation in cognitive and social skill enhancement
    3. Maintaining a daily routine and instituting family and group therapies
    4. Instituting psychopharmacologic prescriptions and supportive communication

17. What is an important aspect of nursing care for a client exhibiting psychotic patterns of thinking and behavior, including withdrawal?
    1. Redirect the client to reality
    2. Involve the client in activities throughout the day
    3. Help the client understand that it is harmful to withdraw from situations
    4. Encourage the client to discuss why interacting with other people is being avoided

See Answers on pages 169-173.

Other Schizophrenia Spectrum Disorders

- Brief psychotic disorder
  - Symptoms less than 1 month
  - Not related to a medical condition, mood disorder, or substance-induced disorder
  - At least one of these: Delusions, hallucinations, disorganized speech, grossly disorganized or catatonic behavior
- Schizophreniform disorder: Symptoms typical of schizophrenia, lasting more than 1 month but less than 6 months; impaired social and work functioning may not yet be evident
- Delusional disorders (see separate section)
  - Characterized by relatively normal behavior, except for delusions
  - Client does not meet criteria for schizophrenia
- Schizoaffective disorder (see separate section)
  - Psychosis with both affective (mood disorder, which can have depressive or manic symptoms, or both) and schizophrenic (thought disorder) symptoms

DELUSIONAL DISORDERS

Etiologic Factors

- Exact physiologic disruption is not understood
- Psychotic disorders thought to involve neurochemicals such as dopamine, serotonin, and norepinephrine; abnormal transmission of neural impulses
- See biologic theories in Schizophrenia section

Behavioral/Clinical Findings

- One or more delusions (fixed false beliefs) present for at least 1 month
  - Client cannot be persuaded that delusion is false
  - These delusions are not bizarre; they are things that could happen in real life
- Clients do not meet the criteria for schizophrenia
- Behavior is relatively normal, except for the delusions; highly organized delusional system but preserves other functions of the personality
- If mood symptoms are present, they are relatively brief
- Symptoms are not the direct result of a substance-induced or medical condition
- If hallucinations are present, they are not a major component
- Delusions do not exhibit the thinking and behavioral disorganization found in the schizophrenia

Types of Delusions

- Erotomanic: Belief that another person is in love with client; idealized, romantic love or spiritual union, rather than sexual attraction
- Grandiose: Belief that client has exceptional abilities, fame, or wealth
- Religious: Belief that client is favored by a higher being or is being instructed by that being
- Somatic: Belief that something abnormal or dangerous is happening to the body
- Paranoid or persecutory: Irrational distrust or suspicion of others; belief that client is being conspired against, spied upon, cheated, followed, poisoned or drugged, maligned, harassed, or obstructed in the pursuit of long-term goals
- Delusions of reference: Belief that certain gestures, comments, environmental cues, book passages, newspaper articles, radio or television commentary, or song lyrics are specifically directed at client
- Delusions of influence: Belief that client can control others

Therapeutic Interventions

- Pharmacotherapy with antipsychotic agents (see Chapter 8)
- Individual psychotherapy

NURSING CARE OF CLIENTS DIAGNOSED WITH DELUSIONAL DISORDER

Assessment/Analysis

- History of onset of disorder
- Delusional ideation; may constitute a danger to self or others
- Absence of odd or bizarre behavior and other criteria related to schizophrenia; client has never met criteria for schizophrenia
- Social and marital functioning

Planning/Implementation

- Provide an environment with some intellectual challenges that do not threaten security
- Accept and recognize client's need for the delusion
- Meet sarcasm and ridicule in a matter-of-fact manner; avoid counteraggression and retaliation
- Set limits on inappropriate behaviors that are derived from delusions
- Accept misinterpretations of events; point out reality but do not challenge delusions directly
- Provide consistency in staff; gradually integrate into unit activities to foster social interaction

Evaluation/Outcomes

- Avoids factors that stimulate delusional thinking
- Continues to function in society

SCHIZOAFFECTIVE DISORDER

Etiologic Factors

- Unrelated to direct physiologic effects of a substance or medication or a general medical condition
- Uninterrupted period of illness, including a major depressive episode or manic episode concurrent with symptoms of schizophrenia (eg, delusions or hallucinations, disorganized speech or behavior, and negative symptoms)

Behavioral/Clinical Findings

- Mixture of symptoms associated with both schizophrenia and mood disorders (mania or depression) with schizophrenic symptoms dominant
- Thought processes and bizarre behavior appear schizophrenic in conjunction with alterations in mood (eg, marked elation, depression)
- Mood disorder symptoms present for most of duration; delusions or hallucinations may also be present
- Loss of social and work functioning

Therapeutic Interventions

- Prognosis is better than for schizophrenia but not as good as for mood disorders
- Antipsychotic and/or mood stabilizers; antidepressants may be used to treat symptoms (see Chapter 8)
- Therapy depends on type and severity of symptoms

Nursing Care of Clients Diagnosed with a Schizoaffective Disorder

- See Nursing Care of Clients Diagnosed with Schizophrenic Disorders in this chapter and Nursing Care of Clients Diagnosed with Mood Disorders (Chapter 11).

APPLICATION AND REVIEW

18. What should a nurse do when caring for a client whose behavior is characterized by pathologic suspicion?
    1. Protect the client from environmental stress
    2. Help the client realize the suspicions are unrealistic
    3. Ask the client to explain the reasons for the feelings
    4. Help the client to feel accepted by the staff on the unit
19. A nurse finds a hospitalized client who has been experiencing persecutory delusions trying to get out the door. The client states, "Please let me go. I trust you. They are going to kill me tonight." Which comment by the nurse is **most** therapeutic?
    1. "You are frightened; come with me to your room, and we can talk about it"
    2. "Come with me to your room; I'll lock the door, and no one will get in to harm you"
    3. "Nobody here wants to harm you, and you know that; I'll come with you to your room"
    4. "Thank you for trusting me; maybe you can trust me when I tell you no one will kill you here"
20. A client is delusional, talking about people who are plotting to do harm. A nurse identifies that the client is pacing more than usual and is concerned that the client is beginning to lose control. What is the **best** nursing intervention?
    1. Advise the client to use a punching bag
    2. Move the client to a quiet place on the unit
    3. Encourage the client to sit down for a while
    4. Allow the client to continue pacing with supervision

See Answers on pages 169-173.

ANSWER KEY: REVIEW QUESTIONS

1. **4 Hyperactivity, auditory hallucinations, and loose associations are positive symptoms associated with schizophrenia; positive symptoms reflect a distortion or excess of normal functions**

   1 Withdrawal, poverty of speech, and inattentiveness are negative symptoms associated with schizophrenia; negative symptoms reflect a lessening or absence of normal functions; **2** Flat affect, decreased spontaneity, and asocial behavior are negative symptoms associated with schizophrenia; negative symptoms reflect a lessening or absence of normal functions; **3** Hypomania, labile mood swings, and episodes of euphoria are symptoms are associated with bipolar disorder or manic episode

   Client Need: Psychosocial Integrity; **Cognitive Level:** Comprehension; **Nursing Process:** Assessment/Analysis

   > 🔑 **Memory Aid:** Positive (**+**) symptoms **add** to the client's perceptions and behaviors; negative (**−**) symptoms **subtract** from the client's interactions and cognitive abilities.

2. **2 Clients acutely ill with schizophrenia frequently do not trust others; feeling trapped may be frightening, causing them to lash out**

   1 There is no indication that voices are speaking to the client in this instance; **3** Clients acutely ill with schizophrenia usually are more concerned with what is happening to them and are not able to be

concerned about others; **4** Although it may be true that the nurse was similar to someone who was previously frightening, it is not likely to be the primary motivation for this behavior
Client need: Psychosocial integrity; **Cognitive level:** Analysis; **Nursing process:** Assessment/analysis

3. **1 The biologic factors, including genetics, neuroanatomy, and abnormal neurotransmitter-endocrine interactions, prevail as the etiology of schizophrenia as the result of studies conducted during the 20th century**
   2 Seasonal perspective is not the primary basis for schizophrenia; **3** Immunologic perspective is not the primary basis for schizophrenia; **4** Psychoanalytic perspective is no longer thought of as the primary basis for schizophrenia
   Client Need: Psychosocial Integrity; **Cognitive Level:** Knowledge; **Nursing Process:** Assessment/Analysis

> **Memory Aid:** To remember that the biologic perspective (based on biologic facts, including genetics, anatomy, and neurotransmitter chemicals) prevails, think about the progress of treatment for schizophrenia throughout history. Now that imaging techniques and genetics have improved so much, there is evidence of the *biologic basis.*

4. **4 The first step in a plan of care should be the establishment of a meaningful relationship because it is through this relationship that the client can be helped**
   1 This client is not getting out of bed; rest periods are not needed; **2** The client has already reduced environmental stimuli by staying in bed; further reduction is not needed; **3** Establishing social relationships is a long-term goal
   Client Need: Psychosocial Integrity; **Cognitive Level:** Application; **Integrated Process:** Caring; **Nursing Process:** Planning/Implementation

5. **1 The initial intervention should be to demonstrate acceptance and work toward developing trust**
   2 Involving the client in occupational therapy and using diversional activities will increase the anxiety of a psychotic client; it is a correct action in the working phase of the nurse-client relationship; **3** Delaying one-to-one client interactions until medications reduce the psychotic symptoms delays the initial stage of the nurse-client relationship; **4** Involving the client in multiple small-group discussions will increase anxiety; it is an acceptable action in the ongoing working phase of a therapeutic relationship, not the initial phase
   Client Need: Psychosocial Integrity; **Cognitive Level:** Application; **Integrated Process:** Caring; **Nursing Process:** Planning/Implementation

6. **1 Stating "It's time for you to go for a walk now" is concise and does not require decision making; it is less likely to increase anxiety**
   2 Asking the client whether he or she wants to take the walk is asking the client to make a decision when a "no" answer is unacceptable; **3** Requiring the client to make a decision when acutely ill may increase anxiety; also, this permits the unacceptable answer of "never"; **4** Stating "You are supposed to be going for your walk now" is somewhat accusatory; it may increase anxiety by placing responsibility on the client
   Client Need: Psychosocial Integrity; **Cognitive Level:** Analysis; **Integrated Process:** Communication/Documentation; **Nursing Process:** Planning/Implementation

7. **3 Saying, "I want to help you; I realize you must be very frightened" demonstrates an understanding of the client's feelings and encourages the client to share feelings, which is an immediate need**
   1 Sitting quietly and not responding to the client's statements probably will increase the client's fears; **2** Listening attentively and assuming a facial expression of disbelief is judgmental and demeaning to the client; **4** Although saying, "Do not become so upset; no one is talking to you; those voices are part of your illness" points out reality, it gives a command that is unrealistic and closes the communication process
   Client Need: Psychosocial Integrity; **Cognitive Level:** Analysis; **Integrated Process:** Caring; Communication/Documentation; **Nursing Process:** Planning/Implementation

8. **1 A firm approach prevents anxiety transference and provides structure and control for a client who is out of control**

    2 A passive approach for a client who may be out of control does not provide structure, which may increase the client's anxiety; 3 Although the nurse should always base a therapeutic response on empathy, an obviously empathetic response may indicate to the client that the behavior is acceptable; 4 A confrontational approach in this situation may escalate the client's agitation and precipitate further acting out

    Client Need: Safety and Infection Control; **Cognitive Level:** Application; **Nursing Process:** Planning/Implementation

9. **2 The client's behavior is escalating and unsafe; the client should be removed from the room and taken to a place where there is decreased environmental stimulation and less chance for the client to act out against others**

    1 Repeating the client's words and asking for clarification accepts the physical abuse, which should never be done; 3 The behavior and the client should never be ignored; the client needs limits set on behavior immediately; 4 When a client is acting out, the nurse must intervene to stop the behavior; discussing the client's feelings can come later when the client is exhibiting more control

    Client Need: Safety and Infection Control; **Cognitive Level:** Application; **Integrated Process:** Caring; **Nursing Process:** Planning/Implementation

10. **2 Stating that the client seems very uncomfortable every time you bring up a new way to cope focuses on a feeling that the client may be experiencing and provides an opportunity to validate the nurse's statement**

    1 Stating "Come back; you agreed that you would discuss other ways to cope" demands that the client stay in an uncomfortable situation without offering any support; 3 Asking "Did you agree to talk about other ways to cope because you thought that was what I wanted" fails to recognize the part anxiety plays in changing behavior; 4 Stating "You walk out each time I start to discuss the hallucinations; does that mean you've changed your mind" seems like an attack on the client; also, although it offers an explanation for the behavior, it fails to convey an understanding that changing behavior is anxiety-producing

    Client Need: Psychosocial Integrity; **Cognitive Level:** Application; **Integrated Process:** Caring; Communication/Documentation; **Nursing Process:** Planning/Implementation

11. **1 An interpersonal relationship based on trust must be established before clients can be helped**

    2 Administering medications on time is an important part of the treatment and care, but it is of lesser importance than a trusting relationship; 3 Socialization comes at a later time in therapy; 4 There is nothing to indicate a need to remove the client from the home

    Client Need: Psychosocial Integrity; **Cognitive Level:** Application; **Integrated Process:** Caring; **Nursing Process:** Planning/Implementation

12. **1 The nurse, demonstrating knowledge and understanding, accepts the client's perceptions even though they are hallucinatory**

    2 Telling the client "It is the voice of your conscience, which only you can control" may increase the client's guilt and fear; 3 Telling the client "Those voices are coming from within you; only you can hear them" may increase the client's fear; 4 Stating "Hearing the voices are a symptom of your illness; don't pay attention to them" presents reality but negates the client's feelings and asks for an unrealistic response

    Client Need: Psychosocial Integrity; **Cognitive Level:** Analysis; **Integrated Process:** Caring; **Nursing Process:** Planning/Implementation

13. **4 Stating "I don't hear anyone else talking, but I can see you are upset" interjects reality and focuses on the client's feelings**

    1 Saying "It seems you heard them before" elicits a yes or no answer and does not foster communication; 2 Telling the client to "try to get control of your feelings" is a directive response that will be perceived as threatening to a disturbed client experiencing hallucinations; 3 Although stating "There is no one

here but me" interjects reality, it is not the most therapeutic response because it does not address the client's feelings

Client Need: Psychosocial Integrity; **Cognitive Level:** Analysis; **Integrated Process:** Caring; Communication/ Documentation; **Nursing Process:** Planning/Implementation

14. **1 The client needs limits to be set; give the client a spoon and suggest that it be used sets limits and rejects the behavior but accepts the client**

    2 Saying in a joking way, "Well, I guess fingers were made before forks" does not help raise the client to a functioning level; **3** Ignoring the behavior and observing additional meals before intervening serves no useful purpose; inappropriate behavior should be addressed when first noted; **4** Removing the food and saying, "You can't have any more until you use your spoon" is a punishing action; it shows no support or acceptance of the client

    Client Need: Psychosocial Integrity; **Cognitive Level:** Application; **Integrated Process:** Caring, **Nursing Process:** Planning/Implementation

15. **4 Command hallucinations are dangerous because they may influence the client to engage in behavior dangerous to self or others**

    1 Although profane language may be a cause for concern, it is not as dangerous as command hallucinations; **2** Although excessive touching of others may be a cause for concern, it is not as dangerous as command hallucinations; **3** Although withdrawn behavior may be a cause for concern, it is not as dangerous as command hallucinations

    Client Need: Safety And Infection Control; **Cognitive Level:** Application; **Nursing Process:** Assessment/Analysis

---

🔑 **Memory Aid:** *Command* hallucinations should *command* your attention because they can interfere with safety.

---

16. **4 Antipsychotic medications reduce or alleviate the signs and symptoms associated with psychoses; conventional or typical antipsychotics block the activity of dopamine; unconventional or atypical antipsychotics block both serotonin and dopamine; the reduction in psychosis will enable the client to participate more in therapy and educational programs**

    1 Although assessing signs and symptoms is an appropriate intervention during the entire hospitalization, teaching regarding this disorder is premature at this time; **2** Encouraging participation in cognitive and social skill enhancement are premature at this time; they may become appropriate after the acute psychotic episode has passed; **3** Although a daily routine is encouraged because it provides structure, it is more beneficial to initiate individual therapy rather than family or group therapy

    Client Need: Psychosocial Integrity; **Cognitive Level:** Application; **Nursing Process:** Planning/Implementation; **Integrated Process:** Communication/Documentation

17. **1 Redirecting the withdrawn client to reality prevents further withdrawal into a private world**

    2 A gradual involvement in selected activities is best; **3** Helping the client understand that it is harmful to withdraw from situations is futile at this time; **4** The client is unable to tell anyone why interacting with other people is being avoided

    Client Need: Psychosocial Integrity; **Cognitive Level:** Application; **Nursing Process:** Planning/Implementation

18. **4 Delusions are protective and can be abandoned only when the individual feels secure and adequate; helping the client to feel accepted by the staff on the unit is the only one directed at building the client's security and reducing anxiety**

    1 Protecting the client from environmental stress is almost impossible; **2** Clients cannot be argued out of a delusion; **3** The client is unable to explain the reason for the feelings

    Client Need: Psychosocial Integrity; **Cognitive Level:** Application; **Integrated Process:** Caring; **Nursing Process:** Planning/Implementation

19. **1 Stating "You are frightened; come with me to your room, and we can talk about it" recognizes the client's feelings and provides assurance that the staff member will be present**

    2 Locking the client in a room will only increase the fear and delusion; **3** The client does not know that no one here wants to hurt the client; if the client did, delusions would not be present; **4** The client is not ready to accept that no one will kill the client here; the client really believes danger is imminent

    Client Need: Psychosocial Integrity; **Cognitive Level:** Analysis; **Integrated Process:** Caring; Communication/ Documentation; **Nursing Process:** Planning/Implementation

20. **2 Clients losing control feel frightened and threatened; they need external controls, such as moving the client to a quiet place on the unit and a reduction in external stimuli**

    1 Advising the client to use a punching bag is helpful for pent-up aggressive behavior but not for agitation associated with delusions; **3** The client is unable, at this time, to sit in one place; the client's agitation is building; **4** The client may get completely out of control if allowed to continue pacing, even with supervision

    Client Need: Safety and Infection Control; **Cognitive Level:** Application; **Integrated Process:** Caring; **Nursing Process:** Planning/Implementation

11

Mood and Adjustment Disorders

MOOD DISORDERS

Terminology

- Mood: The internal manifestation of a subjective feeling state
- Affect: The external expression or manifestation of a feeling state
- Temperament: Observable differences in the intensity and duration of arousal and emotionality
- Emotion: The experience of a feeling state
- Emotional reactivity: The tendency to respond to internal or external events with emotion
- Emotional regulation: The ability to control or modify the occurrence and intensity of feelings
- Range of affect: The span of emotional expression experienced and displayed by an individual

Epidemiology

- Depressive and bipolar disorders, particularly depressive disorders, are common
- According to the National Institute of Mental Health (NIMH), about 9.5% of the U.S. population age 18 or older in any year has one of these disorders
  - Approximately 7% have major depressive disorder
  - Approximately 2.5% have bipolar disorder
- Lifetime prevalence of developing major depressive disorder is 16.2%, with twice as many women as men developing it
- Women's lifetime prevalence of major depressive disorder is 21.3%; prevalence is 8% for persistent depressive disorder
- Men's lifetime prevalence of major depressive disorder is 12.7%; prevalence is 4.8% for persistent depressive disorder; gender differences begin to occur around the age of 13 years
- The most frequent age of onset for depression is between 25 and 44 years
- The average age for the onset of bipolar disorder is late teens to the early 20s
- The risk of developing depression and mania increases if there is a positive family history of these disorders
- Although depression and mania occur throughout the world, ethnicity and culture influence the expression of symptoms; for example, people from Asian countries describe more somatic symptoms of depression, whereas people from Western cultures tend to describe more mood and cognitive changes
- In an increasingly stressful society that is characterized by mobility, family disruptions, and economic stressors, women and younger persons are manifesting depression more than they have in previous generations
- Persons experiencing depression often seek help from their primary care providers for physical symptoms such as fatigue, insomnia, headache, and loss of appetite; primary care providers do not always correctly diagnose depression or treat it appropriately
- The highest suicide rates in the U.S. are among white men who are more than 85 years old (see Chapter 6); four times as many men as women die as a result of suicide, but women attempt suicide two to three times as often as men do
- Depression and bipolar disorder can begin during early childhood and adolescence

- Depressive or bipolar disorders that present during childhood or adolescence:
  - Generate extraordinary distress for young individuals who are not prepared to understand or deal with the resulting feelings, emotions, and behaviors
  - Initiate major difficulties during a time that is essential to psychosocial development
  - Produce tremendous stress and concern for the entire family
  - Affect the educational experience; teachers can become frustrated and not understand the basis for the symptoms, which may result in them treating the child differently
  - Influence biologic processes and brain functioning to create changes that will have lifelong effects
- Symptoms of these disorders in children and adolescents often appear different from those seen in adults
  - Depressed youth often exhibit declining academic performance with school grades dropping for no apparent reason
  - Other indicators include behavioral problems, aggression, difficulty with peer relationships, withdrawal, and moodiness; those symptoms may override depression and sadness as key features
- The diagnosis of early-onset bipolar disorder (EOBD) has gained acceptance; the diagnosis has been made as early as the age of 5 years
  - The symptom profile of EOBD overlaps with that of other childhood psychiatric disorders, some of which may be comorbid
  - It may be difficult to distinguish between EOBD and attention-deficit/hyperactivity disorder (see Chapter 20)
    - Both of these conditions are manifested by hyperactivity, impulsivity, irritability, and inattention
    - One differentiating characteristic seems to be that EOBD symptoms show a cyclic pattern not evident with other disorders, including attention-deficit/hyperactivity disorder
- Late life depression refers to a major depressive episode occurring for the first time in older adults (typically over 50 or 60 years of age)
  - Depression is *not* a normal part of the aging process
  - Older adults with depression, often report symptoms of insomnia, anorexia, fatigue, apathy (loss of interest), rather than symptoms of depression
  - They tend to accept less severe depression as an ordinary life stressor, or a normal part of aging, which often prevents them from seeking professional help
  - Can be misdiagnosed as dementia; pseudodementia is depression appearing as dementia because of cognitive impairment
  - Risk factors in elderly persons include a history of depression, chronic medical illness, alcohol and prescription drug misuse, brain disease, or being female, single, or divorced
  - About 80% of identified cases respond well to treatment that combines psychotherapy with pharmacotherapy

Etiology

- Etiologic factors include biochemical/biologic theories, genetic transmission theories derived from family studies (familial history among close biologic relatives increases risk for disorder), and psychologic theories (feelings of guilt or brooding about the past)
- Note that psychosocial stressors associated with a major loss often play a significant role in first or second depressive onset
- Depression may progress to suicide (see Chapter 6)

BOX 11.1	Selected Medical Conditions and Substances Associated with Mood Disorders

Medical Conditions	Substances
Hypothyroidism/hyperthyroidism	Digitalis
Mononucleosis	Thiazide diuretics
Diabetes mellitus	Reserpine
Cushing's disease	Propranolol
Pernicious anemia	Anabolic steroids
Pancreatitis	Oral contraceptives
Hepatitis	Disulfiram
Human immunodeficiency virus	Sulfonamides
Multiple sclerosis	Alcohol and other substances of abuse
	Marijuana

Modified from Fortinash, K. M., & Holoday, P. A. (2012). *Psychiatric mental health nursing* (5th ed.). St. Louis, MO: Mosby.

- Biologic theories
  - Important biologic theories include those related to altered neurochemicals, neuroendocrine dysregulation, and genetics
  - Individuals with chronic or severe medical conditions are at increased risk (Box 11.1)
- Neurochemical alteration
  - Neurotransmission is a complex activity that includes multiple processes such as neurotransmitter synthesis and release, receptor site function and change, interactions among the various neurotransmitters and hormones, and the action of these transmitters and hormones on genes
  - Neurotransmitter dysregulation includes three key transmitters—serotonin, norepinephrine, dopamine (see Chapter 8)—as well as acetylcholine and gamma-aminobutyric acid (GABA) systems; altered neuropeptides include corticotropin-releasing hormones
  - Brain neurotransmitter functioning affects mood regulation and controls a wide range of behaviors and functions, including appetite, arousal, sleep, cognition, and movement
  - Neurotransmitter availability and receptor change theories have described less-than-normal neurotransmission activity during depression and more-than-normal activity during mania
  - These complex physiologic mechanisms are consistent with theories that propose the development of long-term changes in the brain that occur with these disorders
  - Brain imaging techniques provide additional support for brain disturbances during depression and mania
    - Positron emission tomography (PET scans) enables researchers to examine the brain physiology (glucose and oxygen metabolism) of depressed persons compared with normal control subjects, allowing for comparison of brain functioning during a depressive episode and after recovery
    - Differences are apparent on PET scans among depressed, recovered, and normal control brains and include alterations in blood flow in brains of depressed persons
    - PET scanning has shown that the prefrontal cerebral cortex and the limbic system (including the amygdala) appear to have physiologic and anatomic changes in the brains of persons who are experiencing depression
  - The complexity of the biologic, structural, and physiologic changes that occur with depressive and bipolar disorders continues to pose challenges for researchers

- Neuroendocrine dysregulation
  - Depressive and bipolar disorders have been linked to dysregulation of the limbic hypothalamic-pituitary-adrenal (HPA) axis
  - The hypothalamus, the pituitary, the adrenal glands, and the hippocampus make up the HPA axis, which controls physiologic responses to stress
    - The hypothalamus regulates endocrine functions and the autonomic nervous system; it is also related to the fight-or-flight response, eating, sleep, and sex
  - The hypothalamus and many other sites manufacture serotonin, which is a major neurotransmitter that is implicated in mood disorders; in response to stress, the hypothalamus releases corticotropin-releasing hormone, which stimulates the anterior pituitary to secrete adrenocorticotropic hormone; adrenocorticotropic hormone, in turn, triggers the release of cortisol from the adrenal cortex into the blood
  - The HPA axis is often hyperactive in clients with depression. Clients with moderate to severe depression may exhibit elevated serum cortisol levels
  - Functioning of the HPA axis is related to the 24-hour cycle of circadian rhythms that control physiologic processes
    - Clients with mood disorders have disrupted or irregular cyclic patterns
    - Blood cortisol is normally low during the night and peaks during the day, although constantly higher levels are often apparent in depression
    - Disrupted sleep-wake cycles are associated with mood disorders
    - Clients with mania report a perceived decreased need for sleep, whereas many clients with depression experience hypersomnia (excessive sleep)
    - During depression, clients experience decreased rapid eye movement latency and decreased shallow and slow delta wave sleep, thus fragmenting the sleep-wake cycle
    - Even seasonal patterns appear to have some relationship with mood disorders, with episodes of depression often occurring during periods of decreased light
- Genetic theories
  - Depressive and bipolar disorders tend to occur in certain families; studies of families, twins, adoption, and molecular genetics provide data regarding the heritability of these disorders
  - First-degree relatives of persons diagnosed with bipolar disorder and unipolar depression (depression without mania) have a greater risk for the development of one of these disorders; this risk is particularly high for relatives of persons diagnosed with bipolar disorder, which possibly indicates that genetics plays a greater role in bipolar disorder than in unipolar depression
  - Results of twin research provide additional evidence for the genetic transmission of bipolar and unipolar disorders, with monozygotic twin concordance higher than that of dizygotic twins; both twin types have a higher concordance than individuals in the general population
  - Adoption studies also demonstrate that genetic factors play some role in mood disorders; most studies focus specifically on bipolar disorder and reveal that the biologic parents of adult adoptees who are diagnosed with bipolar disorder have a much higher incidence of the disorder than parents of adoptees with no mood disorders
  - The search for the specific genetic basis of mood disorders continues, with special emphasis on genetic location and genetic processes
  - Genetic expression, the genetic transmission of these disorders, and how these interact with the environment hold the key to advances in understanding, diagnosing, and treating depressive and bipolar disorders
- Psychologic theories

- Psychoanalytic theory
  - The basic premise of psychoanalytic theory is that unconscious processes result in the expression of symptoms, including depression and mania; loss generates intense hostile feelings toward the lost object; the person then turns these feelings inward onto the self, creating guilt and loss of self-esteem; thus depression is linked with loss and aggression
  - Psychodynamically, mania is a defense against depression; clients deny feelings of anger, low self-esteem, and worthlessness and reverse their affect so that there is a triumphant feeling of self-confidence
  - Few data support the psychodynamic theories of depression and mania, but there is evidence that clients with depression have experienced more early childhood loss and trauma than persons without depression
  - The relevance of this theory is in its references to early childhood environment in which loss, disruption, or chaos triggers stress that, in turn, triggers physiologic mechanisms described previously
- Cognitive theory
  - Errors of logical thinking may be one causative factor of depression; this theory suggests that cognitive structures shaped by early life experiences are predisposed to the negative processing of information
  - Automatic thoughts are thoughts that a person responds to but usually does not recognize as a basis for behavior and thinking; they form the person's perception of a situation, and it is this perception—rather than the objective facts about the situation—that results in emotional and behavioral responses; if the perceptions are distorted, inferences and responses will be maladaptive; three types of thinking give rise to the development of depression:
    - Negative, self-deprecating views of the self
    - Pessimistic views of the world, which result in life experiences being interpreted in a negative way
    - The belief that negativity will continue into the future, which promotes a negative view of future events
  - These mindsets result in the misinterpretation of events and situations so that the client sees the self as worthless and views the world and the future as hopeless
  - Faulty cognitive processing leads to assumptions and continued errors of logic that result in depressive symptoms and an ongoing negative view of life
  - Learned helplessness theory is one altered cognition theory whereby uncontrollable stressful events that a person experiences result in a lack of motivation to act in response to the environment, demonstrated by the development of helplessness to the stressful event or aversive situation
  - Learned hopelessness theory is a revision of learned helplessness wherein the individual's inferred negative outcomes and negativity about the self are key elements of depression
- Life events and stress theory
  - Researchers have been interested in the quantity and nature of life events and in the size and perceived support from the client's social network as they relate to depression
  - The person's perception or appraisal of an event is as important as the change in daily life caused by the event
  - Early life stress, including child abuse and loss, influences the development of depression, most likely by disrupting the functioning of the HPA axis
  - Life events most likely influence the development and recurrence of depression through the psychologic and ultimately the biologic experiences of stress

- Researchers have examined the occurrence of stressful life events and depression with regard to gender differences; stressful life events triggered episodes of depression in women that were mediated by genetic risk factors
- There are less data regarding the relationship between stressful life events and bipolar disorder, although studies have suggested a role for disrupted social routines or circadian rhythms

General Nursing Care of Clients Diagnosed with Mood Disorders

- Monitor nutritional intake and elimination
- Keep environment nonchallenging with decreased stimuli; avoid boredom; focus on feelings
- Observe for mood swings, irritability, and depressive episodes
- Protect from suicide or violent acting out; keep under constant observation if necessary; keep communication open and direct; ask if client has a specific plan to commit suicide
- Keep activities simple, uncomplicated, and repetitive and of short duration requiring little concentration
- Base activities on client's status: Psychomotor retardation in depression and hyperactivity in mania; initiate one-to-one interactions with client and eventually expand to one or two other people
- Observe for adverse effects of drugs; monitor therapeutic blood levels if appropriate
- Encourage to continue medications even after symptoms abate
- Provide information regarding special dietary precautions when taking certain medications (eg, monoamine oxidase inhibitors [MAOIs])
- Assist with developing coping strategies; plan for follow-up support and supervision

Depression

- Major depressive disorder
  - Behavioral/clinical findings
    - Recurrent pessimistic thoughts; suicidal ideation with or without a plan (see Chapter 6)
    - Interruption in thinking and concentration that may interfere with occupational and social functioning; difficulty making decisions
    - Diminished interest or pleasure in all activities (anhedonia); apathy
    - Decreased appetite with weight loss or overeating with weight gain
    - Psychomotor retardation; anergia; constipation
    - Anxiety, somatic ailments, tearfulness, fearfulness, and hopelessness
    - Insomnia or hypersomnia
    - Feelings of worthlessness
    - Inappropriate guilt
  - Therapeutic interventions
    - See Depressive Episode of a Bipolar Disorder—Therapeutic interventions
    - Electroconvulsive therapy (ECT)
      - Brief electrical stimulus applied to brain, resulting in a seizure that alters brain chemistry and eventually alters mood
      - Used most often for recurrent depressions, delusions, suicidal ideation, and clients who are resistant to drug therapy
      - A depolarizing muscle relaxant causes paralysis (eg, succinylcholine [Anectine]), which reduces intensity of muscle contractions during tonic/clonic stage of seizure; given after a short-acting barbiturate or other sedative/anesthetic such as propofol; Brevitol is the most common barbiturate given

- Side effects: Fatigue, muscle soreness, mild temporary confusion, and short-term memory loss; headache is common; effects should resolve a few weeks after treatment ends
        - Can be used for depressive episodes of bipolar disorder
    - Nursing care of clients diagnosed with major depressive disorder
        - See General Nursing Care of Clients Diagnosed with Mood Disorders (previously) and Nursing Care of clients during a depressive episode of a bipolar disorder
        - Teach about ECT procedure
            - Informed consent required
            - Never left alone during and after the procedure; remain in recovery for 1 to 3 hours after procedure; criteria for return to unit includes stable vital signs, alert, oriented, able to ambulate without assistance, and ability to swallow and tolerate fluids
            - NPO and fluids for 6 to 8 hours before procedure; patient should void before procedure
            - Asleep at beginning of procedure; short-acting sedative administered
            - Oxygen administered before and after the procedure
            - Full-body muscle response is minimized by medication; muscle-paralyzing agent administered
            - Brief electrical stimulus (no more than 2 seconds) precipitates seizure that eventually causes an elevation in mood
            - May experience disorientation, headache, and muscle aches for about 1 hour after procedure; analgesic given to treat headache
            - May experience temporary memory loss during and for several weeks after completion of therapy
- Persistent depressive disorder (Dysthymia)
    - Description
        - Chronic, but less severe than major depressive disorder
    - Behavioral/clinical findings
        - Depressed mood for most of day
        - Two or more of these symptoms: Depressed appetite or overeating; insomnia or hypersomnia; low energy or fatigue; low self-esteem; concentration or problem-solving difficulties; feelings of hopelessness; anergia
        - Some impairment in social, occupational, and other roles (less than with major depressive disorder)
        - No evidence of manic or hypomanic episodes in present or past history
        - In children/adolescents, symptoms noted are irritability and depression, low self-esteem, poor social skills, pessimism, and impaired school performance and social interactions
        - Duration: At least 2 years in adults; irritable mood for at least 1 year in children and adolescents
    - Therapeutic interventions
        - Often unnecessary; if required, same as those listed under Depressive Episode of a Bipolar Disorder
        - Medications often unnecessary; if required, same as those listed under Depressive Episode of a Bipolar Disorder
    - Nursing care of clients diagnosed with persistent depressive disorder
        - See General Nursing Care of Clients Diagnosed with Mood Disorders (previously) and Nursing care of clients during a depressive episode of a bipolar disorder)

APPLICATION AND REVIEW

1. A client is admitted to the mental health unit because of a progressively increasing depression over the past month. What clinical finding does a nurse expect during the initial assessment of the client?
   1. Elated affect related to reaction formation
   2. Loose associations related to thought disorder
   3. Physical exhaustion resulting from decreased physical activity
   4. Diminished verbal expression caused by slowed thought processes

2. A nurse is planning care for a depressed client. Which approach is **most** therapeutic?
   1. Allowing the client time and placing few demands
   2. Helping the client focus on the family support system
   3. Encouraging the client to perform menial, repetitious tasks
   4. Telling the client repeatedly that the staff views the client as worthwhile

3. What is **most** appropriate for a nurse to say when interviewing a newly admitted depressed client whose thoughts focus on feelings of worthlessness and failure?
   1. "Tell me how you feel about yourself."
   2. "Tell me what has been bothering you."
   3. "Why do you feel so bad about yourself?"
   4. "What can we do to help you when you are here?"

4. A client whose depression is beginning to lift remains aloof from the other clients on the mental health unit. How can a nurse help the client to participate in an activity?
   1. Find solitary pursuits that the client can enjoy
   2. Speak to the client about the importance of entering into activities
   3. Ask the health care provider to speak to the client about participating
   4. Invite another client to take part in a joint activity with the nurse and the client

5. Which activity is **most** appropriate for a nurse to introduce to a depressed client during the early part of hospitalization?
   1. Board game
   2. Project involving drawing
   3. Small aerobic exercise group
   4. Card game with three other clients

6. A withdrawn client refuses to get out of bed and becomes upset when asked to do so. What nursing action is **most** therapeutic?
   1. Require the client to get out of bed
   2. Stay with the client until the client calms down
   3. Give the client the prn antipsychotic that is prescribed
   4. Leave the client alone in bed for as long as the client wishes

7. A depressed client is concerned about many fears that are upsetting and frightening and expresses a feeling of having committed the "unpardonable sin." Which of the following is the **most** therapeutic response?
   1. "Your family loves you very much."
   2. "You do understand that you really are not a bad person."
   3. "You know these feelings are in your imagination and are not true."
   4. "Your thoughts are part of your illness and will change as you improve."

8. A nurse has been assigned to work with a depressed client on a one-to-one basis. The next morning the client refuses to get out of bed, stating, "I'm too sick to be helped, and I don't want to be bothered." What is the nurse's **best** response?
   1. "You will not feel better unless you make the effort to get up and get dressed."
   2. "I know you will feel better again if you could just make an attempt to help yourself."

3. "Everyone feels this way in the beginning as they confront their feelings. ; I'll sit down with you."
4. "I know you don't feel like getting up, but you may feel better if you do. I'd like to help you get started."

9. A frail, depressed client frequently paces the halls, becoming physically tired from the activity. What action should the nurse take to help reduce this activity?
   1. Have the client perform simple, repetitive tasks
   2. Ask the client's health care provider to prescribe a sedative
   3. Restrain the client in a chair, thus reducing the opportunity to pace
   4. Place the client in a single room, thus limiting pacing to a smaller area

10. A nurse sits with a depressed client twice a day, although there is little verbal communication. One afternoon, the client asks, "Do you think they'll ever let me out of here?" What is the nurse's **best** reply?
    1. "We should ask your doctor."
    2. "Everyone says you're doing fine."
    3. "Do you think you are ready to leave?"
    4. "How do you feel about leaving here?"

11. A nurse is working with a client diagnosed with a major depressive episode. What is a long-term goal for this client?
    1. Talk openly about the depressed feelings
    2. Identify and use new defense mechanisms
    3. Discuss the unconscious source of the anger
    4. Verbalize realistic perceptions of self and others

12. What is a therapeutic nursing action when caring for a depressed client?
    1. Playing a game of chess with the client
    2. Allowing the client to make personal decisions
    3. Sitting down next to the client at frequent intervals
    4. Providing the client with frequent periods of time for reflection

13. A client with a diagnosis of major depressive disorder refuses to participate in unit activities because of being "just too tired." What is the nurse's **best** approach?
    1. Plan one rest period during each activity
    2. Explain why the staff believes the activities are therapeutic
    3. Encourage the client to express negative feelings about the activities
    4. Accept the client's feelings about activities calmly, but set firm limits

14. A nurse is assigned to care for a depressed client on a day when the client seems more withdrawn and depressed than usual. Which nursing intervention is **most** appropriate?
    1. Remain visible to the client
    2. Involve the client in group activities
    3. Spend a few extra minutes with the client throughout the day
    4. Ask the client if it would help if you both sat together for a while

15. A nurse is discharging a client from the mental health unit who has been treated for major depressive disorder. Which statement is **most** therapeutic at this time?
    1. "I am going to miss you; we have become good friends."
    2. "I know you are really going to be all right when you go home."
    3. "Call the contact number you were given if you have an emergency."
    4. "This is my phone number; call me to let me know how you are doing."

16. An extremely depressed client signed the consent for ECT but continues to express anxiety about the procedure. What is **most** important for a nurse to emphasize when discussing ECT with the client?
    1. "The procedure may cause a headache."
    2. "The procedure will make you feel better."
    3. "You will not be left alone during the procedure."
    4. "You will have periods of amnesia after the procedure."
17. A nurse is assisting with the administration of ECT to a severely depressed client. What side effect of the therapy should the nurse anticipate?
    1. Loss of appetite
    2. Postural hypotension
    3. Complete temporary loss of memory
    4. Confusion immediately after the treatment
18. When a nurse sits next to a depressed client and begins to talk, the client states, "I'm stupid and useless. Talk with the other people who are more important." Which response is **most** therapeutic?
    1. "Everyone is important."
    2. "Do you feel that you are not important?"
    3. "Why do you feel you are not important?"
    4. "I want to talk with you because you are important to me."
19. A client is admitted to a mental health facility for depression. What action should a nurse take to help the client develop a positive self-regard?
    1. Set limits on the client's negative behaviors
    2. Involve the client in activities that promote success
    3. Demonstrate approval of the client's efforts at every opportunity
    4. Encourage the client to participate in activities with other clients

Bipolar Disorder

- Characterized by a cyclical disturbance of mood, encompassing emotional extremes: Episodes of mania, episodes of despair and lethargy, or a mixture of both (Fig. 11.1)
- Presence of one or more manic or hypomanic episodes with a history of depressive episodes; predominant mood is elevated or irritable, accompanied by one or more of these symptoms: hyperactivity, lack of judgment with no regard for consequences, pressured speech, flight of ideas, distractibility, inflated self-esteem, risky behavior, and hypersexuality
  - Hypomanic: Mood elation with higher than usual activity and social interaction, but not as expansive as full mania; a distinct period of elevated or irritable mood that is different from mania; duration of at least 4 days
  - Mania: Elevated, expansive, or irritable mood accompanied by hyperactivity, grandiosity, and loss of reality
- Divided into Bipolar I and Bipolar II descriptions (NIMH, 2016):
  - Bipolar I disorder—defined by manic episodes that last at least 7 days or by manic symptoms that are so severe that the person needs immediate hospital care; usually depressive episodes occur as well, typically lasting at least 2 weeks; episodes of depression with mixed features (having depression and manic symptoms at the same time) are also possible
  - Bipolar II disorder—defined by a pattern of depressive episodes and hypomanic episodes, but not the full-blown manic episodes described previously

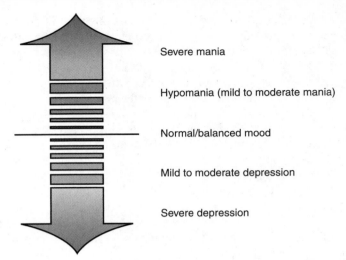

FIG. 11.1 Spectrum of symptoms in bipolar disorders. (Redrawn from National Institute of Mental Health [2008]. *Bipolar disorder.* Washington, DC: U.S. Department of Health and Human Services. In Varcarolis, E. M., & Halter, M. J. [2010]. *Psychiatric mental health nursing: A clinical approach* [6th ed.]. St. Louis, MO: Saunders.)

- Etiology: Neurobiologic perspective
  - Neurotransmitters, or certain chemicals in the brain that regulate mood, have been identified (eg, serotonin, dopamine, norepinephrine, and GABA)
    - Increased levels of norepinephrine, dopamine, and serotonin in acute mania
    - Decreased levels of norepinephrine, dopamine, and serotonin in depression
  - Research suggests this disorder results from complex interactions among chemicals, including neurotransmitters and hormones
  - Family and twin studies suggest a genetic component, but no gene has been identified except in rare, familial forms of the disorder
  - Biologic rhythms and physiology related to depression show abnormal sleep electroencephalogram (EEG), sensitivity to absence of sunlight, and circadian rhythm disturbance
- Etiology: Physiologic theory postulates that mood also may respond to drugs or a variety of physical disorders
  - Drugs associated with depressive status: Alcohol, sedative-hypnotics, amphetamine withdrawal, glucocorticoids, propranolol, risperidone, and steroid contraceptives
  - Drugs associated with manic status: Cocaine, MAOIs, tricyclic and all types of antidepressants, steroids, and levodopa
  - Physical illness, such as brain attack (cerebrovascular accident) and some endocrine disorders (eg, Cushing disease and hypothyroidism), can lead to depressive episodes; hyperthyroidism can cause manic symptoms
  - Obesity is a related factor to depression
- May be response to loss (dysfunctional grieving), increased stress, or change in life events, role, and sleeping and/or eating patterns; overreaction to stress may lead to suicide
- Generally the first onset is between 20 and 40 years of age; however, reported in clients older than 50 years and increasingly in children and adolescents
- Resumption of customary activities and mood between episodes

Depressive Episode of a Bipolar Disorder

- Behavioral/clinical findings
  - Either a depressed mood or loss of interest or pleasure, occurring during a 2-week period, with a change in level of functioning, plus five or more of these:
    - Change in weight
    - Insomnia (especially early morning awakening)
    - Psychomotor agitation or retardation
    - Fatigue
    - Worthless feelings or inappropriate guilt
    - Somatic complaints
    - Diminished hygiene
    - Concentration difficulties
    - Inability to make decisions
    - Social withdrawal
    - Pessimism
    - Suicidal behavior progresses from suicidal ideation, suicide threats, suicide gestures, suicide attempts, to successful suicides; presuicidal behaviors include no interest in the future, giving away personal possessions
  - Orientation and logic unaffected
  - Sex drive (libido) decreased
  - Constipation and urinary retention
  - Anniversary reaction: Depression and suicidal gestures may increase as anniversary of loss of loved object nears
- Therapeutic interventions
  - Antidepressant medications that increase the level of norepinephrine and serotonin (see Chapter 8)
  - Cognitive and behavioral psychotherapy
  - High-protein, high-carbohydrate diet depending on degree of weight loss; dietary supplements if necessary
  - Exercise is an evidence based treatment for mild to moderate depression
  - Transcranial magnetic stimulation is a possible option for clients whose depression resists conventional treatment
  - See Major depressive disorder—Therapeutic interventions for electroconvulsive therapy
- Nursing care of clients during a depressive episode of bipolar disorder

Assessment/Analysis

- Feelings of worthlessness, guilt; often fearful of feelings (Table 11.1)
- Suicidal ideation or acting out; presence of a plan increases the danger of suicide; may be ambivalent about suicide
- Depressed mood, loss of interest or pleasure, and slowing of psychomotor activity
- Weight for recent changes and to establish a baseline
- Changes in sleep patterns
- Changes in ability to concentrate

Planning/Implementation

- See General Nursing Care of Clients Diagnosed with Mood Disorders
- Accept inability to carry out daily routines; assist with ADLs

TABLE 11.1 Bipolar Disorder: Symptoms of Depression

Affect	Cognition	Physiology	Behavior
Apathy	Pessimism	Anorexia	Decreased ADLs
Anhedonia	Worry	Insomnia	Irritability
Anxiety	Poor concentration	Early morning awakening	Agitation
Anger	Slowed thinking	Fatigue	Psychomotor retardation
Guilt	Indecisiveness	Constipation	Social withdrawal
Helplessness	Hypochondriasis	Impotence	Crying
Loneliness	Suicidal ideation	Decreased libido	Self-abusive acts
Low self-esteem	Negative self-appraisal	Hypersomnia and compulsive eating initially in some clients; this changes to anorexia and insomnia as depression worsens	Substance use disorder
Sadness	Psychosis		
Emptiness			
Flat expression			

From Nugent, P. M., Green, J. S., Hellmer Saul, M. A., & Pelikan, P. K. (2012). *Mosby's comprehensive review of nursing for the NCLEX-RN examination* (20th ed.). St. Louis, MO: Mosby.

- Set expectations that can be achieved
- Provide realistic praise whenever possible
- Involve in simple repetitious tasks and activities
- Accept feelings of worthlessness as real; do not deny, condone, or approve feelings
- Spend time with client to demonstrate recognition of client's worth
- Protect from acting on suicidal thoughts, especially when depression begins to lift; suicide is a real and ever-present danger throughout entire illness
- Refer for grief counseling, assertiveness training, and anger management

Evaluation/Outcomes

- Remains free from injury
- Verbalizes feelings
- Verbalizes increased feelings of self-worth
- Continues prescribed treatment regimen
- Returns to preillness level of functioning

Manic Episode of a Bipolar Disorder

- Etiologic factors: See database under Bipolar Disorder
- Behavioral/clinical findings
  - Persistently elevated, expansive, or irritable mood for a duration of 1 week, plus three or more of these symptoms:
    - Grandiosity
    - Insomnia
    - Verbosity (pressured speech)
    - Flight of ideas
    - Hypersexuality
    - Distractibility
    - Social intrusiveness
    - Psychomotor agitation
    - Excessive involvement in pleasurable activities without regard for consequences (eg, shopping, gambling, sexual activity)

- Marked impairment in daily functioning, occupational and social activities, and relationships
- Excessive overactivity requiring hospitalization to prevent harm to self or others
- Symptoms are unrelated to physical illness or physiologic effects of a substance
- Therapeutic interventions
  - High-protein, high-carbohydrate diet; handheld foods should be available; adequate fluids
  - Behavioral and cognitive therapy when medication has decreased mania
  - Pharmacologic approach: Improves productivity by decreasing psychomotor activity or response to environmental stimuli; antimanic and mood stabilizing agents (eg, lithium, anticonvulsants [especially valproic acid]) (see Chapter 8)
- Nursing care of clients during a manic episode of a bipolar disorder

Assessment/Analysis (Table 11.2)

- Progression of manic behavior
- Extent of elevated mood
- Extent of psychomotor agitation
- Impairment in performing ADLs
- Feelings of grandiosity and euphoria
- Nutrition, hygiene, and rest patterns
- Danger to self or others
- Physiologic status

Planning/Implementation

- See General Nursing Care of Clients Diagnosed with Mood Disorders
- Accept client but reject objectionable behavior
- Permit expression of hostility and ambivalence without reinforcement of guilt feelings that usually are precipitated by anxiety
- Approach in a calm, collected manner and maintain self-control
- Set limits for intrusive, aggressive, and hyperactive behavior; channel excess energy into safe, nonstrenuous, noncompetitive activities
- Communicate in a nonargumentative manner

TABLE 11.2 Bipolar Disorder: Symptoms of Mania

Affect	Cognition	Physiology	Behavior
Extroverted	Poor insight	Weight loss or gain if patients eat compulsively	Pressured speech
Irritable/brittle	Impulsive		Increased libido
Overly optimistic	Poor judgment	Dehydration	Spending sprees
Euphoric/high	No introspection	Poor nutrition	Restlessness
Labile	Poor concentration	Lack of sleep	Wastes energy
Lack of shame or guilt	Flight of ideas	Does not feel tired	Legal troubles
Overly humorous	Loose association		Aggressive
Low intimacy	Poor reality testing		Irresponsible
	Distractibility		Inappropriate attire
	Grandiose and persecutory delusions		Socially intrusive
	Weak ego boundaries		

Modified from Nugent, P. M., Green, J. S., Hellmer Saul, M. A., & Pelikan, P. K. (2012). *Mosby's comprehensive review of nursing for the NCLEX-RN examination* (20th ed.). St. Louis, MO: Mosby.

- Use client's easy distractibility to interrupt hyperactive behavior, which may avoid injury and exhaustion
- Advise caregivers to approach client in a consistent manner
- Limit physical exhaustion and maintain physical health; provide foods that can be eaten on the run
- Maintain environmental safety for client, other clients, and staff
- Maintain client's contact with reality by helping with grooming and dressing
- Monitor medications and side effects
- Educate family as to early symptoms of relapse
- Evaluation/outcomes
- Exhibits a decrease in manic behavior
- Verbalizes feelings of increased self-worth
- Maintains adequate nutrition
- Adheres to medication regimen
- Demonstrates an absence of destructive behaviors

Cyclothymic Disorder

- Description
  - Numerous hypomanic episodes dispersed with periods of depressed mood and lack of interest in pleasurable activities
  - No evidence of obvious manic or major depressive episodes
  - Mood disturbance not caused by physiologic effects of substances or a physical illness
  - Symptom-free intervals usually are shorter than 2 months' duration
  - Duration: At least 2 years in adults with symptoms at least half of that time and not disappeared for longer than 2 months
- Behavioral/clinical findings
  - Alternating mood swings between elation and sadness; apparently unrelated to external environment
  - Individual is regarded as temperamental, moody, unpredictable, inconsistent, or unreliable
  - Mood swings do not have obvious emotional intensity
  - See Bipolar Disorder for hypomanic symptoms
- Therapeutic interventions
  - Often unnecessary; if required, same as those listed under Depressive Episode of a Bipolar Disorder or Manic Episode of a Bipolar Disorder
  - Talk therapy helps ease stress for many people
  - Medication often unnecessary; if required, same as those listed under Depressive Episode of a Bipolar Disorder or Manic Episode of a Bipolar Disorder
- Nursing care of clients diagnosed with a cyclothymic disorder
  - See General Nursing Care of Clients Diagnosed with Mood Disorders, Nursing care of clients during a depressive episode of a bipolar disorder, and Nursing care of clients during a manic episode of a bipolar disorder

Prognosis

- Mood disorders are usually lifetime illnesses
- The bipolar disorders historically have been perceived as recurrent, with cycles of mania and depression interspersed with periods of euthymia or normal mood
  - The pattern of cycles varies from person to person, with episodes of depression, mania, and euthymia (neither depressed nor manic mood) varying widely in duration; some individuals experience rapid shifts in mood, which is known as *rapid cycling;* it is often more difficult

to treat individuals who exhibit this pattern; the bipolar disorders have a high rate of recurrence and relapse; many recurrences are controllable with proper treatment and monitoring

- The depression cycle of bipolar disorder may be very difficult to treat, with more sadness, insomnia, cognitive difficulties, and somatic complaints with bipolar disorder than in major depressive disorder

- Major depressive disorder is a serious and recurrent disorder for the majority of clients; nearly two-thirds of people who experience major depressive disorder have at least one recurrence within 10 years
  - Negative long-term effects impair self-care, productivity, social functioning, occupational functioning, and physical health
  - Less than one-third of people who experience depression seek help, putting them at risk for future and more severe depression
  - Education, lifetime monitoring, adherence to treatment, and maintenance treatment for many persons diagnosed with mood disorders can promote health and reduce the risk of recurrence

- Persistent depressive disorder (formerly dysthymia), often continues for years before individuals seek assistance for their symptoms; many people are unaware that the chronic, low-level depression that is draining their energy is a form of depression that is treatable

- With proper treatment, the prognosis for maintaining individual functioning with a mood disorder is favorable

- Failure to seek help, lack of education about the disorder, incorrect diagnosis and inappropriate treatment, not adhering to a treatment plan, and resistance of symptoms to usual interventions result in long-term impaired daily functioning for these clients

ADJUSTMENT DISORDERS

Description

- Life stressors sometimes can lead to adjustment disorders, which are different from major depressive disorder; the main distinction between an adjustment disorder and major depressive disorder is that a specific psychosocial stressor can be identified for adjustment disorder
- Characterized by a short-term disturbance in mood or behavior with nonpsychotic manifestations resulting from identifiable stressors
- Severity of the reaction is not severe enough for a diagnosis of posttraumatic stress disorder (PTSD)
- Problematic response to life events, either developmental or situational
- Interaction of personality, crisis, developmental factors, and cultural influences
- No apparent underlying mental disorder, but there may be low self-esteem and present behavior may be extremely disturbed
- Exhibits capacity to adapt to overwhelming stress when given the time to do so
- Problems with distortions or interruptions in thinking processes and decision-making tend to resolve themselves

Predisposing Factors

- Adjustment disorders or adjustment reactions can occur in response to any type of stressor, including but not limited to loss, personal tragedy, change in lifestyle, maturational crisis, or even success or gain
- Acute symptoms develop within 3 months of a stressor

- Chronic symptoms last more than 6 months after the occurrence of the stressor
- During this time, individuals have difficulty functioning in their roles or interpersonal relationships, and they demonstrate great distress

Epidemiology/Theories

- An adjustment disorder can occur in anyone, regardless of age, gender, or socioeconomic status, when a single stressor or multiple stressors overwhelm a person's coping skills
- There is often no preexisting mental disorder, and the symptoms of adjustment disorder are time limited
- The stress response is highly individualized, and what one person experiences as highly stressful is sometimes perceived as an irritant or a challenge to another person

Behavioral/Clinical Findings

- Any stressor, even life stage stressors, can trigger an adjustment disorder
- Anxiety can be related to low self-esteem
- Onset begins within 3 months of stressors
- Significant impairment in social and occupational functioning
- Duration of disorder lasts no longer than 6 months after stress ceases
- Onset may occur at any age
- Symptoms usually decrease after the stressor is removed.
- In some cases, symptoms disappear outside of the setting that is linked with the stressor, especially when the stressor is specific to a location (eg, the work setting).

Therapeutic Interventions

- Goals:
  - Recognize connection between stressor and response
  - Adapt to feelings and new situation
- See Chapter 12, therapeutic interventions for Anxiety, for more information

NURSING CARE OF CLIENTS DIAGNOSED WITH ADJUSTMENT DISORDERS

Assessment/Analysis

- Individual's perception of problem
- Factors impinging on current situation
- Individual's personal strengths and support systems
- Level of anxiety
- Identification of type(s) of stressors and onset

Planning/Implementation

- Help client and/or parents recognize and accept that a problem exists
- Maintain client safety
- Encourage identification and use of support systems
- Attempt to minimize environmental pressures
- Allow the client time to recover personal resources

Evaluation/Outcomes

- Reorganizes defenses
- Utilizes support systems

- Verbalizes a decrease in anxiety
- Develops more effective coping

APPLICATION AND REVIEW

20. A client is diagnosed with an adjustment disorder with mixed anxiety and depression. What should the nurse anticipate as the client's primary problem?
    1. Low self-esteem
    2. Deficient memory
    3. Intolerance to activity
    4. Disturbed personal identity

21. A client exhibiting manic behavior is admitted to the psychiatric hospital. In which room should the nurse manager place the client?
    1. One that has basic simple furnishings
    2. One with another client who is very quiet
    3. A room that will provide a variety of stimuli
    4. A room with another client exhibiting similar behavior

22. During the orientation tour for three new staff members, a young, hyperactive manic client greets them by saying, "Welcome to the funny farm. I'm Jo-Jo, the head yoyo." Which meaning can the nurse assign to the client's statement?
    1. Trying to fill the happiest-person-in-the-room role
    2. Looking for attention from family
    3. Unable to distinguish fantasy from reality
    4. Anxious over the arrival of new staff members

23. What is the **best** nursing intervention when the language of a client in the manic phase of a bipolar disorder becomes vulgar and profane?
    1. State, "We do not like that kind of talk around here"
    2. Ignore it because the client is using it to gain attention
    3. Recognize that the behavior is part of the illness, but set limits on it
    4. State, "We will talk to you when you can speak in an acceptable way"

24. A client diagnosed with bipolar disorder, manic episode, has a superior, authoritative manner and constantly instructs other clients about how to dress, what to eat, and where to sit. The nurse should intervene because these behaviors eventually will cause the other clients to feel:
    1. angry.
    2. dependent.
    3. inadequate.
    4. ambivalent.

25. A client with the diagnosis of bipolar disorder, manic episode, is extremely active, talks constantly, and tends to badger the other clients, some of whom are now becoming agitated. What is the **best** strategy for a nurse to use with this client?
    1. Humor
    2. Sympathy
    3. Distraction
    4. Confrontation

26. A nurse is caring for a hyperactive, manic client who exhibits flight of ideas and is not eating. What may be the reason why the client is not eating?
    1. Feels undeserving of the food
    2. Is too busy to take the time to eat
    3. Wishes to avoid others in the dining room
    4. Believes that there is no need for food at this time

27. What is essential for the nurse to do when approaching a client during a period of over-activity?
    1. Use a firm but caring and consistent approach
    2. Anticipate and physically control the hyperactivity

   3. Allow the client to choose the activities in which to participate
   4. Let the client know the staff will not tolerate destructive behavior
28. What should the nurse include when developing a plan of care for a client in the manic phase of bipolar disorder?
   1. Focus the client's interest in reality
   2. Encourage the client to talk as much as needed
   3. Redirect the client's excess energy to constructive channels
   4. Persuade the client to complete any task that has been started
29. The nurse assesses a client with the diagnosis of bipolar disorder, manic episode. Which clinical findings support this diagnosis? **Select all that apply.**
   1. Passivity
   2. Dysphoria
   3. Anhedonia
   4. Grandiosity
   5. Talkativeness
   6. Distractibility

ANSWER KEY: REVIEW QUESTIONS

1. **4 As depression increases, thought processes become slower and verbal expression decreases.**
   1 The affect of the depressed person usually is one of sadness, or it may be blank. **2** Loose associations are characteristic of clients diagnosed with schizophrenia, not depressed clients. **3** Decreased physical activity will not produce physical exhaustion.
   Client Need: Psychosocial Integrity; **Cognitive Level:** Application; **Nursing Process:** Assessment/Analysis

2. **1 Routines should be kept simple, and no demands should be made that the client cannot meet. The client is depressed, and all reactions will be slow. Putting pressure on the client will increase anxiety and feelings of worthlessness.**
   2 The client will have to focus on personal strengths, not on family strengths. **3** Encouraging the client to perform menial, repetitious tasks feeds into the client's feelings of unworthiness and frustration. **4** Feelings of worth must come from within the individual; the nurse must reassure the client through actions, not words.
   Client Need: Psychosocial Integrity; **Cognitive Level:** Application; **Nursing Process:** Planning/Implementation

3. **1 Because major depressive disorder is due to the client's feelings of self-rejection, it is important for the nurse to have the client initially identify these feelings before a plan of care can be developed. Later discussion should be on other topics to prevent reinforcement of negative thoughts and feelings.**
   2 Asking the client to explain what is bothering him/her is asking the client to draw a conclusion; the client may be unable to do so at this time. Also, a depression may not be related to external events but to a client's psychobiology. **3** Asking "why" does not let a client explore feelings; it usually elicits an "I don't know" response. **4** Having the client determine how the staff can help is beyond the scope of the client's abilities at this time.
   Client Need: Psychosocial Integrity; **Cognitive Level:** Analysis; **Integrated** Process: Caring; Communication/Documentation; **Nursing Process:** Planning/Implementation

4. **4 Bringing another client into a set situation is the most therapeutic, least-threatening approach.**
   1 At this point in time it is not therapeutic to allow the client to follow solitary pursuits; it will promote isolation. **2** Explanations will not necessarily change behavior. **3** Asking the provider to speak to the client transfers the nurse's responsibility to the health care provider.
   Client Need: Psychosocial Integrity; **Cognitive Level:** Application; **Nursing Process:** Planning/Implementation

5. **2 An art-type project that may be worked on successfully at one's own pace is appropriate for a depressed client.**
   1 A board game requires too much concentration and may increase the client's feelings of despair. **3** This client is probably experiencing psychomotor retardation, and this activity would not be appropriate

at this time. **4** A card game with three other clients requires too much concentration and may increase the client's feelings of despair.

Client Need: Psychosocial Integrity; **Cognitive Level:** Application; **Nursing Process:** Planning/Implementation

6. **2 Staying with the client provides support and security without rejecting the client or placing value judgments on the behavior.**

1 Eventually, limits will have to be set in giving care, but staying with the client and showing acceptance are immediate nursing actions. **3** Although giving the client the prn antipsychotic will calm the client, it does not address the problem. **4** Leaving the client alone ignores the problem; isolation implies punishment.

Client Need: Psychosocial Integrity; **Cognitive Level:** Application; **Integrated Process:** Caring; **Nursing Process:** Planning/Implementation

 Memory Aid: _**PR**_esence _**PR**_ovides support in de_**PR**_ession.

7. **4 The statement "Your thoughts are part of your illness and will change as you improve" points out reality while accepting that the client believes the feelings and thoughts are real.**

1 Saying that the client's family loves him/her is false reassurance; there are no data about the client's family. **2** The client does not know that he or she is not a bad person and believes the opposite to be true. **3** Stating that the feelings are imaginary and not true is reality, but it is not a supportive response.

Client Need: Psychosocial Integrity; **Cognitive Level:** Application; **Integrated Process:** Caring; Communication/Documentation; **Nursing Process:** Planning/Implementation

8. **4 The statement, "I know you don't feel like getting up, but you may feel better if you do. Let me help you get started" acknowledges the client's feelings, offers hope, and assists the client to a higher level of functioning.**

1 Saying "You will not feel better unless you make the effort to get up and get dressed" ignores the client's feelings and may not be true. **2** The statement "I know you will feel better again if you could just make an attempt to help yourself." denies the client's feelings, and feeling better cannot be guaranteed. **3** Saying "Everyone feels this way in the beginning as they confront their feelings. I'll sit down with you." minimizes the client's feelings, and the client is not interested in how others feel.

Client Need: Psychosocial Integrity; **Cognitive Level:** Application; **Integrated Process:** Caring; Communication/Documentation; **Nursing Process:** Planning/Implementation

9. **1 These clients usually can be distracted by planned involvement in repetitious, simple tasks.**

2 Asking the health care provider to prescribe a sedative should be employed only if the client's restlessness cannot be controlled with other measures, and the physical exhaustion creates a danger. **3** Restraining the client is abusive treatment for a client with a need to pace and reinforces the client's belief that punishment is required for redemption. **4** The client may perceive isolation as a punishment, and it will prevent the staff from observing the client.

Client Need: Psychosocial Integrity; **Cognitive Level:** Application; **Nursing Process:** Planning/Implementation

10. **4 The nurse's response urges the client to reflect on feelings and encourages communication.**

1 Saying "We should ask your doctor" is shifting responsibility from the nurse to the health care provider; it is an evasive response. **2** Stating "Everyone says you're doing fine" is not what the client is asking the nurse; it closes the door to further communication. **3** Asking the client "Do you think you are ready to leave?" can elicit a "yes" or "no" answer; it does not encourage communication.

Client Need: Psychosocial Integrity; **Cognitive Level:** Analysis; **Integrated Process:** Communication/Documentation; **Nursing Process:** Planning/Implementation

11. **4 A major part of depression involves an inability to accept the self as it is, which leads to making demands on others to meet unrealistic needs.**

1 A short-term goal is to talk about the client's depressed feelings; a long-term goal is to look at what is causing those feelings. **2** Developing new defense mechanisms is not the priority because they tend to help the client avoid reality. **3** Discussing an unconscious source of anger is not important or crucial to the client's recovery.

Client Need: Psychosocial Integrity; **Cognitive Level:** Analysis; **Nursing Process:** Planning/Implementation

12. **3 Sitting next to the client frequently gives the client the nonverbal message that someone cares and views the client as being worthy of attention and concern.**

1 The concentration required for chess is too much for the client at this time. **2** The client is incapable of making decisions at this time. **4** Depressed clients often have too much thinking time.

Client Need: Psychosocial Integrity; **Cognitive Level:** Application; **Integrated Process:** Caring; **Nursing Process:** Planning/Implementation

13. **4 Fatigue and apathy are symptoms of depression and should be accepted; however, limits should be set to facilitate participation in unit activities.**

1 Planning a rest period during each activity allows the client to manipulate the environment. **2** Explaining why the activities are therapeutic will not change the client's mind about the activities. That response does not show an understanding of the client's needs. **3** Encouraging expression of negative feelings will reinforce negative feelings about participating in the activities.

Client Need: Psychosocial Integrity; **Cognitive Level:** Application; **Integrated Process:** Caring; **Nursing Process:** Planning/Implementation

14. **3 Spending extra time with the client demonstrates that the client is worthy of the nurse's time and that the nurse cares.**

1 Remaining visible to the client does not show the acceptance and care that sitting with the client would. **2** The client may be unable, at this time, to expend energy on anything outside the self. **4** It is unlikely that the client will respond to the nurse because the client feels unworthy and depressed, or the client may just say no.

Client Need: Psychosocial Integrity; **Cognitive Level:** Application; **Integrated Process:** Caring; **Nursing Process:** Planning/Implementation

15. **3 The statement "Call the contact number you were given if you have an emergency" demonstrates an understanding that the newly discharged client needs to have a support system when discharged. Clients need to feel that in a crisis there will be someone there for them.**

1 The role of the nurse was not to become a good friend but to aid the client in becoming a functioning being again. **2** The statement "I know you are really going to be all right when you go home" provides false reassurance; the nurse does not know this. **4** Saying "This is my phone number; call me to let me know how you are doing" is unprofessional and blurs the roles of nurse and client.

Client Need: Management of Care; **Cognitive Level:** Application; **Integrated Process:** Caring; Communication/Documentation; **Nursing Process:** Planning/Implementation

16. **3 The staff's presence provides continued emotional support and helps relieve anxiety.**

1 Although the client should be aware that ECT may cause a headache, it is not the priority information that should be discussed with the client. Also, a mild analgesic will be prescribed if a headache occurs. **2** The treatments may not make the client feel better; to say so is false reassurance. **4** Not all clients experience amnesia, and the amnesia is temporary; placing emphasis on amnesia will increase fear.

Client Need: Reduction of Risk Potential; **Cognitive Level:** Application; **Integrated Process:** Caring; Communication/Documentation; **Nursing Process:** Planning/Implementation

17. **4 The electrical energy passing through the cerebral cortex during electroconvulsive therapy (ECT) results in a temporary state of confusion after treatment.**

1 Loss of appetite is not a usual or expected side effect. **2** Postural hypotension is not a usual or expected side effect. **3** Complete temporary loss of memory is not a usual or expected side effect.

Client Need: Psychosocial Integrity; **Cognitive Level:** Comprehension; **Nursing Process:** Evaluation/Outcomes

18. **4 The response of "I want to talk with you because you are important to me" expresses the nurse's positive thoughts about the client and lets the client know that the nurse is concerned.**

1 Stating that everyone is important demonstrates the nurse's positive thoughts about all people and does not focus on the client specifically. **2** Although asking the client whether he or she does not feel important may promote verbalization of feelings, it does not communicate the nurse's positive regard for the client, which might support a more positive self-esteem. **3** The client may not be aware of what caused feelings of insignificance and may not be able to answer this question.

Client Need: Psychosocial Integrity; **Cognitive Level:** Analysis; **Integrated Process:** Caring; Communication/Documentation; **Nursing Process:** Planning/Implementation

19. **2 Self-esteem and feelings of competence are increased when a person experiences success.**

1 Although setting limits on negative behaviors is a necessary intervention when a depressed client attempts to commit self-harm, it will not promote feelings of self-esteem. **3** Clients recognize unwarranted praise and often interpret these responses as a form of belittlement or pity. **4** Encouraging the client to participate in activities with other clients may or may not increase self-esteem; also, the client may not have the physical or emotional energy to interact with other clients.

Client Need: Psychosocial Integrity; **Cognitive Level:** Application; **Nursing Process:** Planning/Implementation

20. **1 When a client has an adjustment disorder, anxiety may be related to a disturbance in self-esteem, and depression may be related to impaired social interaction.**

2 Problems with memory are not specifically related to an adjustment disorder. **3** Activity intolerance, which is related to oxygenation problems, is not associated with adjustment disorders. **4** A client with an adjustment disorder does not experience a disturbance in personal identity.

Client need: Psychosocial Integrity; **Cognitive Level:** Application; **Nursing Process:** Assessment/Analysis

21. **1 Overactive individuals are stimulated by environmental factors. A responsibility of the nurse is to simplify their surroundings as much as possible.**

2 The quiet client may become the target of this client's overactivity. **3** During this phase the client needs a decrease in stimuli. **4** During this phase the client needs a decrease in stimuli; placing two overactive clients together may produce excessive stimuli.

Client Need: Management of Care; **Cognitive Level:** Application; **Nursing Process:** Planning/Implementation

22. **4 The client's behavior demonstrates increased anxiety. Because it was directed toward the new staff, it was probably precipitated by their arrival.**

1 The client is not filling the happiest-person-in-the-room role; the client is resorting to previous coping behavior in the face of extreme stress. **2** Looking for attention from family is possible, but the remark is more indicative of increased anxiety. **3** The client is aware of what is going on and who everyone is at this time.

Client Need: Psychosocial Integrity; **Cognitive Level:** Analysis; **Nursing Process:** Assessment/Analysis

23. **3 Recognizing the language as part of the illness makes it easier to tolerate, but limits must be set for the benefit of the staff and other clients. Setting limits also shows the client that the nurse cares enough to stop the behavior.**

1 The statement "We do not like that kind of talk around here" shows little understanding or tolerance of the illness. **2** Ignoring the behavior is a form of rejection; the client is not using the behavior for attention. **4** The statement "We will talk to you when you can speak in an acceptable way" demonstrates a rejection of the client and little understanding of the illness.

Client Need: Psychosocial Integrity; **Cognitive Level:** Application; **Integrated Process:** Caring; **Nursing Process:** Planning/Implementation

24. **1 A person with a condescending, superior attitude frequently evokes feelings of anger in others, which helps decrease their anxiety.**

2 It is unlikely that a condescending, superior attitude will produce feelings of dependency in others. **3** It is unlikely that a condescending, superior attitude will produce feelings of inadequacy in others. **4** It is unlikely that a condescending, superior attitude will produce feelings of ambivalence in others.

Client Need: Safety and Infection Control; **Cognitive Level:** Application; **Nursing Process:** Assessment/Analysis

25. **3 During periods of hyperactivity the client has a short attention span and can be distracted easily; distraction is a therapeutic intervention for all the clients.**

1 Humor may increase anxiety, activity, and aggressive behavior. **2** The nurse should be empathetic, not sympathetic. **4** Confrontation may increase anxiety, activity, and aggressive behavior.

Client Need: Psychosocial Integrity; **Cognitive Level:** Application; **Nursing Process:** Planning/Implementation

> 🔑 **Memory Aid:** Just like a child with attention-deficit/hyperactivity disorder, clients with hyperactivity in mania are easily distracted.

26. **2 Hyperactive clients frequently will not take the time to eat because they are overinvolved with everything in their environment.**
    1 Feeling undeserving of the food is indicative of a depressive episode. **3** The client is unable to sit long enough with the other clients to eat a meal; it is not conscious avoidance. **4** The client probably gives no thought to food because of overinvolvement with the activities in the environment.
    Client Need: Psychosocial Integrity; **Cognitive Level:** Comprehension; **Nursing Process:** Assessment/Analysis

27. **1 Using a firm but caring and consistent approach will help reduce the client's anxiety, thereby reducing hyperactivity.**
    2 It is not possible to physically control hyperactivity. **3** The client is not capable of choosing activities at this time. **4** The client may not be capable of controlling overactive behavior; setting verbal limits may not be effective.
    Client Need: Psychosocial Integrity; **Cognitive Level:** Comprehension; **Integrated** Process: Caring; **Nursing Process:** Planning/Implementation

28. **3 The hyperactive client usually is easily distracted, so the excess energy can be redirected into constructive channels.**
    1 There is nothing to indicate that the client is not in touch with reality. **2** The client will talk a great deal with no encouragement. **4** The client will not be able to focus long enough on one task to finish it.
    Client Need: Psychosocial Integrity; **Cognitive Level:** Application; **Nursing Process:** Planning/Implementation

29. **Answers: 4, 5, 6.**
    4 Grandiosity is manifested by extravagant, pompous, flamboyant beliefs about the self, which frequently occur during manic phases of bipolar disorder. **5** As mania increases, the client's rate of speech increases, and speech is delivered with urgency (pressured speech). **6** Clients experiencing a manic episode have difficulty blocking out incoming stimuli, which results in distractibility and responses to irrelevant stimuli.
    1 Passiveness is exhibited when clients turn anger inward and show little emotion. It frequently occurs during the depressive stage of bipolar disorder. **2** Dysphoria, a depressed, sad mood, is associated with the depressive stage of bipolar disorder. **3** Anhedonia, an inability to feel pleasure, is associated with the depressive stage of bipolar disorder.
    Client Need: Psychosocial Integrity; **Cognitive Level:** Comprehension; **Nursing Process:** Assessment/Analysis

Anxiety, Anxiety Disorders, and Obsessive-Compulsive Disorders

12

OVERVIEW

Anxiety

- Anxiety is a normal reaction to stress and can be beneficial in some situations
- Diffuse feeling of uneasiness, uncertainty, and helplessness that occurs as a result of a threat to an individual's self-concept, esteem, identity, or safety (Fig. 12.1)
- Usual response to a real or perceived threat
- Different from fear, which has a specific source or object that can be identified and described
- An emotion that is subjective in nature and without a specific object
- Related to one's culture because culture influences **one's** values
- Causes are uncertain, but research indicates a combination of physical, psychosocial, and environmental factors
- Activates the fight-or-flight response in the autonomic nervous system (see Chapter 5—Adaptation to Stress)

Levels of Anxiety

- Mild—alertness level: Automatic response of the central nervous system (CNS) that prepares the body for danger by regulating internal processes and concentrating all energies for internal activity; perceptual field is increased; may enhance learning
- Moderate—apprehension level: Response to anticipation of short-term threat that prepares the individual for efficient performance; perceptual field is narrowed because focus is on the immediate concern
- Severe—high anxiety level: Focus is on a specific detail, and behavior is aimed at relieving anxiety; needs direction by others to focus on another detail or area; marked reduction in the perceptual field limits cognitive abilities; physiologic symptoms associated with this level include tachycardia, diaphoresis, and chest pain
- Panic—extreme level: Involves disorganization of the personality and is associated with dread and terror; communication abilities and problem solving greatly impaired; loss of rational thought; has great difficulty obeying commands even with direction; perceptual field is distorted; prolonged period of panic may result in exhaustion of the stress response; may act aimlessly or become mute and immobilized ("freeze"); intervention is essential; safety is of utmost concern

Behavioral Defenses Against Anxiety (Table 12.1)

- Consciously directed, task-oriented behaviors that are deliberate attempts to problem-solve, resolve conflicts, and gratify; they tend to involve the individual's deliberate effort to maintain control, reduce tension, and limit anxiety; can be "acting out" behaviors including attack, withdrawal, and compromise behaviors
  - Attack behavior: An attempt to overcome obstacles to satisfy a need
  - Constructive behaviors reflect use of problem solving
  - Destructive behaviors usually are accompanied by feelings of anger and hostility and may violate rights, property, and well-being of others

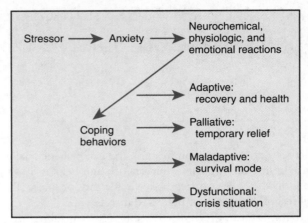

FIG. 12.1   Process of anxiety. (From Keltner, N. L., & Steele, D. [2015]. *Psychiatric nursing* [7th ed.]. St. Louis, MO: Mosby/Elsevier.)

TABLE 12.1   Coping Skills: Affective and Problem-Solving

Affective	Problem-Solving
Pray	Seek advice
Daydream	Obtain another's perspective
Eat, drink, and smoke	Learn new information/skill
Exercise	Set goals
Seek comfort from others	Ask for help
Meditate and do yoga	Do research
Withdraw	Delegate responsibilities
Bathe	Seek alternatives
Sleep	Brainstorm ideas
Make a joke	Draw on past experiences
Cry	Develop new resources
Watch television or go to a movie	Take action
Take a drive	Restructure priorities
Journal	
Breathe deeply	
Practice progressive muscle relaxation	

Modified from Nugent, P. M., Green, J. S., Hellmer Saul, M. A., & Pelikan, P. K. (2012). *Mosby's comprehensive review of nursing for the NCLEX-RN examination* (20th ed.). St. Louis, MO: Mosby.

- Withdrawal behavior: Can be expressed physically or psychologically
  - Physical withdrawal involves removing oneself from the source of threat
  - Psychologic withdrawal occurs when one admits defeat, becomes apathetic, or lowers aspirations; when this behavior isolates the person or interferes with work production, it causes additional problems
- Compromise is essential in situations that cannot be resolved through attack or withdrawal; it occurs by changing usual methods of operating, altering goals, or adjusting personal needs

- Compromise behaviors usually are constructive and are noted in approach-approach and avoidance-avoidance situations
- Compromise solutions can later offer opportunities for renegotiation or adapting different coping mechanisms
- Task-oriented reactions and effective problem solving are influenced by the expectation of some degree of success and drawing on one's past successes to deal with current stressful situations
- Problem-solving perseverance and the belief that one can endure the discomfort help one find the courage to cope with anxiety
- Task-oriented reactions are not always successful in coping with stressful situations; therefore ego-oriented reactions (defense mechanisms) are often used to protect the self

Defense Mechanisms

- Defense mechanisms are (mostly) unconscious cognitive responses that provide protection for the personality from overwhelming anxiety
- Defense mechanisms are most helpful in coping with mild and moderate levels of anxiety because they offer protection from feelings of inadequacy and worthlessness; when used, the individual may have a clear, slightly distorted, or more distorted perception of reality; if used to extreme, they may impede interpersonal relationships and limit productivity (Table 12.2)
- Identifiable patterns of response begin to form when individuals respond to most situations with the same type of behavior
  - Help an individual to cope with reality
  - Used when instincts are a threat to the self
- Can be adaptive or maladaptive
- Commonly used defense mechanisms
  - Compensation: The individual makes up for a perceived lack in one area by emphasizing capabilities in another
  - Identification: The individual internalizes characteristics of an idealized person
  - Rationalization: The individual makes acceptable excuses for behavior, feelings, outcomes; attempts to explain behavior by logical reasoning but does not address underlying feelings
  - Sublimation: The individual substitutes a socially acceptable behavior for an unacceptable instinct

TABLE 12.2 The Use of Defense Mechanisms in Relation to the Perception of Reality

Clear Perception of Reality	Slightly Distorted Perception of Reality	More Distorted Perception of Reality
Fantasy	Compensation	Denial
Identification	Conversion	Dissociation
Introjection	Displacement	Regression
Rationalization	Intellectualization	Repression
Sublimation	Projection	
Substitution	Reaction formation	
Suppression	Splitting	
	Undoing	

From Nugent, P. M., Green, J. S., Hellmer Saul, M. A., & Pelikan, P. K. (2012). *Mosby's comprehensive review of nursing for the NCLEX-RN examination* (20th ed.). St. Louis, MO: Mosby.

- Substitution: The individual replaces an unacceptable emotion or goal by another that is more acceptable
- Compensatory-type defense mechanisms
  - Adaptive when used in moderation; if used to excess, frequently they create greater emotional problems
  - As the use of these compensatory defenses increases and encompasses more of the individual's life, contact with reality is disrupted and distortions begin
  - These patterns of behavior are considered deviations and usually are viewed as signs of emotional stress and mental health problems
    - Conversion: Emotional conflict is unconsciously changed into a physical symptom that can be expressed openly and without anxiety
    - Denial: Emotional conflict is blocked from the conscious mind, and the individual cannot recognize its existence
    - Displacement: Emotions related to an emotionally charged situation or object are shifted to a relatively safe substitute situation or object
    - Dissociation: Separation of any group of mental or behavioral processes from the rest of the individual's consciousness or identity
    - Fantasy: Conscious distortion of unconscious wishes and needs to obtain gratification and satisfaction
    - Intellectualization: Use of thinking, ideas, or intellect to avoid emotions
    - Introjection: Acceptance of another's opinions and values as one's own
    - Projection: Unconscious denial of unacceptable feelings and emotions in oneself while attributing them to others
    - Reaction formation: Unconscious prevention of unacceptable thoughts or behaviors from being expressed by exaggerating opposite thoughts or behaviors
    - Regression: Return to an earlier stage of behavior when stress is overwhelming at the present stage of development
    - Repression: Involuntary exclusion from consciousness of those ideas, feelings, and situations that are creating conflict and causing discomfort
    - Splitting: Viewing others or situations as either all good or all bad; failure to integrate the positive and negative qualities in oneself
    - Suppression: Voluntary exclusion from consciousness of those ideas, feelings, and situations that are creating conflict and causing discomfort
    - Undoing: Act or communication that attempts to compensate for or negate a previous one

Epidemiology

- More than 18% of the U.S. adult population experiences an anxiety disorder within any 12 months
- Anxiety disorders occur more frequently in women and in non-Hispanic whites
- Anxiety disorders are often cooccurring with other emotional illnesses such as affective disorders, substance use disorders, and other anxiety disorders
- About 3% of the adult population has generalized anxiety disorder, with approximately a third of the cases being severe; average age of onset is 31 years
- Less than 1% of the adult population has agoraphobia; 40% of cases are severe, and the average age of onset is 20 years; agoraphobia is associated with a clinical diagnosis or history of panic disorder
- About 1% of the adult population has obsessive-compulsive disorder; half of the cases are severe, and the average age of onset is 19 years

- Of U.S. adults, 2% to 3% have panic disorder, with almost half the cases being severe; average age of onset is 24 years
- Specific simple phobias in U.S. adults affect 8% to 9% of the population, with 22% of cases being severe; specific phobias have an average age of onset of 7 years; most anxiety disorders begin during the bridge to adulthood, but specific phobias usually begin during childhood; lifetime prevalence for specific phobias in 13-year-olds to 18-year-olds is 15%

APPLICATION AND REVIEW

1. A nurse is planning to teach a client about self-care. What level of anxiety will **best** enhance the client's learning abilities?
   1. Mild
   2. Panic
   3. Severe
   4. Moderate
2. A client is scheduled for several diagnostic studies. Which behavior **best** indicates to the nurse that the client has received adequate preparation?
   1. Requests that the tests be reexplained
   2. Checks the appointment card repeatedly
   3. Arrives early and waits quietly to be called for the tests
   4. Paces up and down the hallway the morning of the tests
3. Before discharge of an anxious client, the nurse should teach the client and family that anxiety can be recognized as:
   1. a totally unique feeling.
   2. fears specifically related to the total environment.
   3. consciously motivated actions, thoughts, and wishes.
   4. a pattern of emotional and behavioral responses to stress.

See Answers on pages 213-217.

ANXIETY

Etiology

- Biologic model
  - Darwin identified certain emotions as being universally demonstrated through expression with the use of motor and postural changes
  - During the early 20th century, the endocrine system was linked with emotions, first by establishing the relationship of the adrenal medulla in the production of epinephrine, which results in the fight-or-flight response
  - Hans Selye expanded on the connection between the endocrine system and the central nervous system—particularly the hypothalamus and pituitary gland—and their reciprocal relationship (see Chapter 5—Adaptation to Stress)
  - The autonomic nervous system, particularly the sympathetic nervous system, is responsive to environmental stimuli, including emotional states
  - Imaging techniques, such as positron emission tomography and functional magnetic resonance, have augmented the understanding of the role of stress and brain functioning
  - Fear extinction is the individual's ability to note an environmental cue that may increase anxiety and then use a cognitive response to decrease the fear; individuals with normal brain circuits that contribute to fear extinction can respond to stimuli with the use of a problem-solving approach rather than a fight-or-flight or freeze response

- Genetic considerations are important when assessing individuals diagnosed with anxiety disorders; humans vary in whether they have one or two copies of a short variant of the human serotonin transporter gene as opposed to the long variant of this same gene; the transporter gene helps code protein in the neuronal area that recycles secreted serotonin from the synapse
- Psychodynamic model
  - In psychoanalytic terms, anxiety is a warning to the ego that it is in danger from either an internal or external threat
  - Anxiety is viewed as being involved in the development of personality and personality functioning
  - Symptoms develop in an attempt to defend against anxiety, including somatic symptoms, obsessions, compulsions, and phobias
- Behavioral model
  - In behavioral models that are based on learning theory, the etiology of anxiety symptoms is a generalization from an earlier traumatic experience to a benign setting or object; example: an awkward child's parents ridiculed him when he was bowling; as a result, he associates embarrassment and shame with sports events in indoor facilities and develops panic attacks during basketball games; the same kinds of cognitive operations that link embarrassment with sporting events link the cognition of the expectation of embarrassment with the idea of a sporting event, and the individual begins to experience panic attacks when reading the sports page
  - In this model, anxiety occurs when an individual encounters a signal that predicts a painful or feared event

Clinical Manifestations

- Clinical manifestations of anxiety include biologic, cognitive, behavioral, and affective patterns of behavior
- Review Table 12.3 to help you recognize the manifestations of anxiety on body systems as well as on thought patterns and behavior

Nursing Diagnosis

- Diagnoses are prioritized according to client's needs; diagnoses for clients with anxiety disorders are wide ranging

Outcome Identification

- Outcome criteria differ according to the characteristics of each client's nursing diagnoses and associated DSM-5 diagnoses
- Determining outcomes before implementing the plan will guide both nursing interventions and evaluation
- Nursing diagnoses are associated with outcomes/goals to serve as a guide; in practice, nurses generally determine outcomes by the client's presentation of clinical manifestations

ANXIETY DISORDERS

Generalized Anxiety Disorder

- Etiologic factors of generalized anxiety disorder (GAD)
  - Psychologic, behavioral, and neurobiologic theories are postulated; the latter is most promising

TABLE 12.3	Clinical Manifestations of Anxiety: Symptoms and Responses
Manifestation	**Sympton/Response**
Physiologic	
Cardiovascular system	Palpitations, racing heart, increased blood pressure, fainting, decreased blood pressure
Respiratory system	Rapid and shallow breathing, pressure in the chest, shortness of breath, gasping, lump in the throat
Gastrointestinal system	Loss of appetite or increased appetite, abdominal discomfort or feeling of fullness, nausea, heartburn, diarrhea
Neuromuscular system	Hyperreflexia, insomnia, tremors, pacing, clumsiness, restlessness, flushing, sweating, muscle tension
Genitourinary system	Decreased libido, increased frequency or urgency of urination
Cognitive	Decreased attention, inability to concentrate, forgetfulness, impaired judgment, thought blocking, fear of injury or death
Behavioral	Rapid speech, muscle tension, fine hand tremors, restlessness, pacing, hyperventilation
Affective	Irritability, impatience, nervousness, fear, uneasiness

From Fortinash, K. M., & Holoday, P. A. (2012). *Psychiatric mental health nursing* (5th ed.). St. Louis, MO: Mosby.

- Functions to permit some measure of social adjustment
- Commonly begins in early adulthood as a result of environmental factors and pressures of decision making
- Excessive anxiety and worry involves at least two life situations
- Unrelated to physiologic effects of substances or a medical condition
- Behavioral/clinical findings
  - Persistent anxiety (longer than 6 months) and excessive worry associated with three or more of these symptoms: Restlessness or feeling on edge; becomes easily fatigued; difficulty concentrating; irritability; muscle tension; and sleep disturbance
    - Inability to control the anxiety
    - Impairment in social or occupational relationships
  - Symptoms of autonomic hyperarousal (eg, tachycardia, tachypnea, dizziness, and dilated pupils); however, they are less prominent than in other anxiety disorders
- Therapeutic interventions
  - See General nursing care of clients diagnosed with anxiety disorders
  - Complete diagnostic workup to rule out physical illness
  - Psychotherapy, family therapy, group therapy, cognitive/behavioral therapies
  - Antidepressants (SSRIs and SNRIs) are used in treatment (see Chapter 8)
  - Antianxiety medications (or anxiolytics) are also used (benzodiazepines in the short term and an anxiolytic-like buspirone for longer term)
- General nursing care of clients diagnosed with anxiety disorders
  - Provide an environment that limits demands and permits attention to resolution of conflicts; establish a trusting relationship
  - Identify precipitating stressors and limit them if possible
  - Intervene to protect from acting out on impulses that may be harmful to self or others

- Accept symptoms as real to client; do not emphasize or call attention to them
- Attempt to limit client's use of negative defenses, but do not try to stop them until ready to give them up
- Help client realize when anxiety is developing and escalating
- Help develop appropriate ways of managing anxiety-producing situations through problem-solving and cognitive/behavioral therapies; assist to expand supportive network; assist significant others to understand the client's situation
- Plan a routine schedule of activities
- Manage aggressive behavior progressively using least-restrictive measures when possible (eg, diversion, limit setting, medication administration, seclusion, restraints)
- Collect and document information to assist with determining presence of both an anxiety disorder and depression (comorbidity)
- Encourage to develop a balance between work and relaxation
- Behavioral-based relaxations techniques for overall stress management

Panic Disorder
- Etiologic factors
  - Biochemical and genetic theories are most often cited as the underlying cause; no one gene or biochemical dysfunction has been identified
  - Onset varies, most often noted between late adolescence and mid-30s; infrequently may begin in childhood or after age 45
  - Discrete periods of intense discomfort for more than 1 month in duration
  - Recurrent attacks of severe anxiety may be associated with a stimulus or can occur spontaneously
- Behavioral/clinical findings
  - A panic attack of overwhelming, intense discomfort is the main characteristic of a panic disorder; note that "panic attacks" is not a DSM-5 diagnosis; they are symptoms of many anxiety-related disorders
  - The individual with the diagnosis of panic disorder exhibits sudden, unexpected symptoms of panic attacks such as fear, apprehension, and dread
  - Attack can be accompanied by four or more of these symptoms: palpitations or accelerated heart rate; sweating; trembling or shaking; shortness of breath; feelings of choking, chest pain, or discomfort; nausea or abdominal distress; depersonalization; fear of losing control; fear of dying; paresthesias; and chills or hot flashes
  - Catastrophic or "what if" thinking can trigger responses
  - Persistent fear of having another panic attack may lead the person to make changes to behavior
- Therapeutic interventions
  - Complete diagnostic workup to rule out physical illness
  - Psychotherapy, family therapy, group therapy, cognitive/behavioral therapies
  - Psychotropic medications (see Chapter 8)
    - Antidepressants (SSRIs and SNRIs) are most common for long-term treatment
    - Sedative/hypnotic and antianxiety agents are used short term when client is unable to cope or accomplish daily activities and until healthier coping emerges
- Nursing care of clients diagnosed with panic disorder
  - Assessment/analysis
    - Progression of somatic symptoms
    - Interference in activities of daily living (ADLs) and social and occupational functioning

- Situational triggers that may precipitate the onset of an attack
- Determination whether panic symptoms are related to a phobia (eg, agoraphobia)
  - Planning/implementation
    - See General nursing care of clients diagnosed with anxiety disorders
    - Remain with client during acute and panic levels of an episode; maintain safety
    - Remain calm and in control of the situation; anxiety can be contagious
    - Assign to a private room if hospitalized because it decreases environmental stimuli
    - Administer prescribed medications
    - As client recovers from panic level, exercise is helpful to decrease tension and anxiety
  - Evaluation/outcomes
    - Identifies situations that increase anxiety
    - Demonstrates increased use of anxiety-reducing behaviors
    - Follows prescribed treatment regimen
    - Reports a decreased number of panic attacks

Agoraphobia

- Description: Fear or anxiety triggered by situations in which client feels trapped, helpless or embarrassed , such as being alone or in public places in which help would not be immediately available if necessary (eg, tunnels, bridges, crowds, buses, trains), being in enclosed places, being in a crowd, leaving the home alone
- Behavioral/clinical findings
  - Anxiety and fear disproportionate to threat develops when exposed to a situation that threatens the sense of security
  - Active attempts to avoid the precipitating situation
  - Lifestyle is often greatly limited depending on the situation
  - Able to recognize that the fear is excessive or unreasonable but cannot control it
- Therapeutic interventions
  - Same as those listed under Panic Disorder
  - Behavior modification: A counterconditioning technique to overcome fears by gradually increasing exposure situation (systematic desensitization)
  - Pharmacologic and cognitive therapies
- Nursing care of clients diagnosed with agoraphobia
  - Assessment/analysis
    - Presence, type, and duration of situation producing anxiety
    - Interference in ADLs and social and occupational functioning
    - Avoidance behaviors to prevent exposure to stress-producing situation
    - Presence of behaviors associated with other anxiety disorders
  - Planning/implementation
    - See General nursing care of clients diagnosed with anxiety disorders
    - Identify and accept client's feelings about situation
    - Provide constant support if exposure to situation cannot be avoided
    - Assist with relaxation and cognitive/behavioral techniques to control or diminish anxiety levels
  - Evaluation/outcomes
    - Copes with anxiety-producing situation effectively
    - Continues prescribed treatment regimen
    - Uses relaxation techniques to diminish anxiety

Phobias

- Etiologic factors
  - Anxiety unconsciously transferred to an inanimate object or situation, which then symbolically represents the conflict and can be avoided
  - Anxiety is severe if the object, situation, or activity cannot be avoided
  - Multiple theories as to cause (eg, genetic, psychologic, developmental, and environmental); etiology is unverified
  - Onset begins in childhood; traumatic phobias can occur throughout the life span
- Behavioral/clinical findings
  - Anxiety develops when exposed to a situation that threatens the sense of security
    - A specific phobia is an exaggerated, all-consuming fear that is greater than what other people in similar circumstances would experience
    - The fear is almost always incited by a particular object or situation such as bugs, blood, animals, heights, or flying
    - The situation or object is the stimulus or cue for the person's panic attack
  - Active attempts to avoid the precipitating object/situation
  - For agoraphobia and social phobias, lifestyle is often greatly limited depending on the phobic object/situation
  - Able to recognize that the fear is excessive or unreasonable but cannot control it
- Types
  - Social phobia: Fear of doing something in public that could be embarrassing or cause negative evaluations (eg, speaking, dancing, eating)
  - Specific phobia: Fear of a particular object, animal, or situation
- Therapeutic interventions
  - Same as those listed under Panic Disorder
  - Behavior modification: A counterconditioning technique to overcome fears by gradually increasing exposure to feared object, situation, or animal (desensitization) or by continuous exposure to the feared stimulus until anxiety is extinguished (flooding)
  - Pharmacologic and cognitive therapies
- Nursing care of clients diagnosed with phobic disorders
  - Assessment/*a*nalysis
    - Presence, type, and duration of phobia
    - Interference in ADLs and social and occupational functioning
    - Avoidance behaviors to prevent exposure to phobic object or stress-producing situation
    - Pervasiveness of anxiety and fear
    - Presence of behaviors associated with other anxiety disorders
  - Planning/implementation
    - See General nursing care of clients diagnosed with anxiety disorders
    - Identify and accept client's feelings about phobic object or situation
    - Provide constant support if exposure to phobic object or situation cannot be avoided
    - Assist with relaxation and cognitive/behavioral techniques to control or diminish anxiety levels
  - Evaluation/outcomes
    - Copes with anxiety-producing object or situation effectively
    - Continues prescribed treatment regimen
    - Uses relaxation techniques to diminish anxiety

APPLICATION AND REVIEW

4. A client is diagnosed with generalized anxiety disorder. For what behavior should the nurse assess a client to determine the effectiveness of therapy?
   1. Participates in activities
   2. Learns how to avoid anxiety
   3. Takes medication as prescribed
   4. Identifies when anxiety is developing

5. A nurse is caring for a client diagnosed with a generalized anxiety disorder. Which factor should be assessed to determine the client's present status?
   1. Memory
   2. Behavior
   3. Judgment
   4. Responsiveness

6. A client arrives at the mental health clinic disheveled, agitated, and demanding that the nurse "do something to end this feeling." What clinical manifestation is evident?
   1. Feelings of panic
   2. Suicidal tendencies
   3. Narcissistic ideation
   4. Passive personality

7. A client's severe anxiety and panic are often considered to be "contagious." What action should be taken when a nurse's personal feelings of anxiety are increasing?
   1. Refocus the conversation on some pleasant topics
   2. Say to the client, "Calm down; you are making me anxious, too"
   3. Say, "Another staff member is coming in; I will leave and return later"
   4. Remain quiet so that personal feelings of anxiety do not become apparent to the client

8. A nurse is interviewing a client diagnosed with a phobia. Which treatment should the nurse inform the client has the highest success rate?
   1. Insight therapy to determine the origin of the fear
   2. Systematic desensitization using relaxation techniques
   3. Psychotherapy aimed at rearranging psychotic thought processes
   4. Psychoanalytic exploration of repressed conflicts of an earlier developmental phase

9. An adult reports anxiety, palpitations, and a feeling of impending doom. After a thorough physical examination, the health care provider diagnoses a panic attack. Lorazepam 1.5 mg po stat is prescribed. Lorazepam is available in 0.5 mg tablets. How many tablets should the nurse administer? **Record your answer using a whole number.**
   Answer: _____ tablets

10. A nurse speaks with a client who just experienced a panic attack. Which statement is **most** therapeutic when addressing the client's concerns?
    1. "I would have been upset, too."
    2. "You are concerned that this might happen again."
    3. "Episodes like this can be upsetting even though they do end."
    4. "Your family must have thought you were having a heart attack."

11. A client diagnosed with generalized anxiety disorder says to the nurse, "What can I do to prevent overreacting to stress?" What is the nurse's **best** response?
    1. "Hone your problem-solving skills."
    2. "Improve your time management skills."
    3. "Ignore situations that you cannot change."
    4. "Develop a wide variety of coping strategies."

12. What clinical findings may be expected when a nurse assesses an individual diagnosed with **an anxiety disorder? Select all that apply.**
    1. Worrying about a variety of issues
    2. Acting with grandiose behavior
    3. Regressing to an earlier level of adjustment
    4. Converting the anxiety into a physical symptom
    5. Displacing the anxiety onto a less threatening object
13. How should a nurse expect a client's anxiety to be manifested physiologically?
    1. Constricted pupils
    2. Narrowed bronchioles
    3. Decreased blood pressure
    4. Increased blood glucose level
14. What is an appropriate way a nurse can help a client to decrease anxiety?
    1. Avoid unpleasant events
    2. Prolong exposure to fearful situations
    3. Acquire skills with which to face stressful events
    4. Introduce an element of pleasure into fearful situations
15. A client comes to a mental health center with severe anxiety evidenced by crying, wringing the hands, and pacing. What should be the **first** nursing intervention?
    1. Stay physically close to the client
    2. Gently ask what is bothering the client
    3. Tell the client to try to relax by sitting quietly
    4. Involve the client in a nonthreatening activity

Obsessive-Compulsive Disorder

- Etiologic factors of obsessive-compulsive disorder (OCD)
  - Chronic anxiety disorder with decreased levels of serotonin
  - Control of anxiety with obsessions (intrusive recurring thoughts) or compulsions (repetitive ritualistic behaviors)
  - Symptoms worsen with stress
  - OCD symptoms are similar in adults and children; adults recognize behavior is excessive and interferes with daily activities but cannot be controlled; children do not have this insight
- Behavioral/clinical findings
  - Manifested by symptoms that cause the person to experience either obsessions (persistent recurrent thoughts), compulsions (behavior that relieves the obsessive thought), or both
    - Thoughts persist and become repetitive and obsessive, although people with OCD recognize that their obsessive thoughts are part of their own thinking and do not come from an outside force
    - Obsessions or compulsions consume most of client's waking hours (at minimum more than 1 hour per day) and interfere with ADLs, occupation, social activities, or relationships
  - Major defensive mechanisms are isolation, undoing, and reaction formation; intellectual and verbal defenses are used
  - Demonstrates indecisiveness and a striving for perfection and superiority

- Anxiety and depression present in various degrees, particularly if rituals are prevented
- Limiting or interrupting a ritual increases anxiety
- Therapeutic interventions
  - Diagnostic workup to rule out physical illness
  - Behavior modification to initially allow, then limit length and/or frequency of ritual
  - Cognitive therapy, psychotherapy, family therapy, group therapy
  - Psychotropic medications: SSRIs such as fluvoxamine; clomipramine to control symptoms (see Chapter 8)
- Nursing care of clients diagnosed with obsessive-compulsive disorder
  - Assessment/analysis
    - Type and use of ritual or obsession
    - Level of anxiety (eg, mild, moderate, severe, panic)
    - Level of interference in lifestyle
    - Extent of danger inherent in ritual or obsession
    - Presence of behaviors associated with other anxiety disorders
  - Planning/implementation
    - See General nursing care of clients diagnosed with anxiety disorders
    - Allow performance of the ritual initially unless ritual causes harm and must be stopped (eg, excessive hand washing causing skin damage); eventually attempt to limit length and frequency of the ritual
    - Support attempts to reduce dependency on the ritual
    - Role model appropriate behavior and discuss adaptive responses
    - Relaxation exercises and stress management training
  - Evaluation/outcomes
    - Decreases obsessive thoughts and length and frequency of ritual
    - Follows prescribed treatment regimen
    - Learns new adaptive coping responses

Body Dysmorphic Disorder

- Classified as an Obsessive-Compulsive Disorder in DSM-5
- Etiologic factors
  - Preoccupation (not of a delusional intensity but still intrusive) with a defect in appearance, either imagined or exaggerated, even if there is a slight defect
  - Onset usually during adolescence but can begin in childhood; may continue for years
- Behavioral/clinical findings
  - Excessive grooming, checking the mirror, possible skin picking
  - Possible history of multiple plastic surgeries to correct imagined defects
  - Preoccupation with imagined deficit causes avoidance or impairment in social and occupational relationships
  - Often exhibits symptoms of depression or obsessive-compulsive personality traits
- Therapeutic interventions
  - Same as those listed for OCD
  - Assess for suicidal ideation; high risk for suicide among these clients
- Nursing care of clients diagnosed with body dysmorphic disorders
  - Assessment/analysis
    - Preoccupation with imagined physical defects; ask if client worries about appearance, identify specific worry, and estimate time devoted to it
    - History of medical and surgical therapies to correct imagined defects

- Ability to manage stressful situations
- Level of anxiety
- Planning/implementation
  - See General nursing care of clients diagnosed with anxiety disorders
- Evaluation/outcomes
  - Uses problem solving rather than physical defect to manage anxiety-producing situations
  - Verbalizes that emphasis on physical defect is exaggerated
  - Accepts and is comfortable with self

ADDITIONAL INTERVENTIONS

Pharmacologic Interventions

- Pharmacologic interventions alone or in combination with cognitive behavioral interventions are among the most successful treatments for anxiety and related disorders
- Benzodiazepines have been used widely for the treatment of anxiety disorders; they are relatively safe and effective for short-term use to control the debilitating symptoms of anxiety; however, longer-term treatment with these drugs raises issues of tolerance, misuse, and addiction
- Selective serotonin reuptake inhibitors, antidepressants that are now widely used for the treatment of anxiety disorders, are particularly effective for the treatment of OCD and panic disorders; fluoxetine and fluvoxamine are for OCD; paroxetine is for GAD, OCD, panic disorder, and social phobia; sertraline is for OCD, panic disorder; venlafaxine is for GAD
- Anxiolytic buspirone

Psychotherapy

- Psychotherapeutic intervention takes place in group or individual settings
- Group therapy is the opportunity for the client to learn from the successes and failures of others with similar symptoms
- Behavioral and cognitive behavioral therapies have been widely effective for the treatment of a variety of anxiety disorders
  - Behavioral therapy, including systematic desensitization, is an effective treatment for panic disorder with agoraphobia; therapist and client define the phobic stimulus; the client progressively masters increasing levels of anxiety until s/he encounters the phobic stimulus
  - Cognitive behavioral therapy is used for the treatment of anxiety disorders; success centers on the client's understanding that the symptoms are a learned response to thoughts or feelings about behaviors in daily life; client and therapist identify target symptoms and examine circumstances associated with the symptoms; cognitive behavioral therapy is short-term and demands active participation of both client and therapist
- Additional treatment modalities and collaborative interventions include consultation with occupational therapists, vocational rehabilitation counselors, and psychologists, depending on the particular treatment needs of the client

Prognosis

- Prognosis depends on factors specific to the disorder, the client, and the clinician
- Clients who are treated for panic disorder generally demonstrate some symptoms during the course of their lives after their initial episodes; 6 to 10 years after treatment, 30% of clients are well, 40% to 50% are improved but still symptomatic, and 20% to 30% are the same or slightly worse

- Specific phobias that persist into adulthood are generally chronic; the course of social phobia is often continuous, with onset or reemergence after stressful or humiliating experiences
- The prognosis for OCD is similar to that of anxiety disorders, with increasing and decreasing symptoms related to stressors; however, 15% of clients demonstrate a chronically deteriorating course with the progressive compromise of social and occupational functioning
- Discharge Criteria—the client will:
  - Identify situations and events that trigger anxiety and select ways to prevent or manage them
  - Describe anxiety symptoms and levels of anxiety
  - Discuss the connection between anxiety-provoking situations or events and anxiety symptoms
  - Explain relief behaviors openly
  - Identify adaptive and positive techniques and strategies that relieve anxiety
  - Demonstrate behaviors that represent reduced anxiety symptoms
  - Use learned anxiety-reducing strategies
  - Demonstrate the ability to problem-solve, concentrate, and make decisions
  - Verbalize feeling relaxed
  - Sleep through the night
  - Use appropriate supports from the nursing and medical communities, family, and friends
  - Acknowledge the inevitability of the occurrence of anxiety
  - Discuss the ability to tolerate manageable levels of anxiety
  - Seek help from appropriate sources when anxiety is not manageable, including websites such as www.adaa.org (the website of Anxiety and Depression Association of America)
  - List the medication used to control the symptoms of anxiety as well as the sidef effects, appropriate dosage and scheduled times
  - Continue after care anxiety management, including medication and therapy

APPLICATION AND REVIEW

16. A client believes that doorknobs are contaminated and refuses to touch them, except with a paper tissue. What nursing intervention is **most** therapeutic for this client?
    1. Initially supply the client with paper tissues to help functioning until anxiety is reduced
    2. Have the client scrub the doorknobs with a strong antiseptic so that tissues are no longer needed
    3. Encourage the client to touch doorknobs by removing all available paper tissue until learning how to manage the situation
    4. Explain to the client that the idea about doorknobs being contaminated is part of the illness, so precautions are not necessary
17. A nurse is caring for a client diagnosed with an obsessive-compulsive disorder. What is the psychological or psychoanalytical understanding for the basis for the obsessions and compulsions?
    1. Unconscious control of unacceptable feelings
    2. Conscious use of this method to punish themselves
    3. Acceptance of voices that tell them the doorknobs are unclean
    4. Fulfillment of a need to punish others by carrying out an annoying procedure
18. A nurse is developing a care plan for a client diagnosed with obsessive-compulsive disorder. Which nursing intervention will **most** likely increase the client's anxiety?
    1. Helping the client understand the nature of the anxiety
    2. Limiting the client's ritualistic acts to three times a day

3. Involving the client in establishing the therapeutic plan

4. Providing the client with a nonjudgmental environment

19. Hospitalization or day-treatment centers are often indicated for the treatment of a client diagnosed with an obsessive-compulsive disorder because these settings:

1. prevent the client from completing rituals.

2. allow the staff to exert control over the client's activities.

3. resolve the client's anxiety because decision making is minimal.

4. provide the neutral environment the client needs to work through conflicts.

20. What should a nurse include in the initial plan of care for a client diagnosed with the long-standing, obsessive-compulsive behavior of hand washing?

1. Determine the purpose of the ritualistic behavior

2. Limit the time allowed for the ritualistic behavior

3. Suggest a symptom substitution technique to refocus the ritualistic behavior

4. Develop a routine schedule of activities to reduce the need for the ritualistic behavior

21. A client with a history of obsessive-compulsive behaviors has a marked decrease in symptoms and expresses a wish to obtain a part-time job. On the day of a job interview the client arrives at the mental health center displaying signs of anxiety. What is the nurse's **best** response to the client's behavior?

1. "I know you're anxious, but by forcing yourself to go to the interview, you may conquer your fear."

2. "If going to an interview makes you this anxious, it seems as though you're not ready to go back to work."

3. "It must be that you really don't want that job after all. ; I think you should reconsider going to the interview."

4. "Going for your interview triggered some feelings in you. Perhaps you could call a friend to drive you there."

22. What should a nurse consider when planning care for a client who is using ritualistic behavior?

1. Nurses must attempt to limit the ritualistic behavior

2. Clients need to realize that ritualistic behavior serves no purpose

3. Nurses should try to divert the ritual immediately after it is started

4. Clients do not want to repeat the ritual but feel compelled to do so

23. What is the **priority** discharge criterion for a client who is using ritualistic behaviors?

1. Verbalizes positive aspects about the self

2. Follows the rules of the therapeutic milieu

3. Intervenes to maintain increasing anxiety at a manageable level

4. Recognizes that hallucinations occur at times of extreme anxiety

24. A nurse is caring for a client who uses ritualistic behavior. What common antiobsessional medication does the nurse anticipate will be prescribed?

1. Benztropine

2. Amantadine

3. Fluvoxamine

4. Diphenhydramine

25. A client is using ritualistic behaviors. Why should a nurse allow the client ample time for the performance of the ritual?

1. Denial of this activity may precipitate higher levels of anxiety

2. Anger turned inward on the self should be allowed to be expressed

3. Successful performance of independent activities enhances self-esteem

4. Ample time provides an opportunity to point out the inappropriate behavior

26. A nurse is caring for a client diagnosed with an obsessive-compulsive disorder that involves rituals. What should the nurse conclude about the ritual?
    1. Is under voluntary control
    2. Is performed after long urging
    3. Appears to be performed willingly
    4. Seems illogical but is needed by the person
27. A nurse is preparing to care for a client who engages in ritualistic behavior. What should the plan of care include?
    1. Redirect energy into activities to help others
    2. Teach the client that the behavior is not serving a realistic purpose
    3. Administer antianxiety medications that block out the memory of internal fears
    4. Help the client to understand that the behavior is caused by maladaptive coping to increased anxiety
28. Which is the **best** nursing intervention during the working phase of the therapeutic relationship to meet the needs of individuals who demonstrate obsessive-compulsive behavior?
    1. Restricting their movements
    2. Calling attention to the behavior
    3. Keeping them busy to distract them
    4. Supporting rituals but setting realistic limits

See Answers on pages 213–217.

ANSWER KEY: REVIEW QUESTIONS

1. **1 Mild anxiety motivates one to action such as learning or making changes. Higher levels of anxiety tend to blur the individual's perceptions and interfere with functioning.**

   2 Attention is severely reduced by panic. **3** The perceptual field is greatly reduced with severe anxiety. **4** The perceptual field is narrowed with moderate anxiety.

   Client Need: Psychosocial Integrity; **Cognitive Level:** Comprehension; **Integrated Process:** Teaching/Learning; **Nursing Process:** Assessment/Analysis

2. **3 The client's early arrival indicates an expected degree of anxiety; the quiet waiting indicates that the client has been told what to expect.**

   1 Requesting that the tests be reexplained indicates an inadequate explanation or the inability of the client to remember the explanation that had been given. **2** Checking the appointment card repeatedly indicates a high degree of anxiety that may denote a fear of the tests because they were not adequately explained. **4** Pacing up and down the hallway the morning of the tests indicates a high degree of anxiety that may denote a fear of the tests because they were not adequately explained.

   Client Need: Psychosocial Integrity; **Cognitive Level:** Analysis; **Integrated Process:** Teaching/Learning; **Nursing Process:** Evaluation/Outcomes

3. **4 Anxiety is a human response, causing both physical and emotional changes that everyone experiences when faced with stressful situations.**

   1 Anxiety is experienced to a greater or lesser degree by every person. **2** The fear may be related to a specific aspect of, rather than the total, environment. **3** Anxiety does not operate from the conscious level.

   Client Need: Psychosocial Integrity; **Cognitive Level:** Comprehension; **Integrated Process:** Teaching/Learning; **Nursing Process:** Planning/Implementation

4. **4 Recognition of anxiety or symptoms of increasing anxiety is an indication that the client is improving.**

   1 Participating in activities does not indicate improvement or recognition of feelings; the client may be doing what others expect. **2** Avoidance of anxiety is not a good indication of improvement; there is no

guarantee that anxiety can always be avoided. **3** Taking medication as prescribed does not indicate improvement or recognition of feelings; the client may be doing what others expect.
Client Need: Psychosocial Integrity; **Cognitive Level:** Analysis; **Nursing Process:** Evaluation/Outcomes

> **Memory Aid:** Recognition is key because, like all problems, "You can't fix something if you don't. RECOGNIZE that it's broken!" Or phrased positively, once you recognize a problem, you are capable of fixing it.

5. **2 The client's current behavior is the best indicator of the client's current level of functioning; all behavior has meaning.**
   1 Memory is important and should be assessed, but it is not the best indicator of the client's current level of functioning. **3** Judgment is important and should be assessed, but it is not the best indicator of the client's current level of functioning. **4** Responsiveness is important and should be assessed, but it is not the best indicator of the client's current level of functioning.
   Client Need: Psychosocial Integrity; **Cognitive Level:** Application; **Nursing Process:** Assessment/Analysis

6. **1 The client can no longer control or tolerate overwhelming feelings and is seeking help.**
   2 The client has not indicated plans for self-harm. **3** The behavior is not typical of a narcissistic personality. **4** The behavior does not indicate a passive personality.
   Client Need: Psychosocial Integrity; **Cognitive Level:** Application; **Nursing Process:** Assessment/Analysis

7. **3 The nurse who is anxious should leave the situation after providing for continuity of care; the client will be aware of the nurse's anxiety, and the nurse's presence will be nonproductive and nontherapeutic.**
   1 Refocusing the conversation on some pleasant topics meets the nurse's need; that response may make the client feel guilty that something was said that upset the nurse. The client will be aware of the nurse's anxiety, which will increase the client's own anxiety. **2** Saying to the client, "Calm down; you are making me anxious, too" meets the nurse's need; however, that response may make the client feel guilty that something was said that upset the nurse. The client will be aware of the nurse's anxiety, which will increase the client's own anxiety. **4** The client will probably sense the nurse's anxiety through nonverbal channels, if not through verbal responses.
   Client Need: Psychosocial Integrity; **Cognitive Level:** Analysis; **Integrated Process:** Communication/Documentation; **Nursing Process:** Planning/Implementation

8. **2 The most successful therapy for clients diagnosed with phobias involves behavior modification techniques using desensitization.**
   1 Insight into the origin of the phobia usually is not successful in helping clients overcome phobias. **3** Psychotherapy aimed at rearranging psychotic thought processes may increase understanding of the phobia but may not help the client to cope with the fear; there is no psychotic thought process associated with phobias. **4** Psychoanalysis may increase understanding of the phobia but may not help the client cope successfully with the overwhelming fear.
   Client Need: Psychosocial Integrity; **Cognitive Level:** Comprehension; **Nursing Process:** Planning/Implementation

9. **Answer: 3 tablets. Use the "Desire over Have" formula of ratio and proportion to solve this problem.**

$$\frac{\text{Desire}}{\text{Have}} \frac{1.5\,\text{mg}}{0.5\,\text{mg}} = \frac{\text{x tablet}}{1\,\text{tablet}}$$

$$05\,\text{x} = 1.5\,\text{tabs}$$

$$\text{x} = 1.5 \div 0.5$$

$$\text{x} = 3\,\text{tablets}$$

Client Need: Pharmacologic and Parenteral Therapies; **Cognitive Level:** Application; **Nursing Process:** Planning/Implementation

10 **2 Recurrence of attacks is a common concern.**

1 Stating "I would have been upset, too" redirects the focus to the nurse, which is not therapeutic. **3** Although stating "Episodes like this can be upsetting even though they do end" initially focuses on feelings, it then cuts off communication. **4** The focus should be on the client not what the family believes.

Client Need: Psychosocial Integrity; **Cognitive Level:** Application; **Integrated Process:** Communication/Documentation; **Nursing Process:** Planning/Implementation

11. **4 Suggesting "Develop a wide variety of coping strategies" increases the individual's ability to cope with stress; different defenses can be used in various situations.**

1 The client already has identified the problem. **2** Suggesting the client improve time management skills may or may not be helpful. **3** People should not ignore situations that affect them.

Client Need: Psychosocial Integrity; **Cognitive Level:** Application; **Integrated Process:** Communication/Documentation; **Nursing Process:** Planning/Implementation

12. **Answers: 1, 3, 4, 5.**

1 Excessive anxiety and worry about a number of events, topics, or activities for a 6-month duration are associated with a generalized anxiety disorder. **3** Regression is an attempt during periods of stress to return to behavior that has been satisfying and is appropriate at an earlier stage of development. **4** Converting the anxiety into a physical symptom is an example of a conversion disorder, which decreases anxiety. **5** Displacing the anxiety onto a less threatening object is typical of a phobic disorder, which decreases anxiety.

2 Acting with grandiose behavior is not common in anxiety disorders.

Client Need: Psychosocial Integrity; **Cognitive Level:** Comprehension; **Nursing Process:** Assessment/Analysis

13. **4 The fight-or-flight responses of the sympathetic nervous system are stimulated, causing an increase in blood glucose through glycogenolysis and gluconeogenesis.**

1 The pupils dilate, not constrict, to facilitate the entry of visual stimuli. **2** The bronchioles dilate, not constrict, to facilitate gas exchange. **3** The blood pressure increases, not decreases, to shunt blood to vital centers.

Client Need: Psychosocial Integrity; **Cognitive Level:** Comprehension; **Nursing Process:** Assessment/Analysis

14. **3 Learning a variety of coping mechanisms helps reduce anxiety in stressful situations.**

1 A person must learn to cope with unpleasant events; they cannot be avoided. **2** Prolonged exposure may increase anxiety to possibly uncontrollable levels. **4** Fearful situations can never be viewed as pleasurable.

Client Need: Psychosocial Integrity; **Cognitive Level:** Comprehension; **Nursing Process:** Planning/Implementation

15. **1 By staying physically close, the nurse conveys the message that someone cares enough to be there and that the client is a person worthy of care.**

2 The client is incapable of telling anyone what the problem is. **3** Sitting still will increase the tension the client is experiencing. **4** This is not an initial nursing intervention.

Client Need: Management of Care; **Cognitive Level:** Application; **Integrated Process:** Caring; **Nursing Process:** Planning/Implementation

16. **1 The client is using this compulsive behavior to control anxiety and needs to continue with it until the anxiety is reduced and more acceptable methods are developed to handle it.**

2 Having the client scrub doorknobs will not change the client's behavior; the client cannot stop the compulsive act because it reduces anxiety. **3** Encouraging the client to touch doorknobs will greatly increase anxiety; compulsive behavior is a defense that cannot be interrupted until new defenses are learned. **4** Explaining to the client that the idea about doorknobs being contaminated is part of the illness, so precautions are not necessary, will not change the client's behavior; the client cannot stop the compulsive act because it reduces anxiety.

Client Need: Psychosocial Integrity; **Cognitive Level:** Application; **Integrated Process:** Caring; **Nursing Process:** Planning/Implementation

17. **1 By carrying out the compulsive ritual the client unconsciously tries to control anxiety by avoiding acting on unacceptable feelings and impulses.**

2 The OCD mechanism does not operate on a conscious level. **3** Hallucinations are not part of this disorder. **4** They feel no need to punish others.

Client Need: Psychosocial Integrity; **Cognitive Level:** Comprehension; **Nursing Process:** Assessment/Analysis

18. **2 Limiting the client's ritualistic acts to three times a day sets an unrealistic limit that will increase anxiety by removing a defense the client needs.**

1 Helping the client understand the nature of the anxiety is done in therapy as the client's condition improves. Insight is slowly developed to minimize anxiety. **3** Involving the client in establishing the therapeutic plan will increase self-esteem and self-control, not increase anxiety. **4** Providing the client with a nonjudgmental environment will reduce, not increase, anxiety, because the client will feel free to express feelings.

Client Need: Psychosocial Integrity; **Cognitive Level:** Analysis; **Nursing Process:** Evaluation/Outcomes

19. **4 These clients can work through their underlying conflicts more easily or productively when demands are reduced and the routine is simple.**

1 Preventing these clients from carrying out rituals can precipitate panic reactions. **2** The intent of therapy should be to help the client gain control, not to enable staff to do the controlling. **3** Because anxiety stems from unconscious conflicts, a controlled, neutral environment alone is not enough to effect resolution.

Client Need: Psychosocial Integrity; **Cognitive Level:** Comprehension; **Nursing Process:** Planning/Implementation

20. **4 Knowledge of a schedule allows the client to prepare for transitions; hurrying can increase anxiety and the performance of the ritual. Routines will also decrease anxiety and the need for the ritual.**

1 Determining the purpose of the ritualistic behavior is one of the objectives to be accomplished later during the client's hospitalization, not in the initial phase. Some clients will never be able to identify the purpose of their ritual beyond the fact that it helps decrease their anxiety. **2** Limiting the time allowed for the ritualistic behavior is not an initial intervention because it will increase anxiety. **3** Suggesting a symptom substitution technique to refocus the ritualistic behavior is an appropriate intervention during the working phase of the nurse-client intervention, not the initial phase.

Client Need: Psychosocial Integrity; **Cognitive Level:** Analysis; **Nursing Process:** Planning/Implementation

21. **4 The symptoms are a defense against anxiety resulting from decision-making, which triggers old fears; the client needs support.**

1 Stating "I know you're anxious, but by forcing yourself to go to the interview, you may conquer your fear" ultimately denies the client's overwhelming anxiety and lacks realistic support. **2** Stating "If going to an interview makes you this anxious, it seems as though you're not ready to go back to work" is judgmental; the client should be encouraged to work through symptoms, not avoid risk. **3** Stating "It must be that you really don't want that job after all. I think you should reconsider going to the interview" is judgmental; an increase in anxiety does not necessarily mean the client does not want to attain the goal.

Client Need: Psychosocial Integrity; **Cognitive Level:** Application; **Integrated Process:** Caring; Communication/Documentation; **Nursing Process:** Planning/Implementation

22. **4 The repeated thought or act defends the client against even higher, more severe levels of anxiety.**

1 To deny the client the ritual may precipitate panic levels of anxiety. **2** Usually, these clients recognize that the ritual serves little purpose. **3** To deny the client the ritual may precipitate panic levels of anxiety.

Client Need: Psychosocial Integrity; **Cognitive Level:** Comprehension; **Nursing Process:** Assessment/Analysis

23. **3 Intervening to maintain increasing anxiety at a manageable level will result from teaching the client to recognize situations that provoke ritualistic behavior and from the client learning how to interrupt the pattern.**

1 Verbalizing positive aspects about the self is not a priority; the client probably had little difficulty in this area. **2** Adhering to the rules of the therapeutic milieu is not a priority; the client probably had little difficulty in this area. **4** No evidence was presented to indicate the client was hallucinating.

Client Need: Psychosocial Integrity; **Cognitive Level:** Application; **Nursing Process:** Evaluation/Outcomes

24. **3 Fluvoxamine blocks the uptake of serotonin, which leads to a decrease in obsessive-compulsive behaviors.**

  1 Benztropine is an antiparkinsonian agent, not an antianxiety agent. **2** Amantadine is an antiparkinsonian agent, not an antianxiety agent. **4** Diphenhydramine is an antihistamine, not an antianxiety agent.

  Client Need: Pharmacologic and Parenteral Therapies; **Cognitive Level:** Analysis; **Nursing Process:** Planning/Implementation

25. **1 The repeated act defends the client against severe anxiety; interruption of the ritual will result in increased anxiety.**

  2 The performance of a ritual is not anger turned inward on the self; the ritual reduces anxiety. **3** Rituals are not activities that enhance self-esteem; they control anxiety. **4** Pointing out that the behavior is inappropriate will further increase anxiety. The client does not want to perform the ritual but feels compelled to do so to keep anxiety at a controllable level.

  Client Need: Psychosocial Integrity; **Cognitive Level:** Comprehension; **Nursing Process:** Planning/Implementation

26. **4 The client's exact adherence to carrying out the compulsive ritual relieves anxiety, at least temporarily. Furthermore, it meets a need and is necessary to the client.**

  1 The compulsive act is not under voluntary control. **2** Urging has no effect on trying to have the client start or stop the ritualistic behavior. **3** The person cannot stop the activity; it is not under voluntary control.

  Client Need: Psychosocial Integrity; **Cognitive Level:** Application; **Nursing Process:** Assessment/Analysis

27. **4 Helping clients understand that a behavior is being used to control anxiety usually makes them more amenable to psychotherapy.**

  1 Treatment includes activities to help the client, not others. **2** The client usually already understands that the behavior is not serving a realistic purpose. **3** Administering antianxiety medications that block out the memory of internal fears will only mask symptoms and will not get at the root of what is bothering the client.

  Client Need: Psychosocial Integrity; **Cognitive Level:** Application; **Nursing Process:** Planning/Implementation

28. **4 Accepting these clients and their symptomatic behavior sets the foundation for the nurse-client relationship. Setting limits provides external controls and helps lower anxiety. This intervention is appropriate during the working phase, not the initial phase, of a therapeutic relationship.**

  1 Restricting movements will have no effect other than to increase anxiety. **2** Calling attention to the behavior increases their anxiety and increases their use of the behavior. **3** Keeping them busy to distract them is unrealistic.

  Client Need: Psychosocial Integrity; **Cognitive Level:** Application; **Integrated Process:** Caring; **Nursing Process:** Planning/Implementation

13 Personality Disorders

OVERVIEW

- A personality disorder is a long-standing, pervasive, and maladaptive pattern of inner experiences, behavior, and relating to others that is not caused by another psychiatric disorder such as bipolar disorder or schizophrenia
- These disorders are exaggerations of personality traits or styles that often define the uniqueness of the individual; personality traits are normal; personality disorders are not
- Under stress, individuals manifest patterns of inflexibility, maladaptive emotional responses, and functioning impairments
- Individuals diagnosed with personality disorders typically have persistent and long-standing patterns of behavior that make relating to others extremely difficult and often intolerable
- They often view their surroundings in a negative context and tend to respond negatively and defensively to environmental cues that they believe are threatening to them
- Personality disorders generally begin in adolescence or early adulthood
- Relationship problems develop early in life and often move through predictable stages
- Clients diagnosed with personality disorders have difficulty relating to others at home, at work, and in the community
- The symptoms of a personality disorder are generally not responsive to brief psychotherapy, or medication; the maladaptive symptoms tend to worsen during stress or a crisis, and they persist after the stressor or crisis is resolved
- Premorbid personality of individuals diagnosed with these disorders resembles the compensatory behaviors associated with the pathologic counterpart
- Except for borderline personality disorder, most clients diagnosed with a personality disorder are not hospitalized for it, but rather, for a comorbid condition such as depression or anxiety; however, the personality disorder affects treatment greatly and must be taken into account
- The prevalence for all personality disorders in the U.S. is approximately 9% to 15% in total

Etiologic Theories

- Some etiologic factors are peculiar to just one type of personality disorder; they are listed with that particular disorder
- See Chapter 5 for a review of personality development
- Variations in basic human traits occur for each personality disorder (Table 13.1)

Biologic Theories

- Research evidence suggests that the development of major personality disorders is determined by environmental factors that interact with biologic factors such as inability to tolerate anxiety, aggressiveness, and genetic vulnerability
- Family and twin studies demonstrate a strong genetic influence, suggesting a connection between biologic factors and personality organization
- Study findings suggest a structural brain deficit in antisocial personality disorder that may cause low arousal, low fear, lack of conscience, and deficits in decision making
- Studies on borderline personality disorder indicate that it, too, may have a basis in atypical neurobiological functioning

TABLE 13.1	Relationship of DSM-5 Personality Disorders to the Five-Factor Model Domains				
DSM PD	**Neuroticism**	**Extroversion**	**Openness**	**Agreeableness**	**Conscientiousness**
Paranoid	+			−	
Schizoid		−			
Schizotypal	+		+	−	
Antisocial				−	−
Borderline	+			−	
Histrionic		+			
Narcissistic			+	−	
Avoidant	+	−			
Dependent	+			+	
Obsessive		−			+

PD: Personality disorder
(Modified from Blais, M. A., et al. [2008]. Personality and personality disorders. In T. A. Stern, et al. [Eds.], *Massachusetts General Hospital clinical psychiatry*. Philadelphia: Mosby.)

- Further research is needed to clarify the role of inheritance in relation to brain structure and function in the development of personality disorders

Psychodynamic Theory

- Psychodynamic theory postulates that individuals diagnosed with personality disorders have deficits in psychosexual development or failure to achieve object constancy, the ability to hold the memory of significant others in mind
- There is no specific evidence supporting the psychodynamic theory

Sociocultural Considerations

- Sociocultural factors (isolation and family instability) influence the ability to establish and maintain relationships

Epidemiology and Predisposing Factors

- Biologic factors are not solely responsible for any of the personality disorders
- Social environment and stressful environment are important components
- Psychological vulnerability and negative childhood experiences are also strong influences

Cluster A

- Cluster A is often described as the "odd" or "eccentric" cluster and includes paranoid, schizoid, and schizotypal personality disorders
- Clients diagnosed with disorders in this cluster all have difficulty relating to others; they isolate themselves, and they are unable to socialize comfortably
- Paranoid personality disorder
  - Tends to occur in families who have one or more members diagnosed with schizophrenia
  - Males are diagnosed more often than females
- Schizoid personality disorder
  - Males are diagnosed slightly more often than females

- Families with members who have schizophrenia or schizotypal personality disorder have increased prevalence of this disorder
- Schizotypal personality disorder
  - Individuals diagnosed with schizotypal personality disorder seek treatment for anxiety or depression and not generally for the personality disorder features
  - First-degree relatives of individuals diagnosed with schizophrenia are at increased risk; it is viewed as being on the spectrum of schizophrenia
  - Males are diagnosed slightly more often than females

Cluster B

- Cluster B personality disorders have components of dramatic, emotional, or erratic behavior; it includes antisocial, borderline, histrionic, and narcissistic personality disorders
- Each personality disorder has unique features, but each shares a dramatic quality in the way that the individual lives his or her life
- These individuals share a problem with impulse control and emotional regulation
- Antisocial personality disorder
  - Unstable parent-child environment may lead to delinquency in children
  - History of childhood abuse increases likelihood of antisocial behavior
  - Genetic predisposition; abnormality of monoamine oxidase gene
  - Usually evident before 18 years, but diagnosed at 18 years of age
  - Individuals have a history of conduct disorders before the age of 15 years
  - Males are diagnosed more often than females
  - Characteristics are evident by early childhood in males and by puberty in females
  - Approximately 1% of individuals age 18 years or older in the U.S. are diagnosed with antisocial personality disorder
  - Low heart rate and weak response to stress (low cortisol response); inability to learn from punishment
  - Strong association with substance use disorder
- Borderline personality disorder
  - More likely to occur in those who have close relative with this diagnosis
  - This condition is diagnosed in approximately 1.5% of the general population in the U.S. who are age 18 years or older
  - Diagnosed individuals often have a history of physical and sexual abuse, abandonment, neglect, hostile conflict, early parental loss or separation, and chaos and emotional discord in home as children
  - Females are diagnosed more often than males
  - Multifactorial origin
  - Defects in serotonin function
  - Structural and functional brain changes that affect impulsivity and emotional regulation
- Histrionic personality disorder
  - Females are diagnosed more often than males
- Narcissistic personality disorder
  - Males are diagnosed more often than females
  - Possible emotional arrested development

Cluster C

- Cluster C personality disorders are in the anxious or fearful cluster
- Avoidant personality disorder

- The diagnosis is equal for males and females
- Shyness common in childhood; associated with social phobia
- It is diagnosed in 5.2% of individuals age 18 years or older in the U.S.
- Dependent personality disorder
  - More females are diagnosed than males
  - Symptoms are demonstrated early during life
  - Children or adolescents with chronic physical illness or separation anxiety disorder may be predisposed to this condition
  - Culture implicated as causative factor
- Obsessive-compulsive personality disorder
  - Males are diagnosed twice as often as females
  - Differs from obsessive compulsive disorder
  - Early issues around autonomy, control, and authority may predispose
  - Associated with eating disorders

TYPES OF PERSONALITY DISORDERS

Unspecified Personality Disorders

- The category of unspecified personality disorders describes individuals whose personality pattern meets the general criteria for a personality disorder but not the criteria for any specific personality disorder
- It is also for an individual whose personality pattern meets the general criteria for a personality disorder but not one in the current classification, such as passive-aggressive personality disorder
- Can have features of more than one specific type (mixed disorders)
- Causes functional impairments that are clinically significant beginning in early adulthood

Cluster A Personality Disorders

Paranoid Personality Disorder

- Distrust, fear, irritability, and suspiciousness
- Frequent use of projective mechanisms
- Difficulty adjusting to change
- Sensitivity and argumentation
- Feelings of irreversible injury by others, often without evidence
- Anxiety and difficulty relaxing
- Short temper
- Difficulty with problem-solving
- Lack of tender feelings toward others
- Unwillingness to forgive even minor events
- Jealousy of spouse or significant other, often without evidence

Schizoid Personality Disorder

- Brief psychotic episodes in response to stressful events
- Lack of desire to socialize; enjoys solitude
- Lack of strong emotions
- Detached and self-absorbed affect; daydreaming, use of autistic thinking
- Lack of trust in others; introverted since childhood but fair contact with reality
- Difficulty expressing anger

- Passive reactions to crises
- Research shows that individuals diagnosed with schizotypal personality disorder demonstrate deficits similar to those of individuals diagnosed with schizophrenia, but the deficits are not as severe

Schizotypal Personality Disorder
- Unattached, withdrawn; can have eccentric behavior or appearance
- Incorrect interpretation of external events: cognitive-perceptual disturbances
- Belief that all events refer to self
- Superstition and preoccupation with paranormal phenomena
- Interpersonal disturbances; problems communicating
- Belief in possession of magical control over others
- Constricted or inappropriate affect
- Anxiety in social situations

Cluster B Personality Disorders
- Commonly display projection

Antisocial Personality Disorder
- Chronic lifelong disturbance that conflicts with society's laws and customs; acts out aggressive egocentric impulses on society
- Irresponsibility; failure to honor financial obligations, plan ahead, or provide children with basic needs
- Involvement in illegal activities; impulsive behavior is common
- Inability to postpone gratification; lives only for the moment; lack of guilt
- Difficulty learning from mistakes; does not profit from past experiences or punishment; does not take responsibility for actions and blames others for problems; lacks remorse for unacceptable behavior
- Initial charm dissolves into coldness, manipulation, and blaming others; has the ability to ingratiate self with others but eventually wears them down
- Lack of empathy
- Irritability
- Is in contact with reality but does not seem to care about it or people

Borderline Personality Disorder
- Chronic suicidal ideation; client may extract secondary gain from suicide precautions
- Unpredictable behavior that is potentially self-destructive; self-mutilation
- Impulsivity; tendency to engage in impulsive acts (eg, binge eating, spending money, reckless driving, unsafe sex)
- Intense inappropriate discharge of anger; negative or angry affect; labile (marked mood shifts)
- Feelings of emptiness and boredom
- Difficulty being alone or feeling of abandonment; avoids real or imagined abandonment
- Unstable sense of self; difficulty identifying self, including identifying likes and dislikes, occupational preferences, and self-image; identity disturbances
- Perception of people as all good or all bad; black-or-white (splitting) thinking
- Unstable, intense, and stormy interpersonal relationships; disruptions in cooperation within relationships

Histrionic Personality Disorder

- Theatrical and overreactive
- Use of suicidal gestures and threats when feeling abandoned
- Fluctuation in emotions
- Attention-seeking and self-centered attitude
- Vain and deliberately manipulative
- Sexual seduction and flamboyance
- Attentiveness to own physical appearance
- Dramatic and impressionistic speech style
- Vague logic; a lack of conviction in arguments, often switching sides
- Emotional instability and hyperexcitability
- Extroversion directed toward gaining attention
- Craving for immediate satisfaction
- Complaints of physical illness; somatization

Narcissistic Personality Disorder

- Grandiose, overblown view of self
- Lack of empathy toward others
- Need for attention and admiration
- Preoccupation with fantasies of success, brilliance, beauty and appearance, and ideal love
- Relationships marked by ambivalence

Cluster C Personality Disorders

Avoidant Personality Disorder

- Fearful of criticism, disapproval, or rejection
- Avoidance of social interactions; social discomfort and timidity
- Loner; unwilling to get involved with others
- Tendency to withhold thoughts and feelings
- Negative sense of self and low self-esteem
- Fear of negative evaluation from others

Dependent Personality Disorder

- Dependent; submissiveness and tendency to cling
- Inability to make decisions independently
- Inability to express negative emotions
- Induces others to assume responsibility
- Difficulty following through on tasks
- Lack of self-confidence

Obsessive-Compulsive Personality Disorder

- Rigidity, overly conscientiousness, inordinate capacity for work
- Preoccupation with perfection, organization, structure, and control
- Driven by obsessive concerns
- Procrastination
- Abandonment of projects because of dissatisfaction
- Excessive devotion to work
- Difficulty relaxing
- Rule-conscious behavior

- Self-criticism and inability to forgive own errors
- Reluctance to delegate
- Inability to discard anything
- Insistence on others' conforming to own methods
- Rejection of praise
- Reluctance to spend money
- Background of stiff and formal relationships
- Preoccupation with logic and intellect

APPLICATION AND REVIEW

1. A college student is brought to the mental health clinic by the parents. The diagnosis is borderline personality disorder. Which factors in the client's history support this diagnosis? **Select all that apply.**
   1. Impulsiveness
   2. Labile mood
   3. Ritualistic behavior
   4. Psychomotor retardation
   5. Self-destructive behavior

2. A nurse is working in the orientation phase of a therapeutic relationship with a client diagnosed with borderline personality disorder. What will be **most** difficult for the client at this stage of the relationship?
   1. Controlling anxiety
   2. Terminating the session on time
   3. Accepting the psychiatric diagnosis
   4. Setting mutual goals for the relationship

3. An adult diagnosed with schizotypal personality disorder is likely to display which types of behavior.
   1. Rigid and controlling
   2. Submissive and immature
   3. Arrogant and attention seeking
   4. Introverted and emotionally withdrawn

4. A client has the diagnosis of histrionic personality disorder. Which behavior should the nurse expect when assessing this client?
   1. Boastful and egotistical
   2. Rigid and perfectionistic
   3. Extroverted and dramatic
   4. Aggressive and manipulative

5. A nurse is caring for a client diagnosed with antisocial personality disorder. What client characteristic should the nurse consider when formulating a plan of care?
   1. Suffers from extreme anxiety
   2. Rapidly learns by experience if punished
   3. Usually is unable to postpone gratification
   4. Has a great sense of responsibility toward others

6. The nursing staff is discussing the **best** way to develop a relationship with a new client diagnosed with antisocial personality disorder. What characteristic of clients with antisocial personality should the nurses consider when planning care?
   1. Engages in many rituals
   2. Feels dependent on others
   3. Exhibits lack of empathy for others
   4. Possesses limited communication skills

7. A nurse is working with a client who has the diagnosis of borderline personality disorder. What personality traits should the nurse expect the client to exhibit? **Select all that apply.**
   1. Engaging
   2. Indecisive
   3. Withdrawn
   4. Manipulative
   5. Perfectionistic

See Answers on pages 235-239.

THERAPEUTIC INTERVENTIONS

Overview

- Individual, group, and family psychotherapy may be applicable
- Crisis intervention when necessary
- Vocational and occupational therapy, as well as additional treatment modalities may help

Individual Therapy

- Helps the client explore problem areas, to define new options, and to discuss how the new behavior will help solve the original problem
- With the emphasis in the health care system on short-term therapy, individual therapy is now problem-solving oriented as opposed to explorative with regard to early trauma
- Dialectical behavioral therapy (individual and group): the use of dialogue to help the client learn new patterns of thoughts and behavior

Group Therapy

- Problem-solving oriented
- Based on the repeated dynamics of the individuals in the group
- Especially beneficial for clients diagnosed with a Cluster B personality disorder who are dramatic and require a considerable attention
- Group members help the client understand the effects that the client's behavior has on each of them so that the client is able to use this information when relating to significant people in everyday life

Community Mental Health Centers

- Clients with personality disorders present in both inpatient and outpatient settings such as day treatment facilities, outpatient programs, partial hospital units, clinics, and private office practices
- Because of the time required to change maladaptive social responses, most people who have a personality disorder are treated in community settings not inpatient settings
- Inpatient treatment usually occurs because of a different diagnosis, not the personality disorder; borderline personality disorder is the personality disorder most often seen for inpatient care
- See also Chapter 20 for information about treatment of serious and persistent mental disorders

Additional Treatment Modalities

- A team approach that involves many disciplines provides the most comprehensive interventions for a client with a personality disorder in an inpatient, partial hospitalization, or day treatment setting
- Nurses can encourage and participate in research
  - The more information that the client and the client's family have, the more the choices regarding the use of treatment services and medication adherence make sense
  - Research assists the nurse with providing more comprehensive care, and helps answer questions that drive clinical practice
- See Chapter 8 for additional nonpharmacologic therapies: occupational, art, music, movement, and recreational therapies
- Medication therapy

BOX 13.1 Medication Key Facts: Personality Disorders

- Pharmacologic interventions are symptom oriented, regardless of the type of personality disorder.
- Medications include the short-term use of benzodiazepines and antipsychotics for aggressiveness and impulsivity.
- Mood stabilizers are used for rage, violence, impulsivity, and feelings of losing control.
- Other medications include antidepressants and antianxiety agents.

From Fortinash, K. M., & Holoday, P. A. (2012). *Psychiatric mental health nursing* (5th ed.). St. Louis, MO: Mosby.

- Medications often play a major role in helping the client diagnosed with a personality disorder (Box 13.1)
- Pharmacologic interventions are symptom-oriented
- Clients who are demonstrating violence against others sometimes require medications to gain emotional and behavioral control over their impulses
- Some individuals diagnosed with borderline personality disorder and problems with affect show a reduction in symptoms with the use of a selective serotonin reuptake inhibitor
- If there is an anxiety component with the affective dysregulation, this usually indicates the need for a benzodiazepine, such as clonazepam, along with the selective serotonin reuptake inhibitor
- Mood stabilizers such as lithium carbonate, carbamazepine, and valproate have been successful adjunctive treatments for affective dysregulation
- For individuals who are demonstrating anger and impulsivity, a selective serotonin reuptake inhibitor is the treatment of choice; the clinical practice guideline recommends the use of fluoxetine as the first line of treatment for this symptom
- Clients who are very agitated or who have psychosis sometimes respond to the use of a low-dose antipsychotic class medication
- Clients diagnosed with extreme violence who are unable to control this impulse sometimes receive intravenous or intramuscular sedatives, benzodiazepines, such as diazepam, or antipsychotics
- Monitoring side effects is an important nursing function
- Family therapy
  - Helpful for clients diagnosed with a personality disorder because the dynamics of the family system are often repeated in other relationships in the client's life such as with a boss or spouse
  - Family sessions consist of an assessment of the family system and an exploration of how the current problems that caused the client to seek care affect family dynamics
  - Because of the current philosophy of short-term therapy, the exploration of earlier dynamics or trauma focuses on the current issue
- Milieu therapy
  - When a client is hospitalized in an inpatient psychiatric setting or participates in a partial hospitalization program or a day treatment facility, the client becomes part of that milieu (environment)
  - The purpose of milieu therapy is to re-create a community setting in these units so that the client is able to interact with other client peers to identify and problem-solve issues that occur when relating to others; such relationship issues are discussed in community meetings or other problem-solving groups (eg, a coping skills group)

- Community meetings are for delegating the tasks of the unit such as cleaning off the tables at the end of the meal
  - This meeting is often used to ask each member to think through a daily goal for therapy and to discuss how he or she plans to meet that goal
  - If something happens on the unit (eg, if someone becomes aggressive or brings in drugs or alcohol), then the group discusses these concerns during the community meeting
- Problem-solving groups, such as coping skills groups, often pick a common area of concern, and the group works together to explore the issues and options that are necessary to solve the dilemma
- As in any other community, socializing is an important part of the interaction; in an inpatient, partial hospitalization program or day treatment milieu, socialization groups discuss problems with socializing

Nursing Interventions

- No matter what the coexisting diagnosis is, nurses need be diligent about evaluating and treating the personality disorder as thoroughly as the coexisting disorder in order to ensure safe, comprehensive care

Assessment/Analysis (Box 13.2)

- Overview
  - Level of social and occupational functioning
  - Individual's perception of problem

BOX 13.2 Nursing Assessment Questions: Personality Disorders

These questions involve the nurse's observations of the client's appearance, general nutritional status, and level of observable anxiety manifestations:
1. Does the client appear to be appropriately dressed? Does the client maintain eye contact? Does he or she appear to be properly nourished? Does the client exhibit signs of anxiety such as pacing, foot tapping, sighing, or facial tension? Does the client appear to be hypervigilant (overly watchful)? Does the client appear to be withdrawn?

These questions will help the nurse determine whether there are disturbances in the client's relationships, thought processes, and behaviors:
1. How would you describe yourself? What do you like about yourself? What would you like to change about yourself?
2. Describe your relationships with your spouse or your significant other, your children, your parents, and your other family members. Describe your relationships with your friends. What do you talk about? What types of activities do you do together?
3. How do you feel about your job? Do you get along with your boss and your coworkers?
4. If you have a personal problem, who do you trust to help you with it?
5. What are your main worries? How often do you think about them? Do you talk to anyone about these worries? Does that help?
6. Do you ever feel like hurting yourself or anyone else? Have you ever been suicidal? Have you ever hurt yourself by cutting your skin or burning yourself? If yes, how often does this occur?
7. Have you ever felt hopeless, helpless, worthless, and like a burden? Do you feel this way now? Are you getting any support from friends or family?
8. Do you ever use alcohol or illegal drugs? Have you ever gone to the doctor to get tranquilizers to reduce your nervousness? What did the doctor give you? What are you taking now?
9. What are your religious beliefs and practices?

Modified from Fortinash, K. M., & Holoday, P. A. (2012). *Psychiatric mental health nursing* (5th ed.). St. Louis, MO: Mosby.

- Reason for seeking treatment
- Level of anxiety
- Pending criminal charges
- Drug and alcohol addiction
- History of suicidal gestures and a present risk of violence and level of lethality *to prevent suicide, self-harm, or injury* toward self or others

Planning/Implementation

- The implementation of the care plan for clients diagnosed with personality disorders includes interventions focused on modifying lifelong disruptive and dysfunctional behaviors and thoughts while promoting safety
- Maintain consistency, concern, and a professional relationship
- Accept the individual as is; do not retaliate if provoked; manage countertransference
- Protect the individual from others while protecting others from the individual
- Place realistic limits on behavior; make known what those limits are
- Strive for consistency among health team members; avoid splitting of staff
- Initiate cognitive, behavioral, and dialectic behavioral strategies
- Specific interventions
  - If warranted, place the client on suicide precautions, depending on the person's level of lethality (eg, a client who has verbalized plans to hang himself or herself while in the unit requires close individual observation, even with no means or provisions to carry out the intent) to prevent suicide
  - Encourage the client to attend all group sessions to receive support from peers and to provide opportunities for problem-solving
  - Assess the client for an escalation of anger to rage and possible impulsive actions against self or others (obtain a history of violence, if possible) to prevent harm or injury to self or others
  - Teach the client other options for managing angry and impulsive feelings and behaviors such as leaving the room in which the conflict is occurring or using a quiet area (eg, an unlocked seclusion room) until the impulse to do harm passes; removing the clients from a stimulating and provocative environment will decrease their angry impulses
  - Discuss angry feelings in a group setting that is focused on exploring alternative problem-solving options; alternative actions will distract the client from angry feelings and help focus energy on constructive activities
  - Assess the client for evidence of self-mutilation and self-harm ideation; clients who are self-destructive are likely to repeat such acts and may require further intervention
  - Place the client on individual close watch until the urge to harm self passes or until the client is able to identify another way to obtain emotional relief to protect the client from harmful impulses and to redirect the impulses toward alternative and constructive methods
  - If self-mutilation occurs, attend to the wounds in a matter-of-fact manner to provide the client with safe care in a nonjudgmental manner
  - Encourage the client to keep a journal of the thoughts and feelings that he or she had before experiencing the urge to self-mutilate to help the client acknowledge feelings and thoughts and to help decrease impulsivity
  - Medicate the client with an anxiolytic or antipsychotic medication as ordered to help the client control intense anxiety or rage rather than self-mutilate
  - Use a timeout period, a prn medication, a seclusion room, and physical restraints if all attempts of least restrictive measures have been unsuccessful; document this intervention as per regulatory requirements

- Assist the client with recognizing thought patterns that contribute to impulsive behavior; nurses are able to do this by helping the client understand the role that intense feelings (eg, abandonment, anger, rage, anxiety) play in precipitating impulsive behavior or distorted thinking; the use of a journal to document such feelings and thoughts and receiving feedback during group sessions can be helpful and instructive methods; nurses teach clients to manage their impulsive *behaviors and distorted beliefs through a variety of methods within the setting*
- Suggest alternative behaviors to deal with the intense feelings such as:
  - Recognizing the intense emotional state and writing in a journal or thinking about an action that helps relieve the intensity of the feeling without resorting to impulsive or self-destructive acts
  - Using mindfulness meditation to reduce the intense feelings and to prevent impulsive responses
  - Therapist may suggest talking about the intense feelings when looking into a mirror and telling the mirror what the client would like to express to the object of anger
  - Identifying healthy options for dealing with the anger such as discussing the issue with the person who is involved in the interaction
  - Role-playing with the nursing staff different ways to approach the problem that precipitated the intense feelings
  - Introducing the issue in a problem-solving setting or group meeting to receive feedback from peers
  - Rewarding the self by self-soothing with something that is pleasant and healthful such as buying flowers, going to a movie, playing a video game, or reading a novel
  - Learning alternative ways to cope with intense feelings to reduce anger and anxiety and to provide constructive ways of managing life stressors
- Evaluate the client's family system by observing the family dynamics and determining the client's role within the family; how the client interacts within the family system and the *role that the client takes (eg, victim, placater) offer the nurse insight into the client's self-perception*
- Engage the client in frequent short interactions several times to illustrate the value of interacting with others
- Make use of problem-solving groups and other groups that concentrate on self-care and community responsibilities to help the client understand the value of interacting with others
- Teach the client assertiveness techniques to improve the client's ability to relate to others
- Provide the client with direct feedback about the interaction with others in a nonjudgmental fashion to facilitate the client's ability to learn new social skills
- See Figures 13.1 and 13.2

Evaluation/Outcomes

- Realistic expectations for improvement include a commitment by the client to explore and evaluate thoughts, relationships, and behaviors, especially when under stress
- Two steps:
  - The nurse compares the client's current functioning with the identified outcome criteria
  - The nurse asks questions to determine possible reasons for the outcome criteria not being met
- Criteria:
  - Demonstrates *decreased* episodes of acting out
  - Verbalizes decrease in anxiety

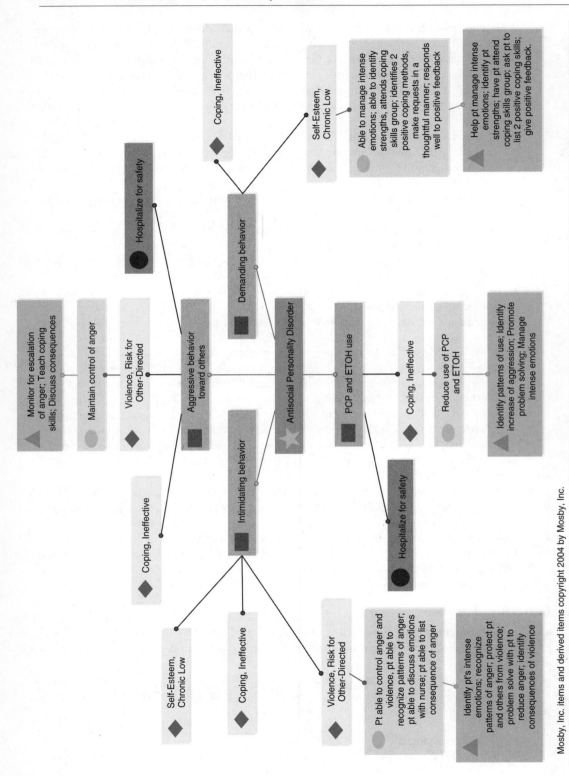

Mosby, Inc. items and derived items copyright 2004 by Mosby, Inc.

FIG. 13.1 Concept map: Antisocial personality disorder. (From Fortinash, K. M., & Holoday, P. A. [2012]. *Psychiatric mental health nursing* [5th ed.]. St. Louis, MO: Mosby.)

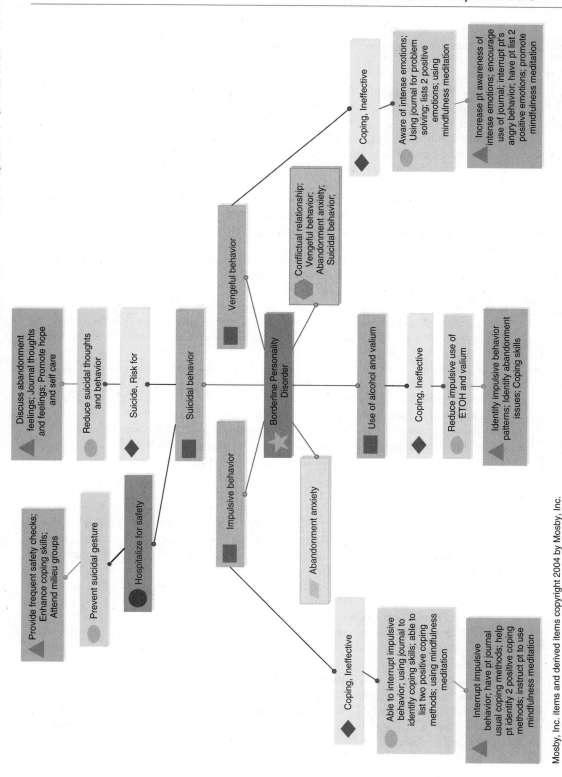

FIG. 13.2 Concept map: Borderline personality disorder. (From Fortinash, K. M., & Holoday, P. A. [2012]. *Psychiatric mental health nursing* [5th ed.]. St. Louis, MO: Mosby.)

Mosby, Inc. items and derived items copyright 2004 by Mosby, Inc.

- Accepts and continues long-term therapy
- Recognizes and *functions* within limits of personality

Prognosis

- When providing nursing care to clients diagnosed with personality disorders, consider the prognosis for improvement, especially during the planning and evaluating phases of the nursing care plan
- Individuals diagnosed with personality disorders have demonstrated pervasive and inflexible behaviors and thoughts that differ from cultural expectations
    - These patterns *first* begin during adolescence or early adulthood, and they are stable over time
    - The prognosis *for* individuals diagnosed with personality disorders is guarded as a result of the ingrained and pervasive nature of these disorders
- The nurse plays a powerful role by providing support, tools for this exploration, and client teaching
    - If the client is not able to use the knowledge of the dysfunctional patterns to predict how he or she will respond when faced with a stressor, the nurse is able to plan innovative options for problem-solving
    - In this way, the *individual* learns new responses and improves functioning
    - This process often needs to be repeated before behavioral and thought patterns change
    - Therefore treatment aimed at problem-solving and cognitive reframing is indicated for these *clients*
- The principal assumption of *dialectical behavioral therapy* is to use dialogue to assist the client with reworking destructive ways of handling crises
    - Dialectical behavioral therapy teaches that there are choices when working through the crisis that decrease suicidal thoughts or emotionally reactive patterns
    - This *therapy* focuses on the client learning new patterns of thoughts and behaviors
    - Research *suggests* that individuals who are treated with dialectical behavioral therapy have a decrease in hospitalizations because of a decrease in suicidal drive and a higher level of interpersonal functioning
- Discharge criteria: Inpatient setting
    - To determine when to discharge a client from an inpatient hospital setting, it is important to consider the risk factors of safety for the client and others; some clients *diagnosed* with personality disorders have suicidal ideas that are part of their day-to-day thought process; in those cases, it is important to determine whether the client has a suicidal plan and if client intends to implement that plan
    - *Individuals* diagnosed with a personality disorder who are hospitalized often have more than one psychiatric diagnosis; their lives are complex and chaotic
        - Psychiatric follow-up care—whether in a partial hospitalization program, a day treatment center, or with an outpatient psychotherapist—is important to help the client work through some of the issues that contributed to the crisis that culminated in the hospital stay
        - Before discharge from the hospital, it is important for the client to have a plan for outpatient follow-up care and the first posthospital appointment established
    - Client *teaching* is a powerful tool to help the client understand the psychiatric problems that the client is experiencing as well as to help prevent a relapse of symptoms; before discharge from the hospital, each client needs to receive education in these areas:
        - The need for follow-up care in an outpatient setting

- The psychiatric symptoms that indicate a need for emergent treatment
- An understanding of any medications that the client is receiving
- Who to call in case of a psychiatric emergency such as the Suicide Prevention Lifeline 1-800-273 TALK (8255)
- This client teaching takes place in a group setting or on an individual basis; if one of the *psychoeducational* activities is a relapse prevention group or a medication group, it is helpful for the nurse to review the material specific to each client before discharge
- Discharge criteria: Outpatient setting
    - If the client is in an outpatient setting, the nurse needs to consider these issues before *discharge* from treatment:
        - The client no longer has active thoughts of wanting to harm self (suicide or self-harm behaviors) or others
        - The client controls self-destructive impulses such as substance misuse when feeling upset or shoplifting when feeling empty
        - The client has an understanding of the symptoms that caused the need for psychotherapy
        - The client understands the types of symptoms that indicate a need for further treatment in the future
    - If *relevant* to his or her problems, the client is able to use community 12-step groups such as Alcoholics Anonymous, Narcotics Anonymous, Co-Dependents Anonymous, Incest Survivors Anonymous, and Overeaters Anonymous
    - The client can identify who to call in case of a psychiatric emergency such as the *Suicide Prevention Lifeline* 1-800-273 TALK (8255)

APPLICATION AND REVIEW

8. A client is diagnosed with a borderline personality disorder. What is a realistic **initial** nursing intervention for this client's care?
   1. Establish clear boundaries
   2. Explore job possibilities with the nurse
   3. Initiate discussion of feelings of being victimized
   4. Spend 1 hour twice a day discussing problems with the nurse

9. A hospitalized client who was diagnosed with a borderline personality disorder consistently breaks the unit's rules. How will confronting the client about this behavior or discussing the behavior with the client help the client?
   1. Controls anger
   2. Reduces anxiety
   3. Sets realistic goals
   4. Becomes more self-aware

10. A client diagnosed with a personality disorder tells a nurse, "I want to tell you something, but you must promise to keep it a secret." Which comment by the nurse could lead to splitting among the staff?
    1. "I am part of a team that shares important information about clients."
    2. "Your comments will be kept confidential because I am your advocate."
    3. "I cannot promise to keep what you say confidential from the rest of the staff."
    4. "Trust me to do what is in your best interests with the information, which includes discussing it with the team."

11. The clients on a mental health unit go on a supervised day trip to a baseball game. When returning to the bus, a client with a narcissistic personality disorder insists on leaving the group to get an autograph from a player. What is the **most** appropriate response by the nurse?
    1. Hold the client by the arm to prevent leaving the group
    2. Instruct the client with a loud voice to get in the bus so the group can go home
    3. Inform the client in a matter-of-fact tone that everyone must remain with the group
    4. Tell the client that the baseball player will not be permitted to give anyone an autograph
12. A nurse begins a relationship with a client diagnosed with the diagnosis of schizotypal personality disorder. What is the **best** initial nursing response?
    1. Set limits on manipulative behavior
    2. Encourage participation in group therapy
    3. Respect the client's need for social isolation
    4. Recognize that seductive behavior is expected
13. A client diagnosed with a borderline personality disorder receives the wrong meal tray for lunch and angrily states, "The next time I see the dietician, I am going to throw this tray at her!" What is the nurse's **most** appropriate response?
    1. Suggest that the client calm down and explain that sometimes trays get mixed up
    2. Inform the client that the behavior is inappropriate and send the client out of the dining room
    3. Tell the client it is frustrating not to get the correct tray, but throwing the tray at the dietician is unacceptable behavior
    4. Inform the client that throwing the tray at the dietician will make matters worse and may result in being placed in seclusion
14. Which nursing intervention is **most** important for a client who has the diagnosis of antisocial personality disorder?
    1. Teach and role-model assertiveness
    2. Use a gentle and reassuring approach
    3. Provide clear boundaries and consequences
    4. Present an empathetic and democratic approach
15. A client with a diagnosis of antisocial personality disorder is being discharged from the hospital. The client asks the nurse, "Can I have your phone number so that I can call you for a date?" What is the nurse's **best** response?
    1. "We are not permitted to date clients."
    2. "It is against my professional ethics to date clients."
    3. "Our relationship is professional; therefore I will not see you socially."
    4. "I'm glad you like me; however, I cannot give out my phone number."
16. A nurse is orienting a new client to the unit when another client rushes down the hallway and asks the nurse to sit down to talk. The client requesting the nurse's attention is manipulative and uses acting-out behaviors when demands are unmet. How should the nurse intervene?
    1. Suggest that the client requesting attention speak with another staff member
    2. Leave the new client, saying, "I'll talk with the other client until things calm down"
    3. Introduce the two clients and suggest that the client join them on a tour of the facility
    4. Tell the interrupting client, "I'll be back to talk with you after I orient this new client"
17. A client with the diagnosis of antisocial personality disorder is is openly discussing interpersonal difficulties with family members and the boss at work from whom money has been stolen. The client presently is facing criminal charges. Which behavior best indicates that the client is meeting treatment goals?
    1. Expression of feelings of resentment toward the employer
    2. Discussion of plans for each of the possible outcomes of a trial

3. Expression of resignation about difficult spousal and children relationships
4. Discussion of the decision to file a grievance against the employer

18. A client with a diagnosis of borderline personality disorder is admitted to the mental health unit. What should the nurse do to maintain a therapeutic relationship with the client? Select all that apply.
   1. Provide an unstructured environment to promote self-expression.
   2. Be firm, consistent, and understanding.
   3. Use an authoritarian approach because this type of client needs to learn to conform to the rules of society.
   4. Record but ignore marked shifts in mood, suicidal threats, and temper displays because these last only a few hours.
   5. Focus on specific behaviors.

19. An adolescent client with a diagnosis of antisocial personality disorder was admitted to the hospital because of a substance use disorder and repeated sexual acting-out behavior. Which client behavior best supports the nurse's evaluation that actions directed toward modifying the behavior of this client are successful?
   1. Promises never to take drugs again
   2. Discusses the need to seduce other adolescents
   3. Recognizes the need to conform to society's norms
   4. Identifies the feelings underlying the acting-out behavior

20. A 22-year-old client with a diagnosis of antisocial personality disorder is being discharged and is to continue psychotherapy on an outpatient basis. When evaluating the chances for improvement, what outcome should the nurse anticipate?
   1. Client's prognosis for adjusting to a limited lifestyle is excellent
   2. Client will not change unless the parents are willing to set and keep firm limits
   3. Client requires intensive psychotherapy along with an anxiolytic drug to produce a remission
   4. Client's ability to change will be limited unless there is a readiness to accept the uncertainty associated with change

See Answers on pages 235-239.

ANSWER KEY: REVIEW QUESTIONS

1. **Answers: 1, 2, 5.**
   1 Clients with a diagnosis f borderline personality disorder often lead complex, chaotic lives because of the inability to control or limit impulses. **2** Extremes of emotions can be displayed over short periods of time and range from apathy and boredom to anger. **5** Impulsive acts, such as reckless driving, spending money, or engaging in unsafe sex, often result in self-destructive consequences.
   3 Ritualistic behavior is associated with obsessive-compulsive disorders. **4** Psychomotor retardation is associated with mood disorders such as depression.
   Client Need: Psychosocial Integrity; **Cognitive Level:** Comprehension; **Integrated Process:** Communication/Documentation; **Nursing Process:** Assessment/Analysis

   Memory Aid: Think of clients diagnosed with *borderline* personality disorder as walking a narrow *borderline* on top of tall wall, which is a reckless act, where one side of the wall represents calmer emotions and one side represents angrier emotions; they may fall off the wall on either side at any moment.

2. **4 Clients diagnosed with borderline personality disorder frequently demonstrate a pattern of unstable interpersonal relationships, impulsiveness, affective instability, and frantic efforts to avoid abandonment; these behaviors usually create great difficulty in establishing mutual goals.**
   1 Although the client diagnosed with a borderline personality disorder may have difficulty in controlling anxiety, it is not the most significant issue. **2** Although the client diagnosed with a borderline personality disorder may have difficulty in terminating the session on time, it is not the most significant issue. **3** Although the client diagnosed with a borderline personality disorder may have difficulty in accepting the psychiatric diagnosis, it is not the most significant issue.
   Client Need: Psychosocial Integrity; **Cognitive Level:** Analysis; **Integrated Process:** Communication/Documentation; **Nursing Process:** Planning/Implementation

3. **4 Clients with a diagnosis of schizotypal personality disorder usually display social inadequacy and lack of emotional contact with others.**
   1 Rigid and controlling behaviors probably reflect an obsessive-compulsive personality disorder. **2** Submissive and immature behaviors probably reflect a dependent personality disorder. **3** Arrogant and attention-seeking behaviors probably reflect a narcissistic personality disorder.
   Client Need: Psychosocial Integrity; **Cognitive Level:** Comprehension; **Nursing Process:** Assessment/Analysis

4. **3 Clients with a diagnosis of histrionic personality disorder draw attention to themselves, are self-centered, and demonstrate emotionality and attention-seeking behavior.**
   1 Boastful and egotistical behaviors are typical of clients with the diagnosis of narcissistic personality disorder. **2** Rigid and perfectionistic behaviors are typical of clients with the diagnosis of obsessive-compulsive personality disorder. **4** Aggressive and manipulative behaviors are typical of clients with the diagnosis of antisocial personality disorder.
   Client Need: Psychosocial Integrity; **Cognitive Level:** Comprehension **Nursing Process:** Assessment/Analysis

5. **3 Individuals with a diagnosis of antisocial personality disorder tend to be self-centered and impulsive. They lack judgment and self-control and are unable to postpone gratification.**
   1 Generally, clients with histrionic personality disorder display the opposite of boastful and egotistical behaviors. **2** Clients with histrionic personality disorder do not usually show rigid and perfectionistic behaviors because they believe that the rules do not apply to them and they do not profit from their mistakes. **4** Clients with histrionic personality disorder do not usually show aggressive and manipulative behaviors because they are too self-centered to have a sense of responsibility to anyone.
   Client Need: Psychosocial Integrity; **Cognitive Level:** Comprehension **Nursing Process:** Assessment/Analysis

6. **3 Self-motivation and self-satisfaction are of paramount concern, and clients with a diagnosis of antisocial personality disorder have little or no concern for others.**
   1 Clients with an obsessive-compulsive disorder, not an antisocial personality disorder, engage in rituals. **2** Clients with dependent personality disorder are extremely dependent on others. They count on others to extricate them from their problems. **4** Clients with antisocial personality disorder usually are charming on the surface and can easily "con" people into doing what they want.
   Client Need: Psychosocial Integrity; **Cognitive Level:** Comprehension; **Nursing Process:** Assessment/Analysis

7. **Answers: 1, 4.**
   1 Clients with a diagnosis of borderline personality disorders initially tend to be engaging and to establish intense relationships. **4** These clients may be manipulative because they are opinionated and they want people to conform to their agenda.
   2 Clients with borderline personality disorders often are decisive and opinionated. **3** Clients with borderline personality disorders have a pronounced intolerance for being alone and usually are quite social. **5** Clients with borderline personality disorders are not perfectionists.
   Client Need: Psychosocial Integrity; **Cognitive Level:** Comprehension; **Nursing Process:** Assessment/Analysis

8. **1 Individuals with a diagnosis of borderline personality disorder are impulsive and have difficulty identifying and respecting boundaries in relation to others.**

   2 Exploration of job possibilities in a meaningful manner can occur only after an ongoing relationship has been established. **3** Feeling victimized is a frequent theme among clients with this disorder; however, they rarely have the insight to initiate discussion of these feelings and usually show resistance when the topic is mentioned. **4** An individual with a borderline personality disorder may not be able to spend this length of time having a meaningful discussion with the nurse; usually they are too impulsive to engage in consistent work until a therapeutic relationship has been established.
   Client Need: Psychosocial Integrity; **Cognitive Level:** Application; **Integrated Process:** Communication/Documentation; **Nursing Process:** Planning/Implementation

9. **4 Clients must first become aware of their behavior before they can change it.**

   1 Confrontation may increase anger and agitation. **2** Confrontation may increase anxiety. **3** The client setting realistic goals occurs after the client is aware of behavior and has a desire to change it.
   Client Need: Psychosocial Integrity; **Cognitive Level:** Application; **Nursing Process:** Planning/Implementation

10. **2 To gain control, clients often try to split the staff apart, separating the nurse from the rest of the treatment team; confidentiality is not expected to be maintained among professionals caring for a client because it is detrimental to the client's therapy.**

    1 The response "I am part of a team that shares important information about clients" reinforces the team approach to care. **3** The response "I cannot promise to keep what you say confidential from the rest of the staff" both reinforces the team approach and avoids providing false assurance that the information will be kept secret. **4** The statement "Trust me to do what is in your best interests with the information, which includes discussing it with the team" does not provide false assurance that the information will be kept secret.
    Client Need: Management of Care; **Cognitive Level:** Application; **Integrated Process:** Communication/Documentation; **Nursing Process:** Planning/Implementation

11. **3 Informing the client in a matter-of-fact tone indicates that negotiation is unacceptable.**

    1 Holding the client by the arm is an inappropriate use of force. The nurse should contact the police if the client continues to refuse to leave. **2** Raising the voice to a client indicates frustration and can be interpreted as threatening. **4** Using the baseball player to meet control issues indicates to the client that the nurse is unable to maintain control of the situation.
    Client Need: Psychosocial Integrity; **Cognitive Level:** Application; **Integrated Process:** Communication/Documentation**Nursing Process:** Planning/Implementation

12. **3 Clients with a diagnosis of schizotypal personality disorder are withdrawn, aloof, and socially distant; allowing distance and** providing **support may encourage the eventual development of a therapeutic alliance.**

    1 Manipulative behavior is typical of clients with the diagnosis of antisocial personality disorder or borderline personality disorder. **2** Group therapy will increase anxiety in the client diagnosed with schizotypal personality disorder; cognitive or behavioral therapy is more appropriate. **4** Seductive behavior is associated with clients with the diagnosis of histrionic personality disorder.
    Client Need: Psychosocial Integrity; **Cognitive Level:** Analysis; **Nursing Process:** Planning/Implementation

13. **3 Validating the client's frustration and correcting behavior are the most appropriate responses; safety is a priority.**

    1 Suggesting that the client calm down and explain that sometimes trays get mixed up does not validate the client's feelings. **2** Sending the client out of the room without offering support and direction is not an appropriate nursing response. **4** Threatening seclusion is an inappropriate nursing intervention.
    Client Need: Safety and Infection Control; **Cognitive Level:** Application; **Nursing Process:** Planning/Implementation

 Memory aid: Be _V_ery _C_autious when giving responses: _V_alidate client's feelings, then _C_orrect behavior.

14. **3 Clients with a diagnosis of antisocial personality disorder interact with others through manipulation, aggressiveness, and exploitation; therefore clear limits must be set with consistently enforced consequences for crossing set boundaries.**

     1 Clients with antisocial personality disorder can be too assertive; a teach and role-model assertiveness approach is appropriate for a client diagnosed with dependent personality disorder. **2** Clients with antisocial personality disorder need a firm, consistent approach with clear and realistic limits on inappropriate behavior; a gentle, reassuring approach should be used with clients who have the diagnosis of avoidant personality disorder. **4** The nurse should provide a neutral, nonemotional approach with clear, realistic boundaries and consequences, not an empathetic and democratic approach.

     Client Need: Psychosocial Integrity; **Cognitive** Level: Application; **Nursing Process:** Planning/Implementation

15. **3 The response "Our relationship is professional; therefore I will not see you socially" sets clear limits on their relationship and maintains a professional rather than a social role.**

     1 The response "We are not permitted to date clients" shifts responsibility from the issue at hand to the institution. **2** The response "It is against my professional ethics to date clients" avoids the real issue and shifts responsibility to the ethical code. **4** The response "I'm glad you like me; however, I cannot give out my phone number" does not clarify the nature of the relationship as professional.

     Client Need: Management of Care; **Cognitive Level:** Analysis; **Integrated Process:** Communication/Documentation; **Nursing Process:** Planning/Implementation

16. **4 Telling the interrupting client, "I'll be back to talk with you after I orient this new client" sets realistic limits on behavior without rejecting the client.**

     1 Suggesting that the client requesting attention speak with another staff member constitutes a rejection of the client rather than the behavior. **2** Saying "I'll talk with the other client until things calm down" will encourage further manipulation by the client. **3** The other client is entitled to a special time with the nurse; suggesting that the client join them on a tour of the facility is inconsistent limit-setting on the part of the nurse.

     Client Need: Psychosocial Integrity; **Cognitive Level:** Application; **Integrated Process:** Communication/Documentation; **Nursing Process:** Planning/Implementation

17. **2 Because the legal difficulties were a precipitating event for hospitalization, if the client can realistically examine the possible outcomes of the trial, then some benefit has been gained from the therapy.**

     1 The client has been freely expressing resentment and victimization by the employer and authority figures; expressing resentment toward the employer does not show improvement or insight. **3** The client has been discussing problems since admission, so expressing resignation about relationships does not indicate the development of insight. **4** Discussion of the decision to file a grievance against the employer after discharge from the hospital indicates unrealistic planning and does not demonstrate the development of insight.

     Client Need: Psychosocial Integrity; **Cognitive Level:** Application; **Nursing Process:** Evaluation/Outcomes

18. **Answers: 2, 5.**

     2 Consistency, limit setting, and supportive confrontation are essential nursing interventions designed to provide a secure, therapeutic environment for this client. **5** Limit setting and supportive confrontation are essential nursing interventions designed to provide a secure, therapeutic environment for this client.

     1 To be therapeutic, the environment needs structure, and the staff must assist the client to set short-term goals for behavioral changes. **3** The use of an authoritarian approach will increase anxiety in this type of client, resulting in feelings of rejection and withdrawal. **4:** Ignoring the client's behavior is nontherapeutic and may reinforce underlying fears of abandonment.

     Client Need: Psychosocial Integrity; **Cognitive Level:** Application; **Nursing Process:** Planning/Implementation; **Integrated Process:** Caring

 Memory Aid: Make the right **C**al**LS** when responding: **C**onsistency and **L**imit **S**etting are keys.

19. **4 Expression of feelings by this individual demonstrates the development of some insight and a willingness to at least begin to look at the underlying causes of behavior.**

1 These words probably will have little meaning to the client. 2 This reflects a continuation of the client's behavior before being hospitalized. 3 These words probably will have little meaning to the client.

Client Need: Psychosocial Integrity; **Cognitive Level:** Application; **Nursing Process:** Evaluation/Outcomes

20. **4 Change is always accompanied by anxiety and uncertainty; without motivation, change will not occur.**

1 The lifestyle of these individuals is rarely limited because they tend to be rather gregarious and outgoing; in reality, they attempt to live by their guile. 2 The effect of the client's parents setting limits is of little influence at this age. 3 Usually these do not work unless the individual is motivated to change; there is no need for an anxiolytic to reduce anxiety.

Client Need: Psychosocial Integrity; **Cognitive Level:** Comprehension; **Nursing Process:** Evaluation/Outcomes

14 Substance Use Disorders

TERMINOLOGY

- Substance refers to any mind-altering chemical
- Substance use disorder (SUD)—maladaptive pattern of drug use leading to impairment or distress, as manifested by one or more of these circumstances occurring within a 12-month period:
  - Failure to fulfill major roles (e.g., social, school, or occupational)
  - Use in hazardous situations
  - Recurring related legal problems
  - Continued use despite social or interpersonal problems
  - Symptoms are not associated with another mental disorder
- Behaviors such as compulsive gambling, compulsive sexual activity, and compulsive overeating are now being treated as addictive disorders
- Substance intoxication: A reversible substance-specific syndrome caused by recent ingestion of or exposure to a substance resulting in maladaptive behavior or psychologic changes from effects on the CNS
- Substance withdrawal: Development of a substance-specific syndrome resulting from cessation or reduction in substance use that has been heavy or prolonged
  - Substance withdrawal is more risky with drugs that are CNS depressants or have a short half-life (eg, alcohol) than those with a long half-life (eg, marijuana); withdrawal is not lethal with some (eg, cocaine)
  - Withdrawal may cause more problems in older adults because they possess less physiologic reserves
- Substance tolerance: The need for greatly increased amounts of the substance to achieve the desired effects or markedly diminished effect with the continued use of the same amount of substance; substance tolerance does not occur with all substances
- Polysubstance use: Use of three or more drugs or of alcohol and drugs
- Potentiation: Two or more substances interact in the body to produce an effect greater than the sum of the effects of each substance taken alone
- Substance dependence/addiction: The continued use of a substance despite significant related problems in cognitive, physiologic, and behavioral components; spending more time in getting, taking, and recovering from the substance; continuous use despite knowledge of physical or psychologic problems or awareness of complications resulting from continued use of the substance; dependency can be both psychologic (needed to enhance coping) and physiologic (discontinuance results in withdrawal signs and symptoms)

ETIOLOGY

Background

- Substance use disorders cause more deaths, illnesses, and disabilities than any other preventable health condition
- The use of alcohol, tobacco, and illicit drugs changes in response to shifts in public tolerance of the behaviors and with various political, economic, and social events

- Alcohol is the most widely available legal drug
- Tobacco use is a major health problem
- Fetal alcohol syndrome is 100% preventable if a pregnant woman abstains from alcohol use
- The treatment of SUDs requires patient perseverance
- Many factors influence substance use disorders
- Dual diagnosis and comorbidities require in-depth assessment followed by the concurrent treatment of both the substance use disorders and the psychiatric diagnoses
- A drug that a particular person prefers is known as his or her "drug of choice"

Biologic Factors

- Research studies, including research conducted among twins and children of alcoholics, have shown that genetic factors influence alcoholism or predispose toward the problematic use of alcohol
  - Children of people with an alcohol use disorder are about four times more likely than the general population to develop alcohol problems
  - Children of people with an alcohol use disorder also have a higher risk for many other behavioral and emotional problems
  - The rate of problems with alcohol increases with the number of relatives with alcoholism, the severity of the disease, and the closeness of the genetic relationship to the person at risk
- Genetics partially determines the rate of metabolism of the substance, the physiologic reactions, the level of tolerance, and the rates of elimination
- However, alcoholism is not determined only by the genes you inherit from your parents
- Note: *More than one-half of all children of alcoholics do not develop a substance use disorder*
- Japanese, Chinese, and Korean people are more likely than Caucasians to have an inactive form of alcohol dehydrogenase, which metabolizes alcohol in the liver; another 40% of this population has active enzymes with decreased activity, which results in an exaggerated response to alcohol that produces flushing, nausea, dizziness, and rapid heartbeat; the lack of this enzyme is protective against alcoholism; Native Americans do not lack this enzyme, so they do not have the benefit of protection

Biochemical Factors

- The gene alleles *ALDH2* and *ALDH3* influence an individual's predisposition to alcohol use disorder, because these genes influence the metabolism of alcohol, which is genetic and varies among individuals
- Dopamine and glutamate are neurotransmitters that occur in various concentrations in different parts of the brain
  - All addicting substances are reinforced via the dopamine pathway; drug use raises dopamine levels in the brain; changes in the brain from continued use make it more difficult to stop
  - Genetics influence the production and regulation of these and other neurotransmitters and play an important role in addiction
- People in some ethnic groups have particular genetic risks for addiction as a result of inherited metabolic patterns

Psychologic Factors

- A person's appraisal and belief systems are factors, as are perceived risk of use and the availability of friends who purchase drugs
- Comorbid mental illness is associated with greater rates of addiction and maladaptive use; posttraumatic stress disorder (PTSD) creates a risk for substance use or relapse; some

individuals begin to use substances maladaptively after exposure to trauma; of persons diagnosed with SUDs, 30% to 60% meet the criteria for comorbid PTSD

- Persons diagnosed with bipolar disorder also have increased risk for SUDs, as do patients diagnosed with anxiety, depression, or schizophrenia disorders
- Researchers have also demonstrated a strong neurobiologic correlation between stress and drug use, especially in relation to relapse; there is a higher rate of problematic substance use in people with borderline or antisocial personality disorders
- Prolonged or chronic stress also fosters the continuation of addiction behaviors
- Stress increases the hormone production of corticotropin-releasing factor (CRF), which in turn initiates the body's biologic response to stressors; after exposure to stress, CRF is in areas of the brain in increased amounts; almost all drugs of abuse also increase CRF levels, which possibly indicates a neurobiologic connection between stress and substance use; withdrawal induces rises in CRF
- Various psychologic theories explain SUDs; although researchers have studied addictive personality attributes carefully, no one unique personality profile is more prone to addiction than another; however, early aggressive behavior and poor social skills are factors that may predispose a person to substance use disorder
- Theories of psychologic causation alone are insufficient to adequately explain the development of substance use disorder

Sociocultural Factors

- Researchers believe a person's risk increases if their family demonstrates these difficulties:
  - A parent with an alcohol use disorder is depressed or has other psychologic problems
  - Both parents have an alcohol or other drug use problem
  - The parents' alcohol use is severe
  - Conflicts lead to aggression and violence in the family
- Additional factors include peer influence, social norms, family influences, and social supports; these factors overlap with other influences
- Children from families in which a member has an SUD tend to become enmeshed in the family system; the multigenerational transmission process traces the recurrence of the disease in the family in subsequent generations; the family conspires to maintain a system that supports addiction
- The term *codependent* describes a person who helps another person maintain the addiction by "enabling" or caring for that person, handling that person's problems, and running interference; on the surface, these efforts appear to be helpful, but they do not permit the affected individual the opportunity to experience the consequences of their behavior, which is an important agent for change
- Healthy parental support is a strong predictor of *decreased* drug use in youth
- Peer group pressures and the need to belong to the group are powerful positive reinforcers for youth; prevention efforts that target situational influences include changing perceptions in groups, promoting positive peer influences, bonding with nonusing peers, and improved parenting skills

Individual Factors

- Age, gender, ethnicity, and other demographic descriptors are in this category
  - The risk for developing an alcohol use disorder increases for those who start drinking before the age of 17 years (approximately 25%) compared with those who start drinking at the age of 21 or 22 years (approximately 10%) or the age of 25 years (approximately 4%)

- The individual's history of drug use, qualities of decision making, positive beliefs about the effects of drugs, availability of drugs, and the money to purchase them along with an individual's physiologic response are all contributing factors to SUD development

Environmental Factors and Access to Psychotropic Medications

- Environmental factors include: an individual's access to and the cost of the desired substance; policies and policy enforcement; and the severity of the punishment of those who engage in illegal behavior to obtain substances or who sell to minors
- Researchers use maps and the mapping of neighborhoods to identify problem areas within communities and to then form action agendas for prevention and intervention
- Reimbursement is often poor for drug and alcohol treatment; the impression that addictions are self-created is partially true, although other diseases have that same potential, and there are no limits regarding the treatment for them (eg, chronic obstructive pulmonary disease, although these patients have smoked for years)
- Reimbursement is available for the consequences of addiction, but prevention and treatment are expensive and not well funded
- The majority of adolescents who use drugs do not develop SUDs; the culture of early adulthood often includes alcohol use and drug experimentation; however, most people stop these behaviors when they enter the workforce and have families and financial obligations

EPIDEMIOLOGY

Alcohol Use Disorder

- An estimated 16 million people in the U.S. have alcohol use disorder (AUD); approximately 15.1 million adults (6.2%) in the U.S., ages 18 and older, had AUD in 2015; this includes 9.8 million men (8.4% of men in this age group) and 5.3 million women (4.2% of women in this age group)
- Adolescents can be diagnosed with AUD as well; in 2015, an estimated 623,000 adolescents between the ages 12 and 17 had AUD

Alcohol Use in the United States

- Prevalence of drinking: According to the 2015 National Survey on Drug Use and Health (NSDUH), 86.4% of people ages 18 or older reported that they drank alcohol at some point in their lifetime; 70.1% reported that they drank in the past year; 56.0% reported that they drank in the past month
- Prevalence of binge drinking and heavy alcohol use: In 2015, 26.9% of people ages 18 or older reported that they engaged in binge drinking in the past month; 7.0% reported that they engaged in heavy alcohol use in the past month
- Alcohol usually is one of the first drugs to be used, as it often begins in teens who are experimenting with the effects of beer and wine for the first time; it is one of the most widely used and most abused substances; about 9.6% of American males and 3.2% of American females are addicted to alcohol
- Accident rates that result from alcohol consumption dramatically influence mortality and morbidity rates in the U.S.; there is evidence that a blood alcohol level as low as 15 mg/dL (0.01), or that which results from about one drink, significantly impairs a person's ability to drive an automobile

Alcohol Use Disorder in the United States

- About 1.3 million adults received treatment for AUD at a specialized facility in 2015 (8.3% of adults who needed treatment); this included 898,000 men (8.8% of men who needed treatment) and 417,000 women (7.5% of women who needed treatment)
- Youth (ages 12–17): According to the 2015 NSDUH, an estimated 623,000 adolescents ages 12 to 17 (2.5% of this age group) had AUD; this number includes 298,000 males (2.3% of males in this age group) and 325,000 females (2.7% of females in this age group)
- An estimated 37,000 adolescents (22,000 males and 15,000 females) received treatment for an alcohol problem in a specialized facility in 2015

Alcohol-Related Deaths

- An estimated 88,000 people (approximately 62,000 men and 26,000 women) die of alcohol-related causes annually
- Box 14.1 illustrates consumption standards for alcohol and classifications for different types of drinkers

Tobacco and Other Drugs

- Tobacco use continues to be the leading cause of preventable death in the U.S.
  - An estimated 25.2% (66.9 million) of Americans age 12 or older were current users of a tobacco product
  - Although tobacco use has declined since 2002 for the general population, this has not been the case for people diagnosed with serious mental illness in which tobacco use remains a major cause of morbidity and early death
  - Approximately 50% of smokers die of smoking-related illnesses; more than 6000 children die each year primarily as a result of sudden infant death syndrome and respiratory infections that are linked to parental smoking and low birth weights associated with smoking during pregnancy
- Illicit drug use estimate for 2014 continues to be driven primarily by marijuana use and the nonmedical use of prescription pain relievers, with 22.2 million current marijuana users age 12 or older (ie, users in the past 30 days) and 4.3 million people age 12 or older who reported current nonmedical use of prescription pain relievers

---

BOX 14.1 Standard Drink and Consumption Levels

A Standard Drink*
12 ounces of beer (5% alcohol content)
8 ounces of malt liquor (7% alcohol content)
5 ounces of wine (12% alcohol content)
1.5 ounces or a "shot" of 80-proof (40% alcohol content) distilled spirits or liquor

Consumption Definitions
Abstinence
No drinking

Moderate Drinking
Women: Up to 1 drink per day
Men: Up to 2 drinks of alcohol per day
Heavy or Excessive Alcohol Use
Women: More than 8 drinks per week or more than 4 drinks per occasion
Men: More than 15 drinks per week or more than 5 drinks or more per occasion
Any drinking by a minor
Any drinking by a pregnant woman

From Centers for Disease Control and Prevention. (2017). *Alcohol and public health: Frequently asked questions.* www.cdc.gov/alcohol/faqs.htm.

- The misuse of prescription drugs is second only to marijuana as the nation's most common drug problem after alcohol and tobacco, leading to troubling increases in opioid overdoses in the past decade
- Also among Americans age 12 or older, the use of illicit drugs has increased over the last decade from 8.3% of the population using illicit drugs in the past month in 2002 to 10.2% (27 million people) in 2014
  - Of those, 7.1 million people met criteria for an illicit drug use disorder in the past year
- Men reported higher rates of illicit drug addiction than did women—3.8% to 1.9%
- American Indians and Alaska Natives have the highest rates of illicit drug addiction at 6%, followed by African Americans at 3.6%; Asian Americans reported the lowest rate at 1%
- About 14% of adults with illicit drug dependence reported receiving treatment in the past year, which did not vary by gender
- Each year, approximately 5000 youth under the age of 21 die as a result of underage drinking
- More than 50% of people age 12 or older in 2011 to 2012 who used pain relievers for non-medical reasons in the past year got them from a friend or relative

ALCOHOL USE DISORDER

Definition

- Alcohol use disorder (AUD) is diagnosed when a patient's drinking causes distress or harm
- The fifth edition of DSM–5 integrates the two DSM–IV disorders—alcohol abuse and alcohol dependence—into a single disorder called alcohol use disorder, or AUD, with mild, moderate, and severe subclassifications
- There are 11 criteria, and a person who meets two of them within a 12-month period is diagnosed with AUD

Background

- Alcohol affects neurotransmitters causing depression of major brain functions (eg, mood, cognition, attention, concentration, insight, judgment, memory, affect)
- Is dose-dependent and ranges from lethargy, unconsciousness, coma, respiratory distress, to death

Physiologic Effects of Use

- Warning signs of alcohol use disorder: Frequent drinking sprees, increased intake, drinking alone or in the early morning, blackouts
- Intoxication: State in which coordination or speech is impaired and behavior is altered
- Episodic excessive drinking: Becoming intoxicated as infrequently as four times a year; episodes may vary in length from hours to days or weeks; may be called binge drinking
- Habitual excessive drinking: Becoming intoxicated more than 12 times a year or being recognizably under the influence of alcohol more than once a week even though not considered intoxicated
- Defense mechanisms of rationalization and denial are often used
  - Blackouts: may fill in gaps in memory with fabricated information (confabulation)
- Alcohol tolerance and addiction: Cessation of drinking results in signs and symptoms of withdrawal (eg, nausea, vomiting, tremor, paroxysmal sweats, anxiety, agitation, headache, impaired orientation/clouding of sensorium, and tactile, auditory, and visual disturbances) (Fig. 14.1)
- Chronic excessive alcohol consumption leads to multisystem physiologic impairments, including cardiomyopathy, hepatopathy, peripheral neuropathy, blackouts, Wernicke encephalopathy, and Korsakoff syndrome

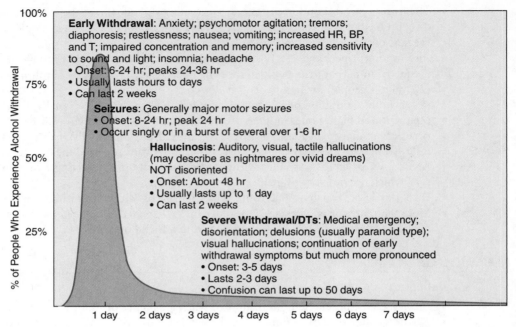

FIG. 14.1 Alcohol withdrawal syndrome. *BP,* Blood pressure; *HR,* heart rate; *T,* temperature. (From Stuart, G. W. [2013]. *Principles and practice of psychiatric nursing* [10th ed.]. St. Louis, MO: Mosby.)

- Alcohol withdrawal delirium: Occurs on days 2 and 3 but may appear as late as 14 days after the last drink or a significant reduction in use; confusion, disorientation, hallucinations, tachycardia, hypertension/hypotension, tremors, agitation, diaphoresis, fever, and seizures
- In most people, moderate to heavy consumption of alcohol can produce euphoria, labile mood, decreased impulse control, and increased social confidence (eg, getting high); such symptoms may appear "hypomanic;" these are often followed the next day with mild fatigue, nausea, and dysphoria (ie, a hangover)
- In the case of addiction to alcohol, the person generally continues to drink, and the subsequent labile mood and lowered impulse control can lead to increased rates of violence toward self and others and may result in suicide
- When those in good health use alcohol sparingly, any changes in body function that occur are usually reversible; likewise, some data reveal that alcohol under certain circumstances has beneficial effects
- When alcohol consumption exceeds two drinks daily or when those in poor physical health drink, damage to body systems is more rapid and pervasive; any amount of alcohol is considered harmful to developing fetuses, children, adolescents, and those recovering from alcohol addiction; it is also harmful to people who are taking medications that interact adversely with alcohol and for those with certain medical conditions or psychiatric disorders
- The liver metabolizes alcohol—the enzyme alcohol dehydrogenase converts alcohol first to acetaldehyde; then the enzyme aldehyde dehydrogenase converts acetaldehyde to acetate, and alcohol is ultimately metabolized into carbon and water
- Effects on the neurologic system
  - Cellular damage and the loss of brain tissue have been documented as a result of alcohol use; some individuals experience symptoms such as intense anxiety, psychoses, depressed

mood, auditory hallucinations, or paranoia with intoxication after ingesting alcohol; most individuals show a clearing of clouded consciousness within a few hours; those with a previous history of severe alcohol use, brain damage, or trauma remain confused for days or weeks

- Nurses should assess alcohol use in all cases of rapidly developing confusion; assessment is imperative in the case of persons diagnosed with mental disorders so that providers do not confuse an alcoholic delirium with dementia or with a worsening mental disorder such as schizophrenia; temporary or permanent signs of confusion are also associated with the direct effects of alcohol and with specific vitamin deficiencies; Korsakoff syndrome symptoms include a severe form of amnesia that is much more profound than that which usually occurs during early dementia; the person also exhibits an inability to learn new skills; Korsakoff syndrome can progress to Wernicke-Korsakoff syndrome, which occurs as a consequence of a thiamine deficiency after many years of excessive alcohol consumption; symptoms of Wernicke-Korsakoff syndrome related to this condition involve neurologic abnormalities, including inflammatory hemorrhagic degeneration of the brain; it can be fatal

- Marchiafava-Bignami disease also occurs as a result of alcohol use disorder; the identification of this condition was rare before the routine use of neuroimaging; atrophy of the corpus callosum and impaired cerebral blood flow characterize this disease; the acute presentation includes dysarthria, impaired consciousness, tetraparesis, and symptoms of interhemispheric dysregulation

- Alcoholic blackouts (also called *anterograde amnesia*) occur in individuals who have consumed sufficient alcohol such that the substance interferes with the acquisition and storage of new memories in the hippocampus portion of the brain; the information is lost from memory within minutes of its occurrence; about one-third of drinkers report having had at least one alcoholic blackout; the history of a blackout experience probably indicates at least one episode of a rapidly consumed excessive amount of alcohol; if there are no other symptoms of alcohol-related problems, a blackout is not indicative of alcohol addiction; persons who have been alcohol dependent for many years have had blackouts after consuming only a small amount of alcohol; blackouts are frightening and unpleasant, regardless of how long the person has been drinking

- Peripheral neuropathy
  - Peripheral nerve deterioration in both hands and feet result from chronic alcohol intake and thiamine deficiency; peripheral neuropathy occurs in about 10% of alcoholics after years of heavy drinking; symptoms include numbness of the hands and feet that is often bilateral and that is often accompanied by tingling and paresthesias; damage does not always improve with abstinence; ulcerations develop from cooccurring circulatory problems related to alcohol use

- Effects on the liver
  - Alcohol metabolism occurs primarily in the liver; as a result, excessive use of alcohol may cause liver damage; increased alcohol use results in the accumulation of fats and proteins in liver cells, which produces a (usually) reversible condition called *fatty liver;* the inflammation of liver cells along with an elevation of some liver function tests and other signs of alcoholic hepatitis, such as fever, chills, nausea, abdominal pain, and jaundice, result in excess deposits of hyaline and collagen near blood vessels, which signals the early signs of cirrhosis of the liver; as damage progresses, normal blood flow through the liver decreases, dilated veins or varices develop, and fluid seeps from the liver and accumulates in the abdomen as

ascites; as liver failure progresses, cognitive impairment also develops as a result of hepatic encephalopathy

- Effects on the gastrointestinal tract
  - Alcohol is associated with ulcers and gastritis (inflammation of the stomach); alcohol stimulates gastric secretions and promotes the colonization of a bacterium identified in the development of ulcers
  - Inflammation of the pancreas occurs as a result of the blockage of pancreatic ducts along with the simultaneous stimulation of the production of digestive enzymes, resulting in acute or chronic pancreatitis
  - Esophageal varices occur in cases of severe alcoholism and result from impaired liver circulation; these dilated and congested veins sometimes rupture and produce a fatal hemorrhage
  - Alcohol has a profound effect on an individual's metabolism of carbohydrates because it impairs the function of the liver and pancreas to respond normally to insulin; this impairment results in very high or low levels of insulin in the blood and has a negative effect on the control of blood sugar in diabetics
  - Alcohol also interferes with the absorption, storage, and distribution of vitamins such as B1, B6, D, and E; vitamins B2, A, folic acid, and K are often deficient in alcoholics
- Effects on the cardiovascular system
  - Heavy consumption of alcohol increases blood pressure and elevates both low-density lipoprotein cholesterol and triglycerides; these changes increase the risk for myocardial infarction and thrombosis; alcohol at high doses also produces a nonreversible deterioration of the heart muscle; wasting of the heart muscle results in cardiac arrhythmias and congestive heart failure or alcoholic cardiomyopathy; higher levels of alcohol consumption are related to an increased risk for hemorrhagic stroke
- Effects on the immune system
  - Researchers estimate that, for some people, alcohol intake of between four and eight drinks per day decreases the production of white blood cells and interferes with the ability of these cells to get to sites of infection; that amount of alcohol also interferes with red blood cell production, significantly increases the average size of red blood cells (ie, the mean corpuscular volume), and impairs the production and efficiency of clotting factors and platelets; a less-effective immune system contributes to an increased risk of developing infectious and noninfectious disease processes
- Sleep disturbance
  - Alcohol intoxication often interferes with sleep; persons under the influence fall asleep more quickly, but they have depressed levels of rapid eye movement and less stage 4 sleep; interruptions between sleep stages, called *sleep fragmentation*, also occur; although some people say that they use alcohol to fall asleep, alcohol often interrupts their sleep architecture, which means that they do not experience the normal pattern of light and deep sleep; the excitatory neurotransmitter glutamate increases as the initial depressant effect of alcohol wanes, thereby causing irritability and an inability to sleep; glutamate rebound is also responsible for many hangover symptoms
- Hormonal changes occur as a result of heavy alcohol consumption; acute intoxication sometimes results in changes in amounts of prolactin, growth hormone, adrenocorticotropic hormone, and cortisol; it also produces a reduction in parathyroid hormone, which is associated with lowered levels of blood calcium and magnesium; some of these changes result in symptoms of menstrual irregularity, decreased sperm production and motility, decreased ejaculate volume, decreased production of testosterone, and impotence

Therapeutic Interventions

- Should be multifaceted (social and medical); involves psychotherapy (eg, group, family, and individual counseling); efforts should be made to engage the person in the recovery process to increase success
- Severity of AUD determines the amount of supervision needed because withdrawal can cause death
- Self-help groups, such as Alcoholics Anonymous (AA), provide support; it is a very useful intervention to change destructive behaviors
    - Relapse or "falling off the wagon" is a symptom of the disease. As with many other chronic illnesses, addiction is subject to periods of relapse. Helping patients recognize beginning warning signs of relapse is part of the recovery process (this change in emphasis decreases stigma and helps caregivers be less judgmental)
- Pharmacologic therapies (Box 14.2)
    - Benzodiazepines during alcohol withdrawal to help prevent seizures and decrease vital signs
    - Negative conditioning with disulfiram appears to help but can never be given without the client's full knowledge, understanding, and consent; the drug interferes with the metabolism of alcohol and causes significant negative physiologic effects (eg, headache, nausea, dyspnea, flushing) if the person drinks after taking the medication
        - Disulfiram inactivates aldehyde dehydrogenase in a person who carries the normal gene for that enzyme, thereby in effect producing the same situation as in the Asians who have the inactive form of the enzyme
        - Acetaldehyde increases in the blood quickly, and the resulting discomfort serves as an effective deterrent to further drinking
    - Naltrexone (or acamprosate) to help overcome the craving for alcohol and decrease the euphoria of intoxication
    - Thiamine to support neurologic functioning and limit peripheral neuropathies
- Relaxation therapy
- Physical needs must be met because of prolonged malnutrition
- Referral of significant others to self-help groups, such as Al-Anon and Adult Children of Alcoholics, to assist with the understanding of the effects of AUD within families and issues of codependency and enabling

NURSING CARE OF CLIENTS WITH AUD

Assessment/Analysis

- History of alcohol use, problematic use, and dependence from client and family if available (eg, type, amount, and frequency)
- Use of the CAGE (or other) questionnaire:
    - Have you ever felt that you ought to Cut down on your drinking
    - Have people Annoyed you by criticizing your drinking
    - Have you ever felt Guilty about your drinking
    - Have you ever had a drink first thing in the morning (Eye opener) to steady your nerves or get rid of a hangover
- Blood alcohol level (BAL) also called blood alcohol concentration (BAC); people with high tolerance to alcohol will appear less intoxicated despite having elevated blood alcohol levels (Table 14.1)

BOX 14.2 Medication Key Facts

Substance-Related Disorders

Alcohol Dependence

Acamprosate calcium for abstinence and disulfiram as a deterrent to alcohol use and abuse
- Cyclic antidepressants may cause neurotoxicity.
- Monoamine oxidase inhibitors may cause delirium and psychosis with combination use.
- Acamprosate is not recommended for children.
- Herbal considerations: St. John's wort may cause alcohol-like reactions.

Alcohol and Opioid Dependence

Naltrexone (Revia, Trexan, Vivitrol) to work as an adjunct in the treatment of alcohol dependence and opiate addiction by decreasing cravings
- The patient must be drug-free before beginning treatment.

Opioid Dependence

Buprenorphine/naloxone and levomethadyl acetate (LAAM)
- Methadone is a substitute drug for narcotic analgesic dependence therapy and the treatment of severe pain.
- Methadone has a high physical and psychologic dependence liability, and withdrawal symptoms will occur with abrupt discontinuation; discontinuation is tapered.
- Alcohol and other CNS depressants may increase CNS or respiratory depression, and hypotension may cause fatal reactions with high doses.
- Monoamine oxidase inhibitors may produce a severe or sometimes fatal reaction; these should not be used together.
- Children are more prone to experience paradoxic excitement. Naloxone and LAAM are not recommended for children who are younger than 16 years old.
- These medications are not recommended for elderly adults.
- Herbal considerations: Valerian, chamomile, kava kava, and poppy may increase CNS depression.

Nicotine Dependence

Bupropion and varenicline for smoking cessation plus nicotine replacement drugs that are tapered

Other Drugs for the Treatment of Alcoholism

Diazepam, clonazepam for alcohol intoxication or withdrawal, and chlordiazepoxide for alcohol withdrawal and anxiety
- These drugs are contraindicated with acute alcohol intoxication and acute angle-closure glaucoma.
- Abrupt or too-rapid withdrawal may result in pronounced restlessness, irritability, insomnia, and seizures.
- Alcohol and CNS depressants increase CNS depression.
- These medications are not indicated for children who are younger than 6 years old.
- Herbal considerations: Cowslip, kava kava, and valerian may increase CNS depression.

Modified from Fortinash, K. M., & Holoday, P. A. (2012). *Psychiatric mental health nursing* (5th ed.). St. Louis, MO: Mosby.

- Data pertaining to substance addiction and psychiatric impairment
- Client's perception of the problem
- Sleep patterns
- Use of assessment scale to assess withdrawal and evaluate medication used to limit withdrawal symptoms
- Physical and emotional status in relation to nutrition, fluid and electrolytes, and safety
- Factors influencing the client's decision to seek treatment
  - Assessment of last use to anticipate potential withdrawal symptoms

TABLE 14.1 Effects of Blood Alcohol Levels

Blood Alcohol Level	Effect on Body
0.02	Slight mood changes
0.06	Lowered inhibition, impaired judgment, decreased rational decision-making abilities
0.08	Legally drunk, deterioration of reaction time and control
0.15	Impaired balance, movement, and coordination
	Difficulty standing, walking, talking
0.20	Decreased pain and sensation
	Erratic emotions
0.30	Diminished reflexes
	Semiconsciousness
0.40	Loss of consciousness
	Very limited reflexes
	Anesthetic effects
0.50	Death

From Nugent, P. M., Green, J. S., Hellmer Saul, M. A., & Pelikan, P. K. (2012). *Mosby's comprehensive review of nursing for the NCLEX-RN examination* (20th ed.). St Louis, MO: Mosby.

Planning/Implementation

- Supervise and prevent injury; institute seizure precautions during withdrawal
- Monitor for CNS and respiratory depression if intoxicated
- Provide support without criticism or judgment
- Accept the smooth facade presented when approaching the lonely and fearful individual inside
- Administer prescribed medications that support nutritional status and limit signs and symptoms of withdrawal
- Provide support during alcohol withdrawal delirium
- Provide support if hallucinations and illusions occur; stay with client; point out reality
- Monitor visitors because they may supply the client with alcohol
- Encourage increased fluid intake, well-balanced diet, and no caffeine
- Provide a well-controlled, alcohol-free environment; explain unit routines
- Plan a full program of activities but provide for adequate rest; environment should be well lit and quiet
- Avoid attempting to talk client out of the problem or making client feel guilty
- Accept hostility and acting-out behaviors without criticism or retaliation; set appropriate limits if hostility is physical or escalates
- Recognize ambivalence and limit the need for decision making
- Maintain the client's interest in a therapy program
- Provide education on alcohol as a disease with negative effects on physical and mental health
- Refer to an appropriate 12-step group such as AA
- Expect and accept lapses as client is changing a long-term habit; accept failures without judgment or punishment; teach how to handle relapses
- Provide family counseling and refer to self-help groups to address effects of drinking and sobriety on the family

Evaluation/Outcomes

- Recognizes, accepts, and seeks treatment for problem
- Accepts responsibility for problem without blaming others
- Achieves optimal physiologic and nutritional status
- Learns new, more self-preserving coping mechanisms
- Verbalizes feelings and situations that pose increased risk for alcohol use
- Enters into and continues with community-based self-help program
- Maintains abstinence from alcohol and chemical substances
- Demonstrates responsibility in meeting own health care needs

APPLICATION AND REVIEW

1. What should a nurse identify as the **most** important factor in rehabilitation of a client addicted to alcohol?
    1. Motivational readiness or willingness to become motivated
    2. Availability of community resources
    3. Accepting attitude of the client's family
    4. Qualitative level of the client's physical state
2. A client with a history of AUD is diagnosed with Wernicke encephalopathy associated with Korsakoff syndrome. What does the nurse anticipate will be prescribed?
    1. Traditional phenothiazine
    2. Judicious use of antipsychotics
    3. Intramuscular injections (or IV infusion) of thiamine
    4. Oral administration of chlorproMAZINE
3. A client with an alcohol dependence problem asks whether the nurse can see the bugs that are crawling on the bed. What is the nurse's initial reply?
    1. "No, I don't see any bugs."
    2. "I will get rid of them for you."
    3. "I will stay here until you are calmer."
    4. "Those bugs are a part of your sickness."
4. A person in recovery joins AA to help maintain sobriety. What type of group is AA?
    1. Social group
    2. Self-help group
    3. Resocializationgroup
    4. Psychotherapeutic group
5. What should a nurse conclude that a client is doing when making up stories to fill in blank spaces of memory?
    1. Lying
    2. Denying
    3. Rationalizing
    4. Confabulating
6. A nurse uses the CAGE Screening Test for Alcoholism to determine the potential an individual has for a drinking problem. Which is one of the four questions included in this test?
    1. "Do you feel you are a normal drinker?"
    2. "Have you ever felt bad or guilty about your drinking?"
    3. "Are you always able to stop drinking when you want to?"
    4. "How often did you have a drink containing alcohol in the past year?"
7. A client in a detoxification unit has an alcohol withdrawal seizure. Diazepam 7.5 mg intramuscularly (IM) stat is prescribed. It is available 5 mg/mL. How many mL should the nurse administer? **Record your answer using one decimal place.**
    Answer: _____ mL

8. While a client is attending an AA meeting, a nurse talks with the client's spouse about the purpose of AA. What is the priority goal of this self-help group?
   1. Change destructive behavior.
   2. Develop functional relationships.
   3. Identify how they present themselves to others.
   4. Understand their patterns of interacting within the group.

9. A client who has just begun attending AA asks a nurse how important it is to attend meetings regularly. What is the nurse's **best** response?
   1. "It's really important if you want to get well."
   2. "It's your decision about whether or not you want to attend."
   3. "Do you think that attending these meetings may not be helpful?"
   4. "Do you feel that it's not worth the effort to keep on attending meetings?"

10. Clients addicted to alcohol often use the defense mechanism of denial. What is the reason why this defense is so often used?
    1. Reduces their feelings of guilt
    2. Creates the appearance of independence
    3. Helps them live up to others' expectations
    4. Makes them look better in the eyes of others

11. A client is admitted to the hospital for acute pancreatitis. The nurse obtains the client's vital signs, performs a physical assessment, and reviews the client's health history. What is the **priority** action by the nurse?

    > **Client Chart**
    > **Vital signs on admission:** T—97.9° F; P—88 beats per minute; R—16 breaths per minute, normal depth; BP—136/88
    > **Health history:** Type 2 diabetes diagnosed 1 year ago; smokes 1 pack daily for 40 years; states the consumption of 5 alcoholic beverages per day for 30 years; divorced for 4 months; laboratory results indicate anemia and leukocytopenia
    > **Physical assessment:** T—99.9° F; P—118 beats per minute; R—24 breaths per minute, shallow; BP—148/96; restlessness and agitation

    1. Reduce environmental stimuli.
    2. Place the client on constant observation.
    3. Assess for alcohol withdrawal symptoms.
    4. Continue to monitor the client's vital signs.

12. What behavior by a client with a long history of AUD is an indication that the client may be ready for treatment?
    1. Drinking only socially
    2. Not drinking for a week
    3. Hospitalization for detoxification
    4. Verbalizing an honest desire for help

13. A nurse is interviewing a client newly admitted to an outpatient program after withdrawal from alcohol. What behavior best indicates that the client has accepted that drinking is a problem?
    1. Participates in scheduled counseling sessions
    2. Attends AA meetings daily
    3. Volunteers to be a sponsor for another alcoholic
    4. Apologizes to family members for causing distress

14. A nurse is discussing AA with a client. What behavior expected of members of AA should the nurse include in the discussion?
    1. Speaking aloud at weekly meetings
    2. Promising to attend at least 12 meetings yearly
    3. Maintaining controlled drinking after 6 months
    4. Acknowledging an inability to control the problem

15. A nurse discusses the philosophy of AA with the client who has a history of AUD. What need must self-help groups such as AA meet to be successful?
1. Trust
2. Growth
3. Belonging
4. Independence

See Answers on pages 266-270.

SUBSTANCE USE DISORDERS

Background

- Misuse of drugs, usually by self-administration, in such a way as to bring about physical, emotional, or behavioral changes and a blurring of reality
- In addition to illegal drugs, many prescription drugs, such as narcotic analgesics and antianxiety agents, may be misused
- Addictive capacity depends on the drug, from lowest potential to highest potential (eg, progressing from codeine, alcohol, and barbiturates to heroin); concurrent use of multiple drugs (polysubstance use) including alcohol

Behavioral/Clinical Findings

- Physical examination reflects type of drug used and route of delivery
- Job or academic failure; marital conflicts; poor reality testing; personality change
- History of violent acting out with disregard for human life or suffering
- History of stealing, selling drugs, and prostitution
- Inability to maintain activities of daily living or fulfill role obligations
- Marked tolerance for some drugs, such as opioids and cocaine, with a progressive need for higher doses to achieve desired effect

TYPES OF DRUGS

Depressants

- In addition to alcohol (see previous section), depressants include anxiolytic/hypnotic drugs (barbiturates, sedatives, benzodiazepines), opioids (including heroin), and cannabis
- Central nervous system (CNS) depressants work in different ways, but they all produce drowsy, calming, and sedating effects to help with sleep disorders and symptoms of anxiety; if an individual uses them over a long period, the body develops tolerance because of the brain's adaptive mechanism called *neuroplasticity*; many of these medications are lethal in overdose situations; patients obtain them by prescription or illegally
- Substances that are shorter acting with rapid onset (eg, alprazolam) have higher addictive potential; individuals often take them to reduce subjective unpleasant anxiety or to manage withdrawal symptoms from other drugs (eg, alcohol, cannabis, heroin, methadone, cocaine, amphetamines)
- CNS depressants' (other than alcohol) use, overdose, and withdrawal are similar to that of alcohol
- Anxiolytic/hypnotics include benzodiazepines, carbamates, barbiturates, barbiturate-like hypnotics, prescription sleeping medications, and almost all prescription antianxiety medications (*except* a nonbenzodiazepine antianxiety agent such as buspirone), and anticonvulsants
  - Carbamates include medications such as meprobamate and tybamate, which are not common in the U.S. but are lethal when taken in overdose amounts; the carbamates also seem to have a higher potential for addiction

- The names of barbiturates all end in -al in the U.S. (eg, phenobarbital, secobarbital)
  - Withdrawal from barbiturates can cause death because of a rebound effect on physiology, causing convulsions and delirium
- Barbiturate-like hypnotics include medications such as ethchlorvynol and glutethimide; hypnotics also includes chloral hydrate
- Benzodiazepines include flurazepam, temazepam, triazolam, chlordiazepoxide, diazepam, lorazepam, clonazepam, and alprazolam
  - Benzodiazepines are relatively safe with regard to the potential for overdose compared with most other types of sedatives and hypnotics
  - When they are used in high doses, benzodiazepines disturb sleep patterns and cause changes in affect
  - Withdrawal from benzodiazepines is lengthy, and the rapid discontinuation after the habitual use of large amounts often causes seizures
  - Midazolam is a popular benzodiazepine that is used for anesthesia induction
- Flunitrazepam is a benzodiazepine that is illegal in the U.S., although it is used in more than 60 countries for sedation, the treatment of insomnia, and as a preoperative anesthetic; it is tasteless and odorless, and it dissolves easily in carbonated beverages, creating a blue hue that can be disguised in dark-colored liquid; when it is used as a drug of abuse, alcohol accelerates its toxic and sedative effects; flunitrazepam causes anterograde amnesia or blackouts; when it is used to victimize others, such as in cases of sexual assault or date rape, as little as 1 mg will impair a person for 8 to 12 hours
- γ-Hydroxybutyric acid (GHB) is an illegal CNS depressant that relaxes or sedates the user; individuals often use it in combination with alcohol, and it is known as a *designer drug*
  - It has been involved in date rapes, poisonings, overdoses, and deaths
  - Individuals use GHB either for its intoxicating, sedative, or euphoria-producing properties or for its growth-hormone–releasing effects, which build muscles
  - The effects last up to 4 hours, depending on the dose
  - In high doses, GHB depresses respirations and heart rates until death occurs
  - Overdose occurs quickly, with nausea, vomiting, headache, and loss of consciousness and reflexes
  - The body metabolizes GHB rapidly, so the drug is difficult to detect in emergency departments
- Opioids include morphine, heroin, oxycodone, hydrocodone, hydromorphone, fentanyl, meperidine, and methadone propoxyphene
  - Opioids are anesthetic agents, antidiarrheal agents, cough suppressants, and pain relievers
  - Heroin is the most widely abused opiate alkaloid; oxycodone misuse is rampant; these pills can be dissolved and injected intravenously, or they may be crushed and snorted or swallowed
  - Those with opioid SUDs have lives that center on acquiring and using drugs; individuals who are dependent on morphine and heroin consume huge amounts (as much as 5000 mg) of the drug each day; fatal overdose is not unusual, and it is often caused by mistakes involving the strength of the drug or the quantity required for the desired effect
  - Physiologic effects: Constricted pupils, drowsiness, euphoria (followed by apathy and dysphoria), slurred speech, psychomotor retardation; needle marks (track marks), particularly on limbs or between toes, which can lead to infections (eg, endocarditis, hepatitis, or human immunodeficiency virus [HIV]); users may wear long-sleeved shirts, even in warm weather; cognitive changes such as drowsiness, coma, and slurred speech are also evident; signs of opioid intoxication include maladaptive behavioral or psychologic changes such as impaired judgment and functioning, which develop during or shortly after use

- Overdose: Respiratory depression, bradycardia, death
- Withdrawal: anxiety, yawning, lacrimation, rhinorrhea, and perspiration; pronounced depression; pupillary dilation; severe abdominal cramps, goose flesh (piloerection), muscle and bone pain, nausea and vomiting if too much time has elapsed between doses
- Drugs that support abstinence: Vivitrol and Subutex
- Because opioids are pain-numbing analgesic drugs, individuals who use them routinely may be unaware of their own serious health problems
  - Intravenous drug users are at risk for subacute bacterial endocarditis and other circulatory compromise created by foreign substances introduced during the process of intravenous use
  - Infection with methicillin-resistant *Staphylococcus aureus* is endemic among intravenous drug users
  - Rates of HIV, HBV and HCV (hepatitis) are also increased
  - Regardless of the setting, nurses need to ask about intravenous drug use whenever a patient presents with fever of unexplained origin
- Cannabis: Marijuana, hashish
  - Marijuana is one of the most widely used drugs; though still considered illegal by the federal government, marijuana is legalized in certain U.S. states
    - Cannabis, the bioactive substance that is extracted from the plant, remains the world's most commonly used illicit drug; it ranks fourth in the world after caffeine, nicotine, and alcohol
    - The active ingredient in these substances is THC, which produces most of the effects that lead to continued use; hashish contains about 10% THC, whereas most marijuana purchased on the street contains from 1% to 5% THC; some forms available today contain up to 40% THC
  - Physiologic effects: Euphoria, anxiety, paranoia, restlessness, talkativeness, increased appetite
    - Symptoms of intoxication vary and include a "high" feeling of euphoria accompanied by inappropriate laughter; feelings of grandiosity, sedation, lethargy, and impaired cognition; distorted sensory perceptions; impaired motor skills and performance; and a sensation of prolonged time sequences
    - The psychoactive effects are followed by other signs within 2 hours of use such as conjunctival injection (ie, bloodshot eye appearance), increased appetite, tachycardia, and dry mouth; if the individual smokes cannabis, the effects develop within minutes and usually last 3 to 4 hours
    - The intensity of symptoms is related to several factors that include the dose, the method of ingestion, and the individual characteristics of the user
  - Overdose: Hallucinations
  - Withdrawal: Restlessness, irritability, decreased appetite, insomnia
  - Individuals smoke cannabis in cigarettes or pipes, although some ingest it in food; others combine it with other drugs such as opium, cocaine, and PCP; cannabis is fat soluble, and high-dose effects sometimes persist for 12 to 24 hours as the drug is released from the tissues; dependence and tolerance can develop over time
  - The federal government declared cannabis to be a schedule I drug (Box 14.3); however, many states have medically legalized its use, and others are debating legislation; the use of cannabis is endorsed for medical conditions, including chronic pain, neurodegenerative and neuromuscular diseases, glaucoma, and many other conditions; ongoing clinical trials are evaluating its use for other medical disorders; the use of any substance has risks, and any misuse of any psychoactive drug is particularly harmful to the developing brain

| BOX 14.3 | United States Drug Enforcement Administration Schedule of Controlled Substances |

Schedule I

Substances in this schedule have no currently accepted medical use in the U.S., a lack of accepted safety for use under medical supervision, and a high potential for abuse.
Examples: Heroin, peyote, methaqualone, marijuana

Schedule II

Substances in this schedule have a high potential for abuse, which may lead to severe psychologic or physical dependence.
Examples: Cocaine, codeine, hydrocodone, methadone, morphine, meperidine

Schedule III

Substances in this schedule have a potential for abuse less than substances in Schedules I or II, and abuse may lead to moderate or low physical dependence or high psychologic dependence.
Examples: Buprenorphine, anabolic steroids, ketamine

Schedule IV

Substances in this schedule have a low potential for abuse relative to substances in Schedule III.
Examples: Alprazolam, diazepam, lorazepam, midazolam, and triazolam

Schedule V

Substances in this schedule have a low potential for abuse relative to substances listed in Schedule IV and consist primarily of preparations containing limited quantities of certain narcotics.
Examples: Only contains cough preparation with codeine up to 200 mg/100 mL, or 100 g and ezogabine.

From the U.S. Drug Enforcement Administration. (2017). *Controlled substance schedules.* https://www.deadiversion. usdoj.gov/schedules.

Stimulants

- Stimulants include caffeine, nicotine (tobacco), ephedrine, cocaine, amphetamines and amphetamine-like substances, methamphetamine, propanolamine, and attention deficit hyperactivity disorder (ADHD) stimulant medications
  - Physiologic effects: Hypervigilance, increased sexual activity, hyperactivity, dilated pupils, euphoria, anorexia and thirst; snorting leads to nasal septum destruction, hoarseness, and throat infections
  - Overdose: Cardiac dysrhythmias, seizures (stimulants lower the seizure threshold), hypertension, paranoid ideation, psychosis with hallucinations
  - Withdrawal: Marked emotional and physical letdown with progression to severe depression and paranoia
  - Stimulants are popular drugs of abuse because of their effects on the brain; people become addicted to the sense of high energy, alertness, and well-being that these drugs produce; these drugs act centrally, which means that their effect is on the CNS mechanisms that control heart rate and respiration
  - Methamphetamine not only creates an immediate surge in dopamine, but it also blocks the reuptake of dopamine, thereby creating more available neurotransmitter in the synaptic

spaces; the efficiency of this drug to produce a stimulating high is also responsible for the eventual depletion and destruction of the neurons that produce dopamine

- Individuals ingest stimulants orally, intranasally, by smoking, or by injection; "ice" is a very pure form of methamphetamine that individuals smoke to produce an immediate and strong stimulant effect; addiction and misuse of this stimulant have recovered from the damage to dopamine receptors substantially after 9 months of abstinence, but they do not recover from impairments in motor skills and memory
- Stimulants such as methylphenidate and dextroamphetamine are used for the treatment of medical disorders such as narcolepsy, ADHD, and obesity; the effects of the stimulants are similar to those of cocaine, but these drugs do not cause local anesthetic effects; in some instances, individuals take them on a regular schedule, similar to what is done for other medications, even when the drugs are being abused; users sometimes binge and have brief drug-free times; these drugs raise the blood pressure and the body temperature to dangerous levels and elevate the heart and respiration rates; aggressive or violent behavior occurs with high-dose use, and anxiety, paranoia, and psychotic episodes occur with the misuse of and dependence on stimulants
- Caffeine is the most widely consumed psychoactive stimulant in the world. It is a methylxanthine, and so are theobromine (in chocolate) and theophylline; more than 80% of adults in the U.S. consume this substance regularly; caffeine produces a wide variety of symptoms, depending on the individual and the level of consumption; tolerance sometimes develops; caffeine is in many beverages, including coffee, tea, chocolate, sodas, and is an additive in some brands of bottled water; caffeine is also in some medications; some people who ingest large amounts of caffeine develop delirium; the cessation of caffeine use causes withdrawal symptoms, including headaches, but because a person's lifestyle is generally not focused on obtaining and using caffeine, it is not typically considered a drug of abuse; however, it is important to ask mental health patients how much caffeine they take because too much can cause anxiety, and caffeine can interfere with the effects of therapeutic psychoactive drugs
- Nicotine/tobacco
  - There is increased recognition of the need for the treatment of tobacco addiction; individuals with other substance-abuse problems, especially alcohol abuse, are typically heavy smokers, as are people with psychiatric illnesses, including those with dual diagnoses; nicotine can interfere with the effects of therapeutic psychoactive drugs
  - The most likely time for addiction to occur is within a month after having smoked the first cigarette; addiction to nicotine occurs within a relatively short time period and usually after the fifth exposure to the drug
  - Brain activity is intense and widespread in response to the nicotine; the reinforcement of smoking and the desire to continue using nicotine results from increases of dopamine, norepinephrine, epinephrine, and serotonin; the body rapidly absorbs nicotine into the circulation, and it reaches the CNS is less than 15 seconds
  - Nicotine has both stimulant and depressive qualities; smoking is also socially reinforcing for some individuals, particularly youth; the body metabolizes nicotine at variable times, which is why some people need cigarettes often but can also go quite some time without nicotine
  - Zyban, varenicline, and nicotine replacement agents are additional pharmacological treatment of withdrawal
- Cocaine is an alkaloid stimulant that is similar in clinical pattern, intoxication, and treatment approaches to that of other stimulants; cocaine is sold on the street as an impure powder that is mixed with glucose, mannitol, or lactose; individuals usually inject the

powder intravenously or snort it nasally; individuals often sprinkle freebase cocaine (which has a lower melting point) over tobacco or smoke it in pipes designed for that purpose; the crystallized form of cocaine, also called crack, has a relatively low melting point, and it is readily soluble in water; freebase or crack cocaine is usually 40% or more pure cocaine, whereas powdered cocaine is less pure; intranasal use has a time to onset of about 3 to 5 minutes, with peak effects occurring in 10 to 20 minutes; the high begins to fade in 45 minutes or less; intravenous use gives a high that lasts 10 to 20 minutes or less; peak blood levels usually develop quickly, within 5 to 30 minutes; the cocaine effects disappear relatively quickly over 2 hours, although some effect will remain for about 4 hours; traces of cocaine are in the urine for at least 3 days, and they may be in the urine for up to 14 days if high doses were used; as with all drugs with high abuse potential, tolerance develops quickly

- Changes, such as euphoria, affective blunting, hypervigilance, agitation, anger, impaired judgment and social functioning, and anxiety, characterize cocaine intoxication; depressant effects, such as sadness, decreased blood pressure, and psychomotor retardation, occur with long-term, high-dose use; the course of intoxication is usually self-limiting to approximately 24 hours, after which withdrawal symptoms occur
- Withdrawal symptoms are often referred to as the *crash*, when the person is depressed and has a potential for suicide; this stimulates a repeat cycle of use, withdrawal, and using again; paranoia is a symptom of withdrawal

Hallucinogens

- Hallucinogens: Lysergic acid diethylamide (LSD), phencyclidine (PCP), mescaline
  - Physiologic effects: Euphoria, visual hallucinations, disorientation, tachycardia, anxiety, dilated pupils, paranoia, impaired judgment, and alterations in time perception
  - Extreme use: Agitation, psychosis, violence, seizures
  - Withdrawal: No symptoms; however, flashbacks of hallucinations and other symptoms of use can occur even after periods of abstinence
  - Many different compounds are included in the class hallucinogens; they alter perception, cognition, and mood; LSD, which is one of the primary drugs in this class, was discovered in 1943; the widespread use of this semisynthetic drug, which was developed by the military for possible use as a chemical warfare agent, led to the widespread use and abuse of hallucinogenic drugs; these drugs were made more cheaply and distributed more easily than the botanical versions such as psilocybin mushrooms and mescaline (peyote cacti); LSD is illegal, but it is available in various forms
  - Other drugs in this class include: 3,4-methylene-dioxymethamphetamine (MDMA; also called *ecstasy*); 3,4-methylenedioxyamphetamine (MDA); and 3,4-methylenedioxy-n-ethylamphetamine (MDEA); these are considered "club drugs" or "designer drugs," and they are neurotoxic; individuals usually take MDA and MDMA orally; the effects of these drugs last between 3 and 6 hours, although confusion, depression, sleep problems, and paranoia often last for weeks
    - The use of MDA and MDMA sometimes results in death caused by neurotoxicity or serotonin syndrome; symptoms include drug-induced anxiety or panic, hyponatremia, and hyperthermia (ie, oral temperatures of greater than 103°F); autopsies show signs of rapid muscle destruction with massive hepatic necrosis, kidney failure, and heat stroke; ecstasy causes neurons to release serotonin, which leads to euphoria; some individuals couple the use of ecstasy with the use of antidepressants that block the reuptake of serotonin from the synaptic space, thereby creating a substantial increase of serotonin in

the brain; this can result in a potentially fatal condition called *serotonin syndrome;* individuals manufacture hallucinogenic drugs illegally in unregulated labs, so purchasers are never certain about the substances that they are ingesting; an analysis of ecstasy has yielded amphetamines, ketamines, and other substances

- Clinical symptoms of hallucinogen use include altered vital signs, panic attacks, flashbacks (ie, the unwanted recurrence of drug effects), psychosis, delirium, altered moods, and states of anxiety; tolerance and addiction occur occasionally
- Hallucinogens are different from other drugs of abuse in that the cessation of use after long-term use does not result in a distinct withdrawal syndrome
- Hallucinogens also place a person at higher risk for suicide and trigger psychiatric disorders after as little as one dose
- Dissociative drugs (ketamine, PCP, DXM, salvia divinorum)
  - Cause their effects by disrupting the actions of the brain chemical glutamate at certain types of receptors—called N-methyl-D-aspartate (NMDA) receptors—on nerve cells throughout the brain; glutamate plays a major role in cognition (including learning and memory), emotion, and the perception of pain (the latter via activation of pain-regulating cells outside of the brain); PCP also alters the actions of dopamine, a neurotransmitter responsible for the euphoria and "rush" associated with many abused drugs
  - Physiologic effects: Numbness, disorientation, confusion, loss of coordination; dizziness, nausea, vomiting; changes in sensory perceptions; hallucinations; feelings of detachment from self and environment; increase in blood pressure, heart rate, respiration, and body temperature; PCP use makes user impervious to pain
  - Extreme use: Hallucinations, memory loss, physical distress (dangerous changes in blood pressure, heart rate, respiration, and body temperature), marked psychologic distress (feelings of extreme panic, fear, anxiety, paranoia, invulnerability, exaggerated strength, and aggression)
  - Use with high doses of alcohol or other central nervous system depressants can lead to respiratory distress or arrest, resulting in death
  - In addition to these general effects, different dissociative drugs can produce a variety of distinct and dangerous effects; eg, at moderate to high doses, PCP can cause a user to have seizures or severe muscle contractions, become aggressive or violent, or even experience psychotic symptoms similar to schizophrenia; at moderate to high doses, ketamine can cause sedation, immobility, and amnesia; at high doses, ketamine users also report experiencing terrifying feelings of almost complete sensory detachment likened to a near-death experience (called a "K-hole," similar to a bad LSD trip); salvia users report intense but short-lived effects—up to 30 minutes—including emotional mood swings ranging from sadness to uncontrolled laughter
  - DXM, which is safe and effective as a cough suppressant and expectorant when used at recommended doses (typically 15–30 milligrams), can lead to serious side effects when misused; eg, use of DXM at doses from 200 to 1500 milligrams can produce dissociative effects similar to PCP and ketamine and increase the risk of serious central nervous system and cardiovascular effects such as respiratory distress, seizures, and increased heart rate from the antihistamines found in cough medicines
  - *Salvia divinorum* works differently; although classified as a dissociative drug, salvia causes its effects by activating the kappa opioid receptor on nerve cells; these receptors differ from those activated by the more commonly known opioids such as heroin and morphine
  - Repeated use of PCP can lead to tolerance and the development of a substance use disorder that includes a withdrawal syndrome (including craving for the drug,

headaches, and sweating) when drug use is stopped; other effects of long-term PCP use include persistent speech difficulties, memory loss, depression, suicidal thoughts, anxiety, and social withdrawal that may persist for a year or more after chronic use stops

- Inhalants: Aromatic hydrocarbons found in aerosol propellants, solvents, glues
- Physiologic effects: apathy; aggressiveness; lethargy; ataxia; euphoria; dizziness; irritation of eyes, nose, throat, and lungs; liver damage; neurotoxic effects
- Extreme use: Depressed reflexes, respiratory compromise, coma
- Withdrawal: No symptoms
- These substances are cheap and easily accessible; inhalants fall into three categories:
  - Solvents (eg, paint thinners, degreasers, gasoline, glues) include toluene, gasoline, ketones, chlorofluorocarbons, and others
  - Gases (eg, refrigerant gases and aerosol gases for whipping cream, spray paints, hair or deodorant sprays, and fabric protectors) include ether, chloroform, nitrous oxide (sold as "poppers"), butane, propane, gasoline, ketones, chlorofluorocarbons, ethyl chloride, and others; a common method of ingestion is the use of "whippets," which are balloons that are filled with an inhalant; the contents of these balloons are breathed in for intoxicating effects
  - Nitrites (eg, aliphatic nitrites, including cyclohexyl nitrite, amyl nitrite, and butyl nitrite [now illegal])
- Inhalants cause effects similar to those of anesthesia, and they slow body functions; depending on the dose, users experience slight stimulation, decreased inhibition, or loss of consciousness; sniffing high concentrations induces heart failure, suffocation, and death; other irreversible effects include hearing loss, peripheral neuropathies or limb spasms, CNS damage, and bone marrow damage; reversible effects include liver and kidney impairment and blood oxygen depletion; long-term use leads to diffuse abnormalities in white brain matter
- Anabolic androgenic steroids
  - Manufactured substances related to male sex hormones; the term *anabolic* refers to muscle building, and *androgenic* refers to increased masculine characteristics
    - Individuals take anabolic steroids orally or by injection, usually in cycles of weeks or months rather than continuously; this type of schedule, called *cycling,* involves taking multiple doses of anabolic steroids over a specific period of time, stopping for a time, and then starting again; users also combine several types of steroids to maximize effectiveness and minimize negative effects, called *stacking;* with the process called *pyramiding,* a person starts with low doses of stacked drugs and then gradually increases the doses for 6 to 12 weeks; during the second half of the cycle, the individual gradually reduces the doses to zero
  - Physiologic effects: Muscle hypertrophy, improved athletic performance
    - Physical changes include breast development and genital shrinking in men plus increased risk for prostate cancer, infertility, and reduced sperm count
    - Women experience masculinization of their bodies, as evidenced by the growth of facial hair, male-pattern baldness, changes in the menstrual cycle, enlargement of the clitoris, and a deepened voice
    - Effects on adolescents are changes in growth hormones, which result in arrested physical development; for all individuals, extreme mood swings occur, and these may be accompanied by violent behaviors; depression, paranoid jealousy, delusions, and impaired judgment all occur as a result of anabolic steroid abuse

- Risks:
  - Higher risks for cardiac events and strokes
  - Increased risk of liver problems among those who ingest oral doses

Therapeutic Interventions

- Treatment for drug overdose
  - Opioid antagonists (see Box 14.2)
    - Naloxone, an opioid antagonist, improves respiratory rate, although it may not affect level of consciousness; respiratory depression can recur when the drug is metabolized before the opioid has been metabolized to a safe level
    - This antagonist completely or partially reverses opioid CNS depression and may produce an acute abstinence (withdrawal) syndrome by blocking euphoric and physiologic effects of the opioid
    - All patients who are taking naloxone need to carry a card or wear a metal bracelet stating that they are taking the drug and that, if they are injured, they will not respond to analgesia from narcotics; this information is critical in the event of a traumatic injury, and it is important for emergency personnel to know
    - Opiate antagonists, such as naloxone and naltrexone, block the effects of heroin and other opioids during rehabilitation and overdose; most patients are then tested periodically for the resumption of opioid use; treatment occurs along with other approaches and has varying degrees of success
    - Gastric lavage may be necessary if substance was taken orally within the past several hours
- Treatment for withdrawal symptoms
  - Antidepressants seem to block the "high" from stimulant abuse and diminish the craving for the substance
  - Methodone is used as a substitution drug that is tapered to facilitate a safe withdrawal
  - Clonidine suppresses some opioid withdrawal signs and symptoms and decreases adrenergic excess while opioid receptors return to normal levels
    - Heroin addicts who are first stabilized on methadone before detoxification respond better than those who go directly from heroin to clonidine
    - Clonidine should not be used in those individuals who also misuse alcohol or those who have unstable psychiatric or cardiovascular conditions
- Methadone maintenance for opioid addiction: Programs change the addiction from an illegal drug to a legal drug, which is administered under supervision; has proven successful only in individuals with long-standing addictions
  - Reduction in dosage can cause withdrawal signs and symptoms
  - Withdrawal signs and symptoms begin to develop in 8 hours and may last as long as 2 weeks
  - Approved for treatment of pregnant opioid addicts
  - Levomethadyl acetate is an alternative to methadone; its 3-day effectiveness increases independence; it is an addictive opioid with effects similar to morphine
  - Vivitrol and Subutex are drugs that support abstinence
- High-calorie, high-protein diet with vitamin supplements
- Treatment in groups led by former addicts
- Therapeutic community setting
- Psychotherapy and family therapy on an outpatient basis

- Vocational counseling
- 12 step programs like Narcotics Anonymous

NURSING CARE OF CLIENTS WITH SUBSTANCE USE DISORDER

Assessment/Analysis

- History of drugs being used (eg, types, amount, and frequency) (Box 14.4)
- Urine toxicology screen and HIV and hepatitis testing
- Drug abuse screening test
- History of length and pattern of drug dependence
- Time since last dose was taken
- Physical status of the client or signs and symptoms of drug dependence; nutritional status
- Signs of drug overdose or withdrawal; use of established scales to help with completeness and consistency of assessment
- Degree of difficulty sustaining role in relation to family members, job, school, etc.
- Why client is seeking treatment at this time
- Pending criminal charges
- Potential for violence toward others or self
- Presence of hallucinations, paranoid ideation, depression, and suicide ideation
- Relationship between substance use and psychiatric disorders (known as dual diagnosis)
- Potential for relapse after period of withdrawal

Planning/Implementation

- Maintain drug-free environment when hospitalized
- Keep atmosphere pleasant and cheerful but not overly stimulating
- Contribute to the client's self-confidence, self-respect, and security in a realistic manner; focus on feelings
- Expect and accept evasion, manipulative behavior, and negativism, but require the maintenance of standards of responsibility; set realistic limits
- Accept client without approving the behavior

BOX 14.4 **Drug Categories Considered During an Assessment**

CNS depressants: Alcohol, anxiolytics/hypnotics, GHB, (and alcohol), opioids, cannabis
- Alcohol: Beer, wine, whiskey, gin, etc.
- Opioids: Heroin, codeine, methadone, oxycodone, hydrocodone, and morphine
- Cannabis: Marijuana, pot, and hashish

CNS stimulants: Amphetamines, caffeine, ephedra, diet pills, nicotine, cocaine
- Nicotine: Cigarettes, chewing tobacco, pipe smoking, snuff, etc.
- Cocaine: Crack and freebase

Hallucinogens: LSD, mescaline, PCP, mushrooms, and peyote; MDMA, MDEA, MDA, GHB, flunitrazepam, and ketamine

Inhalants: Solvents (glue, paint, gasolines), aromatic hydrocarbons (aerosols, gases, hair spray), and nitrites

Anabolic androgenic steroids

Synthetics: Meperidine hydrochloride and propoxyphene hydrochloride

Over-the-counter drugs: Antihistamines, cough syrups, sleeping pills, hormones, laxatives, and herbal products

- Do not permit client to become isolated
- Introduce to group activities as soon as possible; evaluate response to group interaction
- Protect client from self and others
- Refer to appropriate 12-step group such as Cocaine Anonymous and Narcotics Anonymous
- Treat physical effects of substance use
- Provide education related to the disease process, health effects, and the recovery process

Evaluation/Outcomes

- Recognizes, accepts, and seeks treatment for problem
- Accepts responsibility for problem without blaming others
- Achieves optimal physiologic and nutritional status
- Learns new, more self-preserving coping mechanisms
- Verbalizes feelings and emotions
- Enters into and continues with community-based self-help program
- Abstains from all mood-altering chemicals

Prognosis

- Individual, environmental, and situational factors influence the recovery process; one of the most prominent factors that leads an individual to recovery is the patient's recognition that substance use has caused or influenced his or her life's problems and interrupted functioning; the recognition of serious problems takes a long time, partially as a result of impaired frontal lobe function in individuals with addiction; treatment professionals refer to the recognition of serious problems as *hitting bottom*, which means that the individual is often without options for basics such as shelter and food or is unwilling to tolerate his or her lifestyle any longer because of its negative consequences
  - Current trends in treatment emphasize strategies like motivational interviewing as ways to help patient see need for treatment (Fig. 14.2)
- The steps that individuals take differ in detail, but ultimately the goal is to change patterns of functioning to maintain sobriety; sobriety is the goal of complete abstention from drugs, alcohol, and addictive behaviors; the patient has to learn how to prevent or minimize relapses

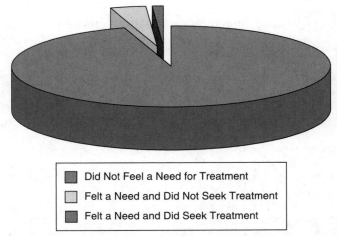

■ Did Not Feel a Need for Treatment

□ Felt a Need and Did Not Seek Treatment

■ Felt a Need and Did Seek Treatment

FIG. 14.2 Perceived need for treatment and effort to receive treatment. (From Keltner, N. L., & Steele, D. [2015]. *Psychiatric nursing* [7th ed.]. St. Louis, MO: Mosby.)

and to get back on course toward achievement and the maintenance of abstinence; *a relapse or slip is not a failure, but an expected part of the recovery process;* addiction is not an intellectual process; some people are intellectually brilliant and still become addicted; addiction is insidious and puzzling; it is a difficult challenge

- During the first year after patients achieve sobriety, they are particularly vulnerable to relapse; individuals with a history of earlier onset of use, higher levels of substance intake, and greater numbers of substance-related problems, who also exhibit a history of tolerance or withdrawal, have a more difficult course of recovery
- Persons diagnosed with serious comorbid mental disorders such as conduct disorders, antisocial personality disorder, untreated major depression, and bipolar disorder are more likely to experience ongoing impairments and, ultimately, a poorer outcome
- A supportive community that includes family and friends—who are often lost during an individual's time of addiction—take time to re-create or replace; recovery groups and their members frequently become the recovering addict's primary social support, at least during the early recovery phases and often for years

APPLICATION AND REVIEW

16. A client who is diagnosed with a polysubstance use disorder is mandated to seek drug and alcohol counseling. What is an appropriate **initial** outcome criterion for this client?
    1. "Verbalizes that a substance use problem exists."
    2. "Discusses the effect of drug use on self and others."
    3. "Explores the use of substances and problematic behaviors."
    4. "Expresses negative feelings about the present life situation."

17. A nurse is caring for a client who is addicted to opioids and who had a major surgery. The client is receiving methadone. What is the purpose of this medication?
    1. Allows symptom-free termination of opioid addiction
    2. Converts opioid use from an illicit to a legally controlled drug
    3. Provides postoperative pain control without causing opioid dependence
    4. Counteracts the depressive effects of long-term opioid use on thoracic muscles

18. A client who is addicted to opioids had emergency surgery. During the postoperative period the health care provider decreases the previously prescribed methadone dose. For what clinical manifestations should a nurse monitor the client?
    1. Constipation and lack of interest in surroundings
    2. Agitation and attempts to escape from the hospital
    3. Skin dryness and scratching under the incision dressing
    4. Lethargy and refusal to participate in therapeutic exercises

19. A client has been receiving oxycodone for moderate pain associated with multiple injuries sustained in a motor vehicle collision. The client has returned three times for refills of the prescription. What behavior, in addition to the client's slurred speech, leads the nurse to suspect opioid intoxication?
    1. Mood lability
    2. Hypervigilance
    3. Constricted pupils
    4. Increased respirations

20. A client is responding within an hour of receiving naloxone to combat respiratory depression from an overdose of heroin. Why should a nurse continue to closely monitor this client's status?
    1. The drug may cause peripheral neuropathy.
    2. Naloxone and heroin when combined can cause cardiac depression.

3. Symptoms of the heroin overdose may return after the naloxone is metabolized.
4. Hyperexcitabilityand amnesia may cause the client to thrash about and become abusive.

21. What is the **primary** nursing concern when caring for a client who is grossly impaired by stimulants?

1. Drowsiness
2. Seizure activity
3. Fluid imbalance
4. Suicidal ideation

22. A client is brought to the emergency department by friends because of increasingly bizarre behavior. Which signs does a nurse identify that indicate the client was using cocaine? **Select all that apply.**

1. Euphoria
2. Agitation
3. Slurred speech
4. Hypervigilance
5. Impaired judgment

23. A client is admitted to the drug detoxification unit for cocaine withdrawal. What is the nurse's **primary** concern when working with clients withdrawing from cocaine?

1. Risk for suicide
2. Potential for seizure
3. Danger of dehydration
4. Probability of injuring others

See Answers on pages 266-270.

ANSWER KEY: REVIEW QUESTION

1. **1 Intrinsic motivation, stimulated from within the learner, is essential if rehabilitation is to be successful. Often clients are most emotionally ready for help when they have "hit bottom." Only then are they motivationally ready to face reality and put forth the necessary energy and effort to change behavior. However, a person can be helped become motivated if willing to do so.**

   2 Availability of community resources is an important factor but not the most important one. 3 Client's family's attitude is an important factor and a helpful one, but not the most important one. 4 The qualitative level of the client's physical state is an important factor but not the most important one.
   Client Need: Psychosocial Integrity; **Cognitive Level:** Comprehension; **Nursing Process:** Assessment/Analysis

2. **3 Thiamine is a coenzyme necessary for the production of energy from glucose. If thiamine is not present in adequate amounts, nerve activity is diminished and damage or degeneration of myelin sheaths occurs.**

   1 A traditional phenothiazine is a neuroleptic antipsychotic that should not be prescribed because it is hepatotoxic. 2 Antipsychotics are avoided; the use of these has a higher risk for toxic side effects in older or debilitated persons. 4 ChlorproMAZINE, a neuroleptic, will not be used because it is severely toxic to the liver.
   Client Need: Pharmacologic and Parenteral Therapies; **Cognitive Level:** Application; **Nursing Process:** Planning/Implementation

3. **1 Stating "No, I don't see any bugs" presents reality and answers the client's question.**

   2 Stating "I will get rid of them for you" is entering into the misperception of reality. 3 Stating "I will stay here until you are calmer" is an intervention that provides comfort and may reduce anxiety, but it should follow the priority intervention of pointing out reality. 4 Stating "Those bugs are a part of your sickness" is an intervention that provides comfort and may reduce anxiety, but it should follow the priority intervention of pointing out reality.
   Client Need: Psychosocial Integrity; **Cognitive Level:** Application; **Integrated Process:** Communication/Documentation; **Nursing Process:** Planning/Implementation

4. **2 Alcoholics Anonymous is a self-help group of individuals who meet together to attain and maintain sobriety.**

   1 A social group centers on building interpersonal relationships through participation in mutual activities. 3 A resocialization group centers on increasing social skills that may be diminished or lacking.

4 A psychotherapeutic group treats mental and emotional disorders by psychologic techniques and always has a member of the health care profession as its group leader.
Client Need: Psychosocial Integrity; **Cognitive Level:** Knowledge; **Nursing Process:** Planning/Implementation

5. **4 The individual is unaware of gaps in memory and therefore uses stories (confabulations) in an attempt to deny or cover up the gaps.**
1 Lying is a deliberate attempt to deceive rather than a face-saving device for loss of memory. **2** Denying is blocking out of conscious awareness rather than a cover-up for loss of memory. **3** Rationalizing is used to explain and justify the behavior rather than to cover up the loss of memory.
Client Need: Psychosocial Integrity; **Cognitive Level:** Comprehension; **Nursing Process:** Assessment/Analysis

> **Memory Aid:** Relate "fib" (to lie) and "fab" to recall that con*fab*ulation is making up stories; con*fib*ulation is misspelled, but writing it that way may help you recall the meaning.

6. **2 The CAGE screening test for alcoholism contains four questions, corresponding to the letters CAGE: C—Have you ever felt you ought to Cut down on your drinking? A—Have people Annoyed you by criticizing your drinking? G—Have you ever felt bad or Guilty about your drinking? E—Have you ever had a drink first thing in the morning (as an "Eye-opener") to steady your nerves or get rid of a hangover?**
1 "Do you feel you are a normal drinker?" is 1 of the 26 questions on the Michigan Alcohol Screening Test (MAST). **3** "Are you always able to stop drinking when you want to?" is 1 of the 26 questions on the Michigan Alcohol Screening Test (MAST). **4** How often did you have a drink containing alcohol in the past year?" is 1 of the 10 questions on the Alcohol Use Disorders Identification Test (AUDIT).
Client Need: Psychosocial Integrity; **Cognitive Level:** Comprehension; **Integrated Process:** Communication/Documentation; **Nursing Process:** Assessment/Analysis

7. **Answer: 1.5 mL. Solve for x by using the "Desire over Have" formula of ratio and proportion.**

$$\frac{\text{Desire}}{\text{Have}} \quad \frac{7.5\,\text{mg}}{5\,\text{mg}} = \frac{x\,\text{mL}}{1\,\text{mL}}$$
$$5\,x = 7.5$$
$$x = 7.5 \div 5$$
$$x = 1.5\,\text{mL}$$

Client Need: Pharmacologic and Parenteral Therapies; **Cognitive Level:** Application; **Nursing Process:** Planning/Implementation

8. **1 The purpose of a self-help group is for individuals to develop their strengths and new, constructive patterns of coping.**
2 Developing functional relationships is just one of the purposes of group therapy. **3** Identifying how they present themselves to others is just one of the purposes of group therapy. **4** Understanding their patterns of interacting within the group is just one of the purposes of group therapy.
Client Need: Psychosocial Integrity; **Cognitive Level:** Comprehension; **Integrated Process:** Communication/Documentation; **Nursing Process:** Planning/Implementation

9. **3 The statement "Do you think that attending these meetings may not be helpful?" reflects the underlying theme in the client's statement and nonjudgmentally encourages the client to verbalize further.**
1 The statement "It's really important if you want to get well" is a judgmental response that may cut off further communication. **2** Although "It's your decision about whether or not you want to attend" is a true statement, it does not promote further communication, nor does it promote continued attendance. **4** The question "Do you feel that it's not worth the effort to keep on attending meetings?" is an inaccurate conclusion based on incomplete information; also, it is judgmental and may cut off further communication.

Client Need: Psychosocial Integrity; **Cognitive Level:** Application; **Integrated Process:** Communication/Documentation; **Nursing Process:** Planning/Implementation

10. **1 These clients often use denial as a defense against feelings of guilt; this will reduce anxiety and protect the self.**

2 Denial may make a client seem more stable to others, not independent. **3** Denial deals more with a client's own expectations. **4** Making them look better in the eyes of others may be part of the reason, but the bigger motivating factor is to decrease guilt feelings.

Client Need: Psychosocial Integrity; **Cognitive Level:** Comprehension; **Nursing Process:** Assessment/Analysis

11. **3 Alcohol, a depressant, will result in rebound agitation with elevated vital signs when there is acute abstinence. A further assessment is indicated, and then the health care provider should be notified of the client's status.**

1 Although reducing environmental stimuli may be done eventually, reducing environmental stimuli is an insufficient initial intervention. **2** Although placing the client on constant observation may be done eventually, constant observation is an insufficient initial intervention. **4** Although continuing to monitor the client's vital signs may be done eventually, monitoring the client is an insufficient initial intervention in light of the client's elevated vital signs and changing status.

Client Need: Physiological Integrity; **Cognitive Level:** Analysis; **Nursing Process:** Assessment/Analysis

 Memory Aid: (first A-A-A-A): **A**lcohol **A**cute **A**bstinence = **A**gitation

12. **4 When clients with alcohol problems voice a desire for help, it usually signifies they are ready for treatment because they are admitting they have a problem.**

1 Adherence to an alcohol treatment program requires abstinence. **2** Not drinking for a week is too short a time to signal readiness for treatment. **3** Hospitalization alone is not an indication that the client is really ready for treatment, because many factors can influence admission.

Client Need: Psychosocial Integrity; **Cognitive Level:** Application; **Nursing Process:** Assessment/Analysis

13. **2 Attendance at AA meetings on a daily basis usually indicates an acceptance of the problem and a desire for help.**

1 Attendance at counseling sessions is helpful but is not specific to the problem of alcoholism. **3** Clients with alcohol problems should not sponsor other clients until a long period of sobriety is maintained. **4** Clients with alcohol problems may say they are sorry many times but still not take responsibility for their drinking problem.

Client Need: Psychosocial Integrity; **Cognitive Level:** Analysis; **Nursing Process:** Assessment/Analysis

14. **4 A major premise of AA is that to be successful in achieving sobriety, clients with alcohol abuse problems must acknowledge their inability to control their drinking.**

1 There are no rules about speaking at meetings, although members are strongly encouraged to do so. **2** There are no rules of attendance at meetings, although members are strongly encouraged to attend as often as possible. **3** Maintaining controlled drinking after 6 months is not part of AA; AA group strongly supports total abstinence for life.

Client Need: Psychosocial Integrity; **Cognitive Level:** Comprehension; **Nursing Process:** Planning/Implementation

15. **3 Self-help groups are successful because they support a basic human need for acceptance. A feeling of comfort and safety and a sense of belonging may be achieved in a nonjudgmental, supportive, sharing experience with others.**

1 AA may not meet the need for trust. **2** AA may not meet the need for growth. **4** AA meets dependency needs rather than focusing on independence.

Client Need: Psychosocial Integrity; **Cognitive Level:** Application; **Integrated Process:** Caring; **Nursing Process:** Planning/Implementation

16. **1 The client must first acknowledge that a substance abuse problem exists and is creating chaos; verbalizing that a problem exists indicates that the client is not in denial and is demonstrating the first step toward a readiness to change.**

    2 Once a problem is identified, then the numerous ways that drug use has controlled the client's life can be explored. **3** Once a problem is identified, then the client can explore the use of substances and the resulting lifestyle problems. **4** Once a problem is identified, the nurse can assist the client to express and process negative feelings.

    Client Need: Psychosocial Integrity; **Cognitive Level:** Analysis; **Nursing Process:** Evaluation/Outcomes

17. **2 Methadone can be legally dispensed; the strength of this drug is controlled and remains constant from dose to dose, which is uncertain with illicit drugs.**

    1 Methadone is used in the medically supervised withdrawal period to treat physical dependence on opiates; it substitutes a legal for an illegal drug. Methadone may be administered long term to replace illegal opioid use. If methadone treatment is abruptly stopped, there will be withdrawal symptoms. **3** Methadone is a synthetic opioid and can cause dependence; it is used in the treatment of heroin addiction but may be prescribed for people who have chronic pain syndromes. It is not used for acute postoperative pain. **4** Methadone is not known to counteract the depressive effects of long-term opioid use on thoracic muscles.

    Client Need: Pharmacologic and Parenteral Therapies; **Cognitive Level:** Comprehension; **Nursing Process:** Planning/Implementation

18. **2 When methadone is reduced, a craving for opioids may occur, anxiety will increase, agitation will occur, and the client may try to leave the hospital to secure drugs.**

    1 Constipation and lack of interest in surroundings are not related to methadone reduction. **3** Skin dryness and scratching under the incision dressing are not related to methadone reduction. **4** Lethargy and refusal to participate in therapeutic exercises may occur with methadone overdose.

    Client Need: Pharmacologic and Parenteral Therapies; **Cognitive Level:** Application; **Nursing Process:** Evaluation/Outcomes

19. **3 Constricted pupils is a physical response to opioid intoxication; the pupils will dilate with opioid overdose.**

    1 Opioids cause apathy or a depressed, sad mood (dysphoria); lability of mood is associated with the use of anabolic androgenic steroids. **2** Opioids cause drowsiness and psychomotor retardation; alertness is associated with the use of stimulants such as caffeine and amphetamines. **4** Opioids depress the respiratory center of the brain, causing slow, shallow respirations; increases in temperature, pulse, respirations, and blood pressure are associated with cocaine use.

    Client Need: Pharmacologic and Parenteral Therapies; **Cognitive Level:** Application; **Nursing Process:** Assessment/Analysis

20. **3 When naloxone is metabolized and its effects are diminished, the respiratory distress caused by the original drug overdose returns.**

    1 There are no reports of peripheral neuropathy. **2** A combination of these drugs does not cause cardiac depression. **4** There are no reports of hyperexcitability and amnesia.

    Client Need: Pharmacologic and Parenteral Therapies; **Cognitive Level:** Comprehension; **Nursing Process:** Evaluation/Outcomes

21. **2 Stimulants increase the excitatory neurotransmitters (eg, adrenaline and dopamine), which will lower the seizure threshold.**

    1 A person who is under heavy influence of stimulants will be unable to rest and sleep because of stimulation of the sympathetic nervous system. **3** Although dehydration can occur, it is not the priority concern. **4** Suicidality is of greatest concern during stimulant withdrawal, not when grossly impaired by stimulants.

    Client Need: Safety and Infection Control; **Cognitive Level:** Application; **Nursing Process:** Planning/Implementation

Memory Aid: Stimulants can start seizures.

22. **Answers: 1, 2, 4, 5.**
    1 Cocaine is an alkaloid stimulant; euphoria or affective blunting is associated with cocaine intoxication.
    2 Cocaine is an alkaloid stimulant; agitation or anger is associated with cocaine intoxication.
    4 Cocaine is an alkaloid stimulant; hypervigilance is associated with cocaine intoxication. **5** Cocaine is an alkaloid stimulant; impaired judgment and impaired social functioning are associated with cocaine intoxication.
    3 Slurred speech is associated with opioids.
    Client Need: Psychosocial Integrity; **Cognitive Level:** Analysis; **Nursing Process:** Assessment/Analysis

23. **1 The greatest risk in cocaine withdrawal is risk for suicide**
    2 The risk for seizure is increased when under the influence of cocaine, not during withdrawal.
    3 Although dehydration can occur during cocaine use and withdrawal, it is not the priority concern.
    4 People in cocaine withdrawal, although irritable, are more apt to hurt themselves than others.
    Client Need: Safe Effective Care Environment; **Cognitive Level:** Application; **Nursing Process:** Planning/Implementation

Somatic Symptom and Dissociative Disorders $\boxed{15}$

ETIOLOGY

Biologic Theory

- Changes in the structure and function of the brain caused by prolonged stress or trauma can result in a somatic symptom disorder by altering the individual's perceptions and interpretations of bodily functions
- Some persons develop an anxiety disorder and others develop a somatic symptom disorder; many clients experience both
- Somatic symptom disorders may be caused in part by a misinterpreted cortical perception of distress; speculation is that there may be a disruption in the physical sensation signals that are part of the cortical symptom
- Neurotransmitters such as serotonin and norepinephrine are closely involved with depression and anxiety, but they are also known to modulate pain; individuals who experience severe pain generally have abnormal levels of neurotransmitters, particularly serotonin

Behavioral Theory

- Behaviorists believe that some individuals learn to use somatic symptoms to communicate helplessness and to manipulate others
- Attention from others tends to exacerbate somatic symptoms in these individuals
- Nurses and doctors in the U.S. are trained to respond to clients who report pain
    - In DSM-5, *pain disorder* is not a major category in somatic symptom and related disorders, but it is included as part of somatic symptom disorder category

Cognitive Theory

- Cognitive theorists believe that clients with somatic symptoms misinterpret the meaning of body functions and sensations and become overly alarmed by them
- Cognitive therapy is used to help clients reinterpret the meaning of body sensations

Epidemiology

- Somatic symptom disorders tend to run in families
- Somatic symptom disorder
    - Widely variable lifetime prevalence; 1% to 7% of the general population
    - Seen in 5% to 10% of primary care outpatients
    - Occurs in all cultures; up to 60% to 80% of a population may have at least one somatic symptom without a known organic cause
    - Puts individuals at risk for excessive testing and treatment because *organic* causes must be ruled out
- Conversion disorder (Functional neurological symptom disorder)
    - Widely varied prevalence; reported in up to 3% of outpatient referrals to mental health clinics
    - Conversion symptoms identified in 1% to 15% of *general* medicosurgical patients
- Illness anxiety disorder
    - Previously called hypochondriasis; occurs in 4% to 15% of general population

- Factitious disorder
  - Limited information about prevalence, because this disorder generally involves deception, which can be difficult to recognize
  - More common among females than males
    - Munchausen is the most chronic and severe form, in which a person feigns illness or injures oneself to gain sympathy; more common among males
  - Higher prevalence in specialized treatment settings

SOMATIC SYMPTOM AND RELATED DISORDERS

Overview

- DSM-5 categorizes somatic symptom and related disorders under the major headings discussed in this chapter: *Somatic symptom disorder, Illness anxiety disorder, Conversion disorder, and Factitious disorder*
- The unifying characteristic for somatic symptom disorders is that there is no known organic cause

General Nursing Care of Clients Diagnosed with Somatic Symptom and Related Disorders

- The treatment for somatic symptom and related disorders is multidisciplinary and usually involves more than one treatment modality
  - The inpatient treatment of somatic symptom disorders is usually the result of suicidal risk and the failure of treatment in an outpatient setting
  - The nursing role in the treatment of clients diagnosed with somatic symptom and related disorders varies; common to all treatment settings is the nurse's role in client and family education about the disorders and their treatment
  - Nursing care plans for clients with symptoms of somatic symptom disorders reflect the understanding that managing anxiety effectively is part of daily living
  - Nurses actively participate in behavioral interventions that are structured to decrease the somatic responses
- General nursing interventions (Box 15.1) (Table 15.1)
  - Identify when anxiety or depressed mood is translated into physical illness or bodily complaints (somatization)
  - Establish a trusting relationship
  - Provide an environment that limits demands on and permits attention to resolution of conflicts
  - Identify pattern of recurring clinically significant somatic symptoms; accept that symptoms are real to client
  - Attempt to limit client's use of negative defenses, but do not try to stop them until ready to give them up
  - Help develop appropriate ways of managing anxiety-producing situations through problem solving and cognitive therapies
  - Accept physical symptoms but do not talk about, emphasize, or call attention to them
  - Minimize sick-role behavior; encourage independence within abilities; avoid providing secondary gains
  - Encourage to develop a balance between work and relaxation
  - Help identify and label needs met by symptoms

BOX 15.1 Key Nursing Interventions for Somatic Disorders

1. Use a matter-of-fact, caring approach when communicating with clients.
   Rationale: To decrease secondary gains
2. Ask clients how they are feeling, and ask them to describe their feelings.
   Rationale: To increase verbalization about feelings (especially negative ones), needs, and anxiety rather than about somatization
3. Assist clients with developing more appropriate ways to verbalize feelings and needs.
   Rationale: To increase adaptive coping through assertiveness
4. Use positive reinforcement, and set limits by withdrawing attention from clients when they focus on physical complaints or make unreasonable demands.
   Rationale: To decrease complaining behavior
5. Be consistent with clients, and have all requests directed to the primary nurse providing care.
   Rationale: To decrease attention-seeking or manipulative behaviors
6. Use diversion by including clients in milieu activities and recreational games.
   Rationale: To decrease rumination about physical complaints
7. Do not push awareness of or insight into conflicts or problems.
   Rationale: To prevent an increase in anxiety and the need for physical symptoms

From Keltner, N. L., & Steele, D. (2015). *Psychiatric nursing* (7th ed.). St. Louis, MO: Mosby.

TABLE 15.1 Basic Level Interventions for Somatic Symptom Disorders

Intervention	Rationale
Offer explanations and support during diagnostic testing.	Reduces anxiety and rules out organic illness
After physical complaints have been investigated, avoid further reinforcement (eg, do not take vital signs each time client complains of palpitations).	Directs focus away from physical symptoms
Spend time with client at times other than when client summons nurse to voice physical complaint.	Rewards behaviors not related to illness and encourages repetition of desired behavior
Observe and record frequency and intensity of somatic symptoms. (Client or family can give information.)	Establishes a baseline and later enables evaluation of effectiveness of interventions
Do not imply that symptoms are not real.	Acknowledges that psychogenic symptoms are real to the client
Shift focus from somatic complaints to feelings or to neutral topics.	Conveys interest in client as a person rather than in client's symptoms; reduces need to gain attention via symptoms
Assess secondary gains "physical illness" provides for client (eg, attention, increased dependency, and distraction from another problem).	Allows these needs to be met in healthier ways and thus minimizes secondary gains
Use matter-of-fact approach to client exhibiting resistance or covert anger.	Avoids power struggles; demonstrates acceptance of anger and permits discussion of angry feelings

Continued

TABLE 15.1 Basic Level Interventions for Somatic Symptom Disorders—cont'd

Intervention	Rationale
Have client direct all requests to case manager.	Reduces manipulation
Help client look at effect of illness behavior on others.	Encourages insight; can help improve intrafamily relationships
Show concern for client but avoid fostering dependency needs.	Shows respect for client's feelings while minimizing secondary gains from "illness"
Reinforce client's strengths and problem-solving abilities.	Contributes to positive self-esteem; helps client realize that needs can be met without resorting to somatic symptoms
Teach assertive communication.	Provides client with a positive means of getting needs met; reduces feelings of helplessness and need for manipulation
Teach client stress reduction techniques such as meditation, relaxation, and mild physical exercise.	Provides alternate coping strategies; reduces need for medication

Modified from Varcarolis, E. M., & Halter, M. J. (2010). *Psychiatric mental health nursing: A clinical approach* (6th ed.). St. Louis, MO: Saunders.

- Pharmacologic interventions for somatic symptom disorders and factitious disorder are symptom oriented; medications include:
  - Antidepressants, especially SSRIs, for associated depression and for intense focus on somatic concerns
    - SSRIs decrease the client's awareness to body sensations.
  - Antipsychotics for any underlying psychosis

Somatic Symptom Disorder
- Overview
  - Preoccupation with belief that there is a serious illness because of misinterpretation of physical symptoms
  - Can occur across the life span but usually begins in young adulthood
  - Diagnostic evaluation does not support beliefs and does not allay client fears
  - Psychosocial stresses influence development of this disorder
  - Individuals diagnosed with somatic symptom disorder frequently seek and obtain medical treatment for multiple and clinically significant somatic complaints
  - The symptoms have no known source
    - Clients who present with chronic debilitating diseases such as multiple sclerosis or lupus erythematosus *do not have a somatic symptom disorder because their symptoms are caused by their disease process*
    - Clients are not in control of their symptoms; they are involuntary
    - Client expresses emotions by somatizing them into symptoms
  - Nurses in a general hospital or clinical practice setting are more likely to encounter clients diagnosed with a somatic symptom related disorder than those who are working in inpatient psychiatric units

- Behavioral/clinical findings
  - Misinterpretation and exaggeration of physical symptoms
  - Inability to accept reassurance even after exhaustive testing and therapy; leads to "doctor shopping"
  - History of repeated absences from work
  - Adoption of sick role and lifestyle
- Therapeutic interventions: See those listed under Conversion Disorder

NURSING CARE OF CLIENTS DIAGNOSED WITH SOMATIC SYMPTOM DISORDER

Assessment/Analysis

- Level of preoccupation with symptoms
- Duration and degree of impaired functioning associated with symptoms
- History of psychosocial precipitant stressors
- Confirm that symptom is not related to underlying medical condition

Planning/Implementation

- See General Nursing Care of Clients Diagnosed with Somatic Symptom and Related Disorders

Evaluation/Outcomes

- Accepts that there is no physical basis for the symptoms
- Uses more effective coping mechanisms to manage anxiety
- Continues therapy even after condition has improved

Conversion Disorder (Functional Neurological Symptom Disorder)

- Overview
  - Anxiety unconsciously converted to physical symptoms that are not under voluntary control; usually localized to one area of the body; symptoms permit avoidance of an unacceptable activity or stressful situation
  - Symptom or deficit is not related to an underlying medical condition, to substances, or to a cultural norm; distinguishes conversion from other disorders associated with tissue changes
  - Symptoms permit some measure of social adjustment
  - Onset before 30 years of age; may recur
  - Pressures of decision making regarding lifestyle in early adult years may act as precipitating factors
- Behavioral/clinical findings
  - Symptoms or deficits that affect voluntary motor or sensory function (eg, paralysis, blindness, deafness)
    - Symptoms appear to be related to a neurologic or general medical condition; however, they are not caused by a general medical condition or a substance (drugs or medication), nor are they influenced by a culturally approved behavior
    - Symptoms not intentionally produced as in factitious disorder (see Factitious Disorder) and not limited to pain or sexual dysfunction
    - Symptoms cause clinically significant distress or impairment in social, occupational, or other important areas of functioning
    - Common symptoms are blindness, paralysis, deafness, seizures, anesthesia, or abnormal motor movements

- Conflicts or stressors (usually dependence versus independence) precede initiation or exacerbation of symptoms or deficits
  - Psychological factors associated with symptom onset or exacerbation
- Noticeable lack of concern about problem ("la belle indifference") that is inconsistent with the problem
- Impairment may vary over different episodes and may not follow anatomic structure (eg, paralysis or numbness may circle foot or arm [stocking-and-glove anesthesia])
- Therapeutic interventions
  - Complete diagnostic workup to rule out physical problems
  - Psychotherapy, family therapy, group therapy as necessary to resolve severe emotional problems
  - Psychotropic medications: antidepressants (selective serotonin reuptake inhibitors [SSRIs])
- Nursing care of clients diagnosed with conversion (functional neurologic symptom) disorders

Assessment/analysis

- Presence of physical symptoms with no pathophysiologic basis
- Level of concern regarding physical symptoms
- Degree of impairment
- Level of anxiety

Planning/implementation

- See General Nursing Care of Clients Diagnosed with Somatic Symptom and Related Disorders

Evaluation/outcomes

- Uses problem-solving rather than physical symptoms to manage anxiety-producing situations
- Decreases episodes that use physical symptoms to manage anxiety

Illness Anxiety Disorder

- Like somatic symptom disorder, these clients have a preoccupation with belief that there is a serious illness because of misinterpretation of physical symptoms
- If present, *somatic symptoms are mild*
- Diagnostic evaluation does not identify a medical condition
- Client feels anxious about symptoms despite reassurance that they are not reflective of an actual disease
- Behavioral/clinical findings
  - Persistent preoccupation and fixation with belief that there is a serious illness because of misinterpretation of physical symptoms, despite evidence to the contrary
  - Despite reassurances, client's beliefs and anxiety persists to the extent that they interfere with the client's daily functioning
- Therapeutic interventions
  - Same as those listed in Conversion Disorder
- Nursing care of clients diagnosed with illness anxiety disorder
  - See Nursing Care of Clients Diagnosed with Somatic Symptom Disorder

APPLICATION AND REVIEW

1. A nurse considers that, in a conversion (functional neurological symptom) disorder, symptoms such as paralysis or blindness:
   1. Are conscious methods for getting attention
   2. Will subside if the client is helped to focus on getting healthy
   3. Are generally necessary for the client to cope with a stressful situation
   4. Will usually resolve when the client learns to cope with ongoing family conflicts

2. An anxious client reports experiencing pain in the abdomen and feeling empty and hollow. A diagnostic workup reveals no physical causes of these clinical findings. What term best reflects what the client is experiencing?
   1. Dissociation
   2. Somatic symptom disorder
   3. Stress response
   4. Anxiety reaction

3. A client newly diagnosed with a conversion (functional neurological symptom) disorder is manifesting paralysis of a leg. The nurse can expect this client to:
   1. Demonstrate a spread of paralysis to other body parts
   2. Require continuous psychiatric treatment to maintain independent functioning
   3. Recover the use of the affected leg but, under stress, develop similar symptoms again
   4. Follow an unpredictable emotional course in the future, depending on exposure to stress

4. A nurse is caring for a client who has a diagnosis of conversion (functional neurological symptom) disorder with paralysis of the lower extremities. Which is the most therapeutic nursing intervention?
   1. Encouraging the client to try to walk
   2. Explaining to the client that there is nothing wrong
   3. Avoiding focusing on the client's physical symptoms
   4. Helping the client follow through with the physical therapy plan

5. What characteristic uniquely associated with psychophysiologic disorders differentiates them from somatic symptom disorders?
   1. Emotional cause
   2. Feeling of illness
   3. Restriction of activities
   4. Underlying pathophysiology

6. A nurse is caring for a client diagnosed with a somatic symptom disorder. What should the nurse anticipate that this client will do?
   1. Redirect the conversation with the nurse to physical symptoms
   2. Monopolize conversations about the anxiety being experienced
   3. Write down conversations to assist in remembering information
   4. Start a conversation asking the nurse to recommend palliative care

7. A nurse plans care for a client diagnosed with a conversion (functional neurological symptom) disorder based on the understanding that it is:
   1. A physiologic response to stress
   2. A conscious defense against anxiety
   3. An intentional attempt to gain attention
   4. An unconscious means of reducing stress

8. A health care provider refers a 52-year-old male client to the mental health clinic. The history reveals that the man's wife died from colon cancer 6 months ago, and since that time he has seen his health care provider seven times with the concern that he has colon cancer. All tests prove negative. Recently, he has stopped seeing friends, dropped his hobbies, and stayed home to rest. Which disorder should the nurse identify as consistent with the client's preoccupation with the fear of having a serious disease?
   1. Conversion disorder
   2. Somatic symptom disorder
   3. Illness anxiety disorder
   4. Body dysmorphic disorder

9. A client is admitted to the psychiatric unit of the hospital with a diagnosis of conversion (functional neurological symptom) disorder. The client is unable to move either leg. Which finding should the nurse consider consistent with this diagnosis?
   1. Feeling depressed
   2. Appearing composed
   3. Demonstrating free-floating anxiety
   4. Exhibiting tension when discussing symptoms

10. A client is admitted and diagnosed with a conversion (functional neurological symptom) disorder. What is the **primary** nursing intervention?
   1. Talk about the physical problems
   2. Explore ways to verbalize feelings
   3. Explain how stress caused the physical symptoms
   4. Focus on the client's concerns regarding the symptoms

11. A client has a history of a conversion reaction that involves a weakness in the right arm that periodically progresses to paralysis. This client is hospitalized on the mental health unit of the local community hospital. While listening to instructions for a group project, the client experiences a feeling of weakness and is unable to move the right arm. After assessing the client, what should the nurse ask?
   1. "Exactly when did the weakness begin?"
   2. "Is this similar to what you usually experience?"
   3. "Would you like to leave the group for a while?"
   4. "What emotion were you feeling before you felt the weakness?"

12. A client with a history of stabbing pain in the eyes and blurring and gradual loss of vision is examined by an ophthalmologist, a neurologist, and an internist, all of whom find no organic cause. When eye complaints increase, the client is admitted to a mental health unit. After keeping the patient safe, what is the **priority** nursing intervention?
   1. Encouraging involvement in group activities
   2. Requesting a description of the eye discomfort
   3. Exploring feelings about possible impending blindness
   4. Focusing on daily activities but avoiding discussion of the eye discomfort

13. A client is diagnosed with conversion (functional neurological symptom) disorder. What is a typical characteristic of the client's reaction to the physical symptom?
   1. Anger   3. Anxiety
   2. Apathy   4. Agitation

14. What characteristic of anxiety is associated with a diagnosis of conversion (functional neurological symptom) disorder?
   1. Free floating   3. Consciously felt by the client
   2. Relieved by the symptom 4. Projected onto the environment

See Answers on pages 286–289.

Factitious Disorder

- Overview
  - Falsification of signs and symptoms of a medical disorder in oneself or others
  - Munchausen syndrome: Intentionally causing own illness; this may involve self-mutilation, fever, hemorrhage, hypoglycemia, seizures, nonhealing wounds, and abdominal or back pain
    - Munchausen syndrome by proxy: Parent creates an illness in the child through simulation or production of illness; frequent symptoms include bleeding, seizures, apnea, diarrhea, vomiting, fever, and rash

- No identifiable predisposing factor
- Manipulation of the health care system for personal gain
- Health care knowledge may be used to aid in deception
- Behavioral/clinical findings
  - Physical or psychologic symptoms are intentionally produced or feigned to enable one to assume the sick role and for other secondary gains; reports of back pain and recurrent headaches are most common
  - "Doctor shopping," or seeking treatment in multiple emergency departments; little or no improvement is made in comfort or symptom management after treatment
  - Must be distinguished from a true medical condition through a medical diagnostic workup
  - When under supervision of other caretakers, the child who is abused by Munchausen syndrome by proxy exhibits no symptoms
  - Comorbidity: Some persons also have symptoms of depression, somatic symptom disorder, anxiety, borderline personality disorder, and other disorders
- Therapeutic interventions
  - Psychiatric treatment
  - Supervision of child who is a victim of Munchausen syndrome by proxy
  - Munchausen syndrome by proxy reported to child protective services
- Nursing care of clients diagnosed with factitious disorder

Assessment/Analysis

- Level of preoccupation with symptoms that keep recurring despite treatment
- Absence of symptoms when client is closely observed
- Past and present degree of interference with functioning related to symptoms
- Duration and degree of disability associated with symptoms
- History of psychosocial stressors

Planning/Implementation

- Report suspected Munchausen syndrome by proxy to child protective services
- Recognize negative feelings toward the client; remain nonjudgmental when establishing nurse–client relationship
- Keep lines of communication open and direct; the nurse needs to confront any feelings directed toward the client that are not therapeutic and work to establish a therapeutic relationship
- Supportive, empathetic relationship helps the client change the maladaptive behaviors
- A multidisciplinary team approach of both medical and psychiatric practitioners, with one practitioner responsible for the care of the client, provides consistent comprehensive care and has the greatest success in reducing the symptoms of factitious disorder
- See General Nursing Care for Clients Diagnosed with Somatic Symptom and Related Disorders

Evaluation/Outcomes

- Uses more effective coping mechanisms to cope with anxiety rather than feigning illness
- Accepts need for psychotherapy
- Avoids causing harm to self or others

Dissociative Disorders

- Characterized by a sudden or a gradual disruption in integrated functions of consciousness, memory, identity, or perception of the environment

- May be transient or become a well-established pattern
- Etiologic factors: Related to increased stress or traumatic event(s) such as sexual abuse during childhood
- Types
  - Dissociative identity disorder: Coexistence of two or more distinct personalities within an individual
  - Dissociative amnesia: Inability to recall important personal information, usually of a traumatic or stressful nature, as distinguished from ordinary forgetfulness
  - Depersonalization/derealization disorder: Persistent or recurrent feeling of being detached from one's mental processes or body that is accompanied by intact reality testing
- General behavioral/clinical findings
  - Inability to recall important personal information, usually of a traumatic or stressful nature
  - Gaps in recalling aspects of one's life history, usually related to traumatic episodes
- Therapeutic interventions
  - Complete diagnostic workup to rule out possibility of organic causes (eg, brain tumor)
  - Psychotherapy (eg, individual, family)
  - Development of more effective and satisfying ways to manage anxiety

Dissociative Identity Disorder

- Initially labeled multiple personality disorder and subsequently changed to dissociative identity disorder, which more accurately describes its primary symptoms
- Located in the trauma and stressor category that identifies its origins
- To meet the diagnostic criteria of dissociative identity disorder, the individual must demonstrate two or more distinct identities or personality states, each with its own relatively enduring pattern of perceiving, relating to, and thinking about the environment and the self; also, two of these personality states must recurrently take control of the person's behavior
- The person is unable to recall important personal information to a degree that it is too extensive for ordinary forgetfulness (eg, dissociation)
- These behavior patterns and thoughts are not substance or medically induced, and in children, they are not part of imaginary or fantasy play
- Risk and prognosis for dissociative identity disorder are related to all types of physical and sexual abuse
- Risk for suicide is high, and nurses need to be diligent in their assessing for suicide in all clients diagnosed with symptoms of this disorder
- Comorbidity: A large number of persons diagnosed with dissociative identity disorder present with a coexisting disorder; nurses and other health care personnel should be cognizant of treating the dissociative identity disorder as well as the coexisting disorder, because ignoring it could further damage the client's morale
- Over 70% of individuals diagnosed with dissociative identity disorder have attempted suicide; multiple suicide attempts and other self-injurious behavior are common
- Suicide assessment is difficult due to the amnestic nature of the disorder and the separate identities experienced by the individual
  - An individual may not remember past suicidal behavior, and the present identity may not feel suicidal
  - This complex diagnosis presents a huge challenge for caregivers and family members in preventing self-harm or injury for these individuals

Dissociative Amnesia

- Individuals with dissociative amnesia experience one or more episodes of inability to recall important personal information that is usually stressful or traumatic in nature, and the loss or memory is too extensive for ordinary forgetfulness (eg, dissociation)
  - The disturbance does not occur exclusively during the course of dissociative identity disorder and does not result from the effects of a substance (eg, blackouts or intoxication) or a general medical condition (eg, amnesia after head trauma)
- Prevalence: Dissociative amnesia is seen in all age groups
  - Children are the most challenging to diagnose due to the difficulty they have in understanding questions about amnesia and the close resemblance dissociative amnesia has with other disorders (eg, anxiety, oppositional behavior, learning disabilities, and inattention)
  - It is critical that parents or caregivers ask for feedback from other sources such as teachers, therapists, or nurses
- Risk and prognosis: Dissociative amnesia is associated with experiences such as childhood sexual and physical abuse, war, disaster, genocide, and imprisonment in a concentration camp; the more severe and frequent the abuse, the greater the chance for this disorder to emerge
- Comobidity: A wide variety of affective and mood disturbances are possible, and the nurse needs to diligently conduct a suicide assessment on all clients with symptoms of this disorder

Depersonalization/Derealization Disorder

- Essential features of depersonalization/derealization disorder are persistent or recurrent episodes of feelings of *detachment* or estrangement from one's self, sensations of being outside of one's body or mental processes, or of being an observer on one's body
- Various types of sensory anesthesia, lack of affective response, and a sense of losing control of one's actions or speech are often present
- The individual demonstrates intact reality testing and awareness of the situation
- Depersonalization is a common experience, and the diagnosis is made only if the experience occurs exclusively during the course of another mental disorder (eg, schizophrenia, panic disorder, acute stress disorder, another dissociative disorder) or if it is caused by the physiologic effects of substance use or a general medical condition
- Risk and prognosis: The prognosis varies and ranges from a rapid, complete recovery to episodic and more chronic courses
  - It may reemerge during periods of stress, or during a relapse of substance misuse
  - Clients may be at risk for suicide; therefore the nurse needs to diligently conduct a suicide assessment on all clients with symptoms of this disorder
- Prevalence: Symptoms of this disorder are common in the general population and can last from hours to days in various forms; precise estimates are not available
- Comorbidity: Depressive and anxiety disorder are prevalent with this disorder, with fewer posttraumatic stress disorder (PTSD) and personality disorders observed

Nursing Care of Clients Diagnosed with Dissociative Disorders

- Overview
  - Individuals with this challenging disorder are often treated in an outpatient facility with the use of several different modalities (eg, individual therapy; psychotherapy; group therapy; family therapy; art therapy; and medications as needed)

- Inpatient hospitalization is typically available for only brief periods of time for clients who are at imminent risk of harm to themselves or others or who have debilitating cooccurring illnesses
- The nurse can provide clients and family with information about treatment alternatives and be actively involved in discharge planning

Assessment/Analysis

- Identity, memory, consciousness
- Physical condition
- Psychosocial component to discover fundamental anxiety source
- History of emotional trauma in childhood
- Suicidal risk and self-harm risk
- Recent use of alcohol or drugs
- The nurse needs to rule out neurologic disorders, substance-related disorders, and other co-occurring psychiatric disorders in order to link the symptoms with a dissociative disorder
- The nurse uses several components of the mental status examination (MSE), including the psychosocial and psychiatric history, family history, stressors and losses, childhood history, thoughts, perceptions, and insight (Box 15.2)
- Objective Data: Studies to rule out head trauma and other medical issues
  - Physical examination
  - Electroencephalogram (EEG)
  - Imaging studies (x-rays)

Planning/Implementation

- Assist with treatment plan to alleviate symptoms
- Reinforce effective coping skills
- Assist with problem-solving
- Encourage involvement in individual long-term therapy and family therapy
- General nursing interventions *(with rationale)* (Table 15.2)
  - Identify the degree of suicidal ideation and depressive symptoms for clients diagnosed with dissociative disorder and related disorders; *a thorough evaluation of these clients will help prevent suicide or other destructive behaviors; safety is the highest priority!*
  - Monitor your own level of anxiety or other concerns you may have about working with clients diagnosed with dissociative disorders, and do not be influenced by stories and movies that tend to be overly dramatic; *fear and anxiety are readily transferrable, and clients may not respond openly if they sense that the nurse is uncomfortable*
  - Recognize the client's heightened anxiety, the emergence of a panic attack, or a dissociative state, and help the client identify triggers that provoke these states; *identifying triggers that provoke anxiety and dissociative states can help prevent or reduce them*
  - Promote stress and anxiety reducing exercises such as Mindfulness Meditation, Progressive Relaxation, or slow deep breathing techniques; *these exercises help reduce stress and anxiety and provide relief and comfort for the client*
  - Engage the client in brief individualized interactions; *individual interactions at appropriate intervals help reduce or manage episodes of anxiety, impulsivity, panic, or dissociation that may occur at different times throughout the day*
- Client and family teaching guidelines for dissociative identity disorders
  - Educate the client and family about the importance of identifying environmental cues or words that may trigger the client's dissociative behaviors

| **BOX 15.2** | Assessment Questions for Possible Dissociative Disorder |

"What kinds of symptoms do you have that brought you to the hospital?"
"Have you had any stressors in your life in the past, or recently?"
"Please describe those stressors as best you can."
"When did you first notice you were having problems?"
"Do you consider yourself different now from the way you were before your problem?"
"How would you describe those differences?"
"Have you ever been diagnosed with a mental illness before?"
"Have you ever had a problem with alcohol or drugs, or had a head injury?"
"Have you ever had symptoms of amnesia, such as forgetting periods of time?"
"Do you sometimes find yourself in a place, and can't recall how you got there?"
"Tell me what your childhood was like (eg, happy, sad, troubling)?"
"How are you getting along at home (fair, good, poor)?"
"What do you think is the cause of any problems at home?"
"Does your family notice anything different about you?"
"If yes, how do they describe the differences that they see?"
"How are you getting along at school (to a student) or at work (to an employed adult)?"
"Has anyone at school or at work noticed anything different about you?"
"How do they describe the differences that they see?"
"Do you sometimes have trouble identifying familiar faces of family or friends?"
"Do you find yourself daydreaming or fantasizing, and believe it is real?"
"What have you noticed that is different about your personality, if anything?"
"How would you describe those differences in your personality?"
"Do you sometimes feel as if you were two or more different people?"
"Do you feel as if some other identity has taken over your own identity?"
"Describe your feelings when that happens (eg, frightened, panicky, empowered)?"
"Who are the people you can count on for support and safety?"
"What do you want to happen, from your treatment in this facility?"

Note: Questions may vary depending on the examiner and the responses of the client, and they are not all asked in one interview or in one setting. It is up to the nurse to assess the client's comfort level, degree of shame or embarrassment, and give the client as much time as he or she needs to explain the problem.

Modified from Fortinash, K. M., & Holoday, P. A. (2012). *Psychiatric mental health nursing* (5th ed.). St. Louis, MO: Mosby.

- Inform the family or caregivers to address the client by his or her given name, and not to use names of other personalities or identities
- Teach the client to use "I" messages to meet needs or voice concerns (eg, "I need to talk to my therapist" or "I feel overwhelmed right now")
- Explain to the client and family that using "I" messages empowers the client and ensures that he or she is addressing his or her own identity rather than other personalities or identities
- Teach the client and family the importance of adhering to the medication regimen and the need to take medication as prescribed

Evaluation/Outcomes

- Dissociative disorders are chronic and enduring conditions; it takes patience and support for the client to change his or her patterns of behavior and incorporate methods that promote recovery

TABLE 15.2 Basic Level Interventions for Dissociative Disorders

Intervention	Rationale
Ensure client safety by providing safe, protected environment and frequent observation.	Sense of bewilderment may lead to inattention to safety needs; some subpersonalities may be thrill seeking, violent, or careless
Provide undemanding, simple routine.	Reduces anxiety
Confirm identity of client and orientation to time and place.	Supports reality and promotes ego integrity
Encourage client to do things for self and make decisions about routine tasks.	Enhances self-esteem by reducing sense of powerlessness and reduces secondary gain associated with dependence
Assist with other decision making until memory returns.	Lowers stress and prevents client from having to live with the consequences of unwise decisions
Support client during exploration of feelings surrounding the stressful event.	Helps lower the defense of dissociation used by client to block awareness of the stressful event
Do not flood client with data regarding past events.	Memory loss serves the purpose of preventing severe to panic levels of anxiety from overtaking and disorganizing the individual
Allow client to progress at own pace as memory is recovered.	Prevents undue anxiety and resistance
Provide support during disclosure of painful experiences.	Can be healing and minimize feelings of isolation
Help client see consequences of using dissociation to cope with stress.	Increases insight and helps client understand own role in choosing behaviors
Accept client's expression of negative feelings.	Conveys permission to have negative or unacceptable feelings
Teach stress reduction methods.	Provides alternatives for anxiety relief
If client does not remember significant others, work with involved parties to reestablish relationships.	Helps client experience satisfaction and relieves sense of isolation

From Varcarolis, E. M., & Halter, M. J. (2010). *Psychiatric mental health nursing: A clinical approach* (6th ed.). St. Louis, MO: Saunders.

- General outcomes: The client will:
  - Recall and identify past experiences accurately
  - Verbalize increased satisfaction with family and work relationships
  - Cease incidents of being absent without explanation
  - Develop more effective coping mechanisms to manage anxiety
  - Contact the nursing staff members if experiencing thoughts or desires that are suicidal or harmful toward self or others
  - Identify situations and events that trigger dissociative episodes, and select learned strategies to prevent or manage them
  - Describe feelings that occur during a heightened anxiety state, and verbalize ways to prevent them from reaching a panic state

- Explain the connection between anxiety-provoking situations or events and dissociative episodes
- Identify adaptive exercises and strategies that relieve anxiety and limit or reduce focus on dissociative episodes
- Demonstrate behaviors that promote a means of reassociation to original identity when experiencing a dissociative state (eg, using assertive-response behaviors such as identifying self with "I" messages such as "I am Jessica," "I know who I am"), and making sure that others address you by your given name rather than other identities they are aware of
- Use learned anxiety-reducing exercises such as mindfulness meditation
- Sleep through the night for 6 to 8 hours
- Learn to manage anxiety at mild or tolerable levels without dissociating
- Seek help from appropriate sources at the earliest sign of dissociative symptoms
- Verbalize feeling of relaxation and ability to control dissociative states
- Demonstrate the ability to concentrate, make decisions, and solve problems as treatment and condition progresses
- List the medications that are used to control the symptoms, as well as appropriate doses and scheduled times
- Continue aftercare symptom management, including medication and other therapies
- Continue to use appropriate supports from the nursing and medical community, family, and friends
- Discharge Criteria—the client will:
  - Alert the contact person or therapist or use a hotline when feeling suicidal or having self-harm ideation
  - Identify periods of increasing levels of anxiety
  - Identify situations and events that trigger dissociative states, and select adaptive ways to prevent or manage these situations
  - Demonstrate behaviors that represent reduced dissociative states
  - Respond to given name when addressed by staff member or significant other
  - Refer to self in the first-person pronoun (eg, "I think . . .; I feel . . .")
  - Use assertive-response behaviors to meet needs
  - Inform others of problems or dissatisfaction in an assertive manner
  - Keep a written journal to identify stressors and when dissociation emerges
  - Identify when to use prn (as needed) medication to decrease an increasing anxiety response to an environmental cue
  - Contact the therapist at the first sign of increasing symptoms

APPLICATION AND REVIEW

15. A nurse identifies that a client is falsifying signs and symptoms of a medical disorder. What does this behavior usually indicate?
    1. Psychosis
    2. Factitious disorder
    3. Out of contact with reality
    4. Use of conversion defenses
16. Shortly after admission an adolescent falls to the floor and has tonic-clonic movements. There is no verbal response, but a nurse observes that the client is still chewing gum. What should the nurse do next?
    1. Remove the chewing gum
    2. Document the observation
    3. Send another client for help
    4. Insert a tongue blade between the teeth

17. A child has been hospitalized repeatedly for illnesses with unknown etiologies. Finally, the health care provider makes the diagnosis of Munchausen syndrome by proxy. What is the nurse's most therapeutic approach with the involved parent?
    1. Confrontation
    2. Open communication
    3. Health teaching about child rearing
    4. Validation of the child's physical status
18. A nurse is assessing a client for the use of defense mechanisms. Which defense mechanism separates certain mental processes from consciousness as though they belonged to another?

    1. Projection
    2. Conversion
    3. Dissociation
    4. Compensation

    See Answers on pages 286-289.

ANSWER KEY: REVIEW QUESTIONS

1. **3 The client is experiencing a psychological conflict that is manifested by a change in body function. Paralysis or blindness justifies the inability to move in any direction.**

   1 A conversion disorder is an unconscious method of solving a conflict. **2** It is necessary for the client to focus on the problem causing the disorder, not on the cure. **4** It is more important that the client learn how to manage personal feelings before addressing family conflicts that may or may not exist.

   Client Need: Psychosocial Integrity; **Cognitive Level:** Comprehension; **Nursing Process:** Assessment/Analysis

---

 Memory Aid: *Conversion* disorder *converts* anxiety into a physical disorder.

---

2. **2 Somatic symptom disorder involves erroneously attributing an anxious feeling to a body system or part.**

   1 Dissociation is separating an overwhelming event from one's consciousness. **3** The stress response results from exposure to a threatening stimulus. **4** An anxiety reaction is the body's reaction to a stressful event.

   Client need: Psychosocial Integrity; **Cognitive Level:** Comprehension; **Nursing process:** Assessment/Analysis

3. **3 The conversion type of defense tends to be a learned behavioral response that the individual will use when experiencing excessive stress.**

   1 Demonstration of a spread of paralysis to other body parts is not a likely occurrence. **2** Psychiatric treatment may be needed at different times throughout life but usually not on a continuous basis. **4** Based on studies of this disorder, its course is somewhat predictable; it usually returns when the client is under severe stress.

   Client Need: Psychosocial Integrity; **Cognitive Level:** Comprehension; **Nursing process:** Assessment/Analysis

4. **3 The physical symptoms are not the client's major problem and therefore should not be the focus for care. This is a psychologic problem, and the focus should be in this domain.**

   1 Encouraging the client to try to walk is focusing on the physical symptom of the conflict; the client is not ready to give up the symptom. **2** The disorder operates on an unconscious level but is very real to the client; explaining that there is nothing wrong denies the client's feelings. **4** Psychotherapy is needed at this time, not physical therapy.

   Client need: Psychosocial Integrity; **Cognitive Level:** Application; **Nursing Process:** Planning/Implementation

5. **4 The psychophysiologic response (eg, hyperfunction or hypofunction) creates actual tissue change. Somatic symptom disorders are unrelated to organic changes.**

   1 There is an emotional component in both psychophysiologic and somatic symptom disorders. **2** There is a feeling of illness in both psychophysiologic and somatic symptom disorders. **3** There may be a restriction of activities in both psychophysiologic and somatic symptom disorders.

   Client Need: Psychosocial Integrity; **Cognitive Level:** Comprehension; **Nursing Process:** Assessment/Analysis

6. **1 Clients diagnosed with a somatic symptom disorder are preoccupied with the symptoms that are being experienced and usually do not want to talk about their emotions or relate them to their present situation.**

   2 Clients diagnosed with a somatic symptom disorder do not seek opportunities to discuss their feelings. **3** Memory problems are not associated with somatic symptom disorders. **4** These clients want and seek treatment, not palliative care.

   Client Need: Psychosocial Integrity; **Cognitive Level:** Comprehension; **Nursing Process:** Assessment/Analysis

7. **4 When emotional stress overwhelms an individual's ability to cope, the unconscious seeks to reduce stress. A conversion disorder removes the client from the stressful situation, and the conversion reaction's physical/sensory manifestation causes little or no anxiety in the individual. This lack of concern is called *la belle indifference*.**

   1 No physiologic changes are involved with this unconscious resolution of a conflict. **2** The conversion of anxiety to physical symptoms operates on an unconscious level. **3** The conversion of anxiety to physical symptoms operates on an unconscious level.

   Client Need: Psychosocial Integrity; **Cognitive Level:** Comprehension; **Nursing Process:** Assessment/Analysis

8. **3 Preoccupation with fears of getting or having a serious disease is called illness anxiety disorder. The condition usually exists for 6 months or longer, causes preoccupation with illness despite negative medical tests and reassurance, and results in social or occupational impairment.**

   1 Conversion disorder is characterized by the presence of one or more symptoms related to a neurologic problem that has no organic cause. **2** Somatic symptom disorder is characterized by many physical problems being reported by the client, usually beginning before age 30; physical problems may include pain, gastrointestinal symptoms, sexual or reproductive problems, and at least one symptom that suggests a neurologic disorder. **4** Body dysmorphic disorder is characterized by preoccupation with some imagined defect in appearance that causes marked distress and significant impairment in social and occupational functioning (see **Chapter 12**).

   Client Need: Psychosocial Integrity; **Cognitive Level:** Analysis; **Nursing Process:** Assessment/Analysis

9. **2 The client with a conversion disorder literally converts the anxiety to the symptom. Once the symptom develops, it acts as a defense against the anxiety, and the client is diagnostically almost anxiety free.**

   1 In a conversion disorder, the reactions the nurse should expect to encounter are not in proportion to the disability; therefore, clients usually are not depressed. **3** The conflict is resolved by the paralysis of the legs; therefore, the anxiety is under control. **4** The opposite is true; these clients usually are calm and composed when discussing symptoms.

   Client Need: Psychosocial Integrity; **Cognitive level:** Application; **Nursing Process:** Assessment/Analysis

10. **2 The priority is to get the client to express feelings appropriately rather than through the use of physical symptoms.**

    1 Focusing on symptoms will encourage their use. **3** An expression of feelings, not an intellectual understanding of the cause of the symptoms, is required. Avoidance of feelings resulted in the symptoms. **4** Clients diagnosed with a conversion disorder rarely are concerned about the associated physical problem, which is known as *la belle indifference*.

    Client Need: Psychosocial Integrity; **Cognitive Level:** Application; **Nursing Process:** Planning/Implementation; **Integrated Process:** Caring

11. **4 Asking "What emotion were you feeling before you felt the weakness?" focuses the client on the relationship between emotion and physical symptoms in a nonthreatening, accepting manner**
    1 The nurse knows when the weakness began, so it is unnecessary to ask. **2** Asking "Is this similar to what you usually experience?" does not identify what the person was feeling when the weakness happened. **3** Asking "Would you like to leave the group for a while?" will provide a secondary gain; it implies sympathy, and the client avoids an undesired activity.
    Client Need: Psychosocial Integrity; **Cognitive Level:** Analysis; **Nursing Process:** Planning/Implementation; **Integrated Process:** Caring

12. **4 The client's eye problems are a conversion reaction. Not discussing the physical problems prevents the client from using this topic to avoid an exploration of feelings. Focusing on the safe topic of activities may eventually progress to a discussion of emotion-laden topics such as feelings.**
    1 It is too early for encouraging involvement in group activities; the client is too introspective to become involved with group activities at this time. **2** Focusing on the physical problem allows the client to avoid feelings. **3** The data do not indicate that the client has an organic problem and is going blind.
    Client Need: Management of Care; **Cognitive Level:** Application; **Nursing Process:** Planning/Implementation

13. **2 Development of the symptom is an unconscious method of reducing anxiety. Because the symptom is meeting this need, it does not create anxiety itself but is passively accepted (*la belle indifference*).**
    1 There is no anger; symptoms are passively accepted. **3** There is no anxiety; the conflict is resolved by the physical symptom. **4** There is no agitation; symptoms are passively accepted.
    Client Need: Psychosocial Integrity; **Cognitive Level:** Comprehension; **Nursing Process:** Assessment/Analysis

14. **2 The client's anxiety results from the inability to choose psychologically between two conflicting actions. The conversion to a physical disability removes the choice and therefore reduces the anxiety.**
    1 The anxiety is not free-floating or diffuse, but rather localized and converted to a physical disability. **3** The conversion of the anxiety to a physical disability occurs on an unconscious level; the original anxiety no longer exists, and the client generally is not anxious about the physical disability. **4** The anxiety is internalized into a physical symptom, not projected onto the environment.
    Client Need: Psychosocial Integrity; **Cognitive Level:** Comprehension; **Nursing Process:** Assessment/Analysis

15. **2 When the individual falsifies signs and symptoms of a medical disorder in oneself or others, it is characteristic of factitious disorder.**
    1 People who are psychotic experience delusions, hallucinations, and disorganized thoughts, speech, or behavior. **3** A person out of contact with reality is unable to pretend to be ill. **4** The use of conversion defenses is not a conscious act.
    Client Need: Psychosocial Integrity; **Cognitive Level:** Comprehension; **Nursing Process:** Assessment/analysis

 Memory Aid: In a *f*actitious disorder, the *f*acts of a medical disorder are *f*alsified.

16. **2 If seizures were physiologically based, the client would not be able to continue to chew gum. This "attack" should be reported as a behavioral response, with the characteristics of the situation noted.**
    1 The chewing gum is not a danger when the client is not having a true seizure. **3** It is not necessary to send another client for help. **4** It is not safe to insert a tongue blade between the teeth; it is not used in a true seizure.
    Client Need: Psychosocial Integrity; **Cognitive Level:** Application; **Integrated Process:** Communication/Documentation; **Nursing Process:** Assessment/Analysis

17. **2 Maintaining open communication is important for any therapeutic nurse-client relationship.**
    1 Confrontation will put the parent on the defensive and close off communication. **3** Health teaching at this time is premature; the parent is not ready for this approach. **4** Validation of the child's physical status focuses on the physical symptoms, which will reinforce the parent's behavior.
    Client Need: Psychosocial Integrity; **Cognitive Level:** Application; **Integrated Process:** Communication/Documentation; **Nursing Process:** Planning/Implementation

18. **3 With dissociation, there is separation of certain mental processes from consciousness as though they belonged to another; a dissociative-type reaction is expressed as amnesia, dissociative identity disorder, depersonalization, and other behaviors.**

   1 Projection occurs when people assign their own unacceptable thoughts and feelings to others. **2** The defense mechanism is called conversion because the individual reduces emotional anxiety by converting it to a physical disability. **4** Compensation is a mechanism used to make up for a lack in one area by emphasizing capabilities in another.

   Client Need: Psychosocial Integrity; **Cognitive Level:** Comprehension; **Nursing Process:** Assessment/Analysis

> **Memory Aid:** In the ***dissociation*** defense mechanism and in dissociative disorders, mental processes ***"dis-associate"*** or separate from each other.

16 Anger, Aggression, Abuse, Assault, Violence

TERMINOLOGY AND BACKGROUND

Anger

- Anger is defined as an emotional reaction characterized by extreme displeasure, rage, indignation, or hostility
  - Expressions of anger vary widely in different individuals and cultures
- This powerful emotion primarily comes from the amygdala (in the limbic system)
- It can be constructive (adaptive) if it motivates positive action or destructive (maladaptive) when it leads to aggression or violence
- It arouses the sympathetic nervous system and the associated physiologic changes (increased heart rate and breathing, pupil dilation, decreased digestion, etc.)
- Anger lowers inhibitions
- Anger is seen in many mental health disorders, including posttraumatic stress disorder (PTSD), depression, anxiety, psychosis, and personality disorders
- Positive ways to cope with anger include exercise, talking to others, and counting to 10 (or higher!) to give time to engage the cerebral cortex and consider inhibitions
- Ways to decrease stress that may lead to anger include avoiding drugs and alcohol, getting enough sleep, meditation or the relaxation response, and taking care of oneself, which includes taking a break if stressed

Anger Management and Assertiveness Training

- Anger management is a form of therapy that focuses on clients with a history of hostile or aggressive behavior
- How an individual handles anger is first learned from one's family; learning plays a role in the maladaptive response to anger
- Anger management can be relearned through anger management therapy
- Anger management therapy teaches clients to first assume responsibility for hostile actions, then identify anger triggers, and learn new methods of responding; teaching should not take place when the client is angry as that may increase agitation
- Anger management therapy
  - Teach clients enhanced communication skills
  - Teach clients relaxation techniques
  - Encourage cognitive therapy strategies to redefine anger triggers and responses
- Assertiveness training
  - Clients learn the differences among aggressive, nonassertive, passive-aggressive, and assertive communication and behavior
  - Techniques include role playing, cognitive restructuring, and fogging/clouding (concurs with another's statement without being defensive or agreeing to change)
  - Nursing care associated with assertiveness training
    - Teach differences among aggressive, nonassertive, passive-aggressive, and assertive communication and behavior
    - Role model assertive communication and behavior

- Provide positive reinforcement for assertive communication and behavior
- Be aware that anger may be a defense against anxiety

Aggression

- Aggression is a forceful behavior, action, or attitude that is expressed physically, verbally, or symbolically; it can be an attitude or a behavior or both; it may arise from innate drives or occur as a defense mechanism, often resulting from a threatened ego; it is manifested by either constructive or destructive acts directed toward oneself or others
- Destructive aggression is intended to threaten or injure an individual or that individual's self-esteem; constructive aggression can be used for self-defense or defense of others

Bullying

- Bullying is the abuse of power over another person through repeated aggressive behaviors; these behaviors can be verbal, such as teasing, or physical; they are intentionally hurtful and unprovoked
- Studies of the prevalence of bullying estimate that 20% to 90% of children are bullied
- Because of its connection to violent and aggressive behaviors that result in serious injury to the self and to others, bullying is now considered a major public health issue; once viewed as a ritual of childhood and adolescence, bullying has now captured media headlines
- For bullies, power may arise from physical strength and maturity, from a higher status within a peer group, from knowing another child's weakness, or from recruiting the support of other children; as bullies age, they rely less on physical means to intimidate their victims and turn to indirect forms that entail verbal abuse and social exclusion
- Bullying can occur in both direct and indirect ways; males and females tend to differ with regard to the ways that they bully; girls are less likely to bully physically and more often engage in relational aggression; this type of bullying involves a deliberate isolation and exclusion of the victim from friendship, using tools such as slander, spreading rumors, and manipulation; the relational bully also engages other students' assistance in the scheme with the use of threats of exclusion if they do not comply
- A bullied person is one who is exposed repeatedly to negative actions on the part of one or more persons
- Victimization is of great concern as a result of the potentially debilitating effects of chronic peer rejection, including increased anger and depression, low self-esteem, and social withdrawal
  - Children form their interpersonal and self-schemas on the basis of their social interactions
  - Not all bullies develop psychiatric disorders, but a persistent pattern of antisocial behavior during childhood and adolescence can be predictive of future difficulties
  - At-risk personality traits in children include aggression toward animals or other children, a lack of empathy, and the destruction of property
- Cyberbullying is bullying via electronic means such as texting, e-mail, or social networking sites; it can be through images (real or modified) or words; about 20% of U.S. schoolchildren have been cyberbullied

Assault and Battery

- Assault is an unlawful act that places another person, without that person's consent, in fear of immediate bodily harm or battery; it is the threat of bodily harm or injury
- Battery is the unlawful use of force on a person

Violence

- Violence is great force, either physical or emotional, usually exerted to damage or abuse someone or something
- It can also be described as abusive or unjust exercise of power over another
- Violence may be overt or covert; violence as an overt event is experienced at the local level in homes, neighborhoods, schools, and workplace settings
- Interpersonal violence can have serious deleterious effects on mental health, and these are most notably expressed as instances of PTSD, dissociative symptoms, and enduring personality changes
- Nurses deal with violence regularly; in the U.S., more than 2 million emergency visits are related to assault annually
- Nurses also are at greater risk for violence while working as nurses

Abuse

- Abuse is physical or verbal attack or injury
- There are many types of abuse:
  - Child abuse (maltreatment): The physical, sexual, or emotional maltreatment/victimization of a minor
  - Physical abuse: One or more episodes of aggressive behavior, usually resulting in physical injury with possible damage to internal organs, sense organs, the central nervous system, or the musculoskeletal system of another person
  - Neglect: Failure by a parent or guardian of a child or other dependent person (such as an elderly or disabled person) to provide minimal physical and emotional care for that person
  - Sexual assault: The forcible perpetration of an act of sexual contact on the body of another person, male or female, without consent; legal criteria vary among different communities
  - Rape: Sexual assault, homosexual or heterosexual, the legal definitions for which vary from state to state; rape is a crime of violence or one committed under the threat of violence, and its victims are treated for medical and psychological trauma; note that rape is not sexual in motivation; rather, it is sexual expression of power and anger
  - Statutory rape: Sexual intercourse with a person younger than the age of consent, which varies from state to state
  - Sexual abuse: The sexual mistreatment of another person by fondling, rape, or forced participation in unnatural sex acts or other behavior; victims tend to experience a traumatic feeling of loss of control of themselves
    - Sexual abuse can be of children, adults, or elders (see later in this chapter)
  - Incest: Sexual intercourse between persons too closely related to marry legally
    - Research on intrafamilial sexual abuse indicates that incest families are highly dysfunctional, although they may appear to be normal; studies do not find a correlation with incest and characteristics such as socioeconomic status, culture, race, and ethnicity; rather, incest seems to cross all boundaries
    - Within incestuous families, multiple forms of abuse are likely to be present, including physical and other forms of psychologic and emotional abuse; most incestuous families are described as enmeshed, which means that they are relatively isolated from those outside of the family and that they tend to focus most of their energies on relationships within the family; boundaries within the family are poorly defined, and members are characterized by excessive dependency on each other for physical, social, and psychologic needs; individual members have little to no autonomy; role reversals often occur

Assault Cycle

- The five-phase assault cycle includes the following:
  - *Triggering phase: The stress-producing event occurs, initiating the stress responses. Escalation phase: Responses represent escalating behaviors that indicate a movement toward the loss of control; also known as preassaultive phase. Crisis phase: During this period of emotional and physical crisis, loss of control occurs. Recovery phase: In this period of cooling down, the person slows down and returns to normal responses. Postcrisis depression phase: In this period, the person attempts reconciliation with others.*

(Keltner, 2015)

- Nursing interventions can be based on the assault cycle (Table 16.1)

APPLICATION AND REVIEW

1. A client with a history of violence is becoming increasingly agitated. Which nursing intervention will **most** likely increase the risk of acting out behavior?
   1. Being assertive
   2. Responding early
   3. Providing choices
   4. Teaching relaxation
2. What is an early objective for clients in relation to anger management?
   1. Expressing remorse over aggressive actions
   2. Taking responsibility for the hostile behavior
   3. Developing alternative methods to release feelings
   4. Teaching others how to avoid triggering the angry behavior
3. A nurse leads an assertiveness training program for a group of clients. Which client statement demonstrates that the treatment has been effective?
   1. "I know I should put the needs of others before mine."
   2. "I won't allow it, so I told my boss he's a jerk and to leave me alone."
   3. "It annoys me when people call me 'Dearie,' so I told him not to do it anymore."
   4. "It is easier for me to agree up front and then just do enough so that no one notices."
4. A client with a history of aggressive, violent behavior is admitted to the psychiatric unit involuntarily. The nurse, who understands the need to use deescalation approaches during the preassaultive stage of the violence cycle, monitors the client's behavior closely for progression of signs of impending violence. List these client assessments in order of escalating aggression from the lowest risk to the highest risk.
   1. Pacing in the hall
   2. Increasing tension in facial expression
   3. Engaging in verbal abuse toward the nurse
   4. Having difficulty waiting to take turns during a group project
   5. Pushing another client when waiting in line to the dining room

See Answers on pages 323-325.

Etiology/Predisposing Factors to Violent Behavior

- There is no single etiology, but many theories have been proposed, with much support for generational transmission of violence

TABLE 16.1 Interventions Based on Assault Cycle

Phase	Behaviors	Nursing Interventions
Triggering phase: +1 to +2 level of anxiety	Muscle tension, changes in voice quality, tapping of fingers, pacing, repeated verbalizations, restlessness, irritability, anxiety, suspiciousness, perspiration, tremors, glaring, changes in breathing	Convey empathic support. Encourage ventilation. Use clear, calm, simple statements. Ask patient to maintain control. Facilitate problem solving by discussing alternative solutions. If needed, ask patient to go to a quiet area. Offer safe tension reduction measures. If needed, offer oral medications (prn).
Escalation phase: +2 to +3 level of anxiety	Pale or flushed face, screaming, anger, swearing, agitation, hypersensitivity, threats, demands, readiness to retaliate, tautness, loss of reasoning ability, provocative behaviors, clenched fists	Take charge with calm, firm directions. Direct patient to a quiet room for "time out." Offer oral medications (prn), if ordered. Ask the staff to be on standby at a distance. Prepare for a "show of concern."
Crisis phase: +3 to +4 level of anxiety	Loss of self-control, fighting, hitting, rage, kicking, scratching, throwing things	Use involuntary seclusion, restraints, or IM medications (prn), if ordered. Initiate intensive nursing care.
Recovery phase: +3 to +2 level of anxiety	Accusations, recriminations, lowering of voice, decreased body tension, change in conversational content, more normal responses, relaxation	Continue intensive nursing care. Process the incident with staff and other patients. Assess patient and staff injuries. Evaluate patient's progress toward self-control.
Postcrisis depression phase: +2 to +1 level of anxiety	Crying, apologies, reconciliatory interactions, repression of assaultive feelings (which might later appear as hostility, passive aggression)	Process incident with patient. Discuss alternative solutions to the situation and feelings. Progressively reduce the degree of restraint and seclusion. Facilitate reentry to unit.

IM, Intramuscular; *prn*, as needed.

Data from Maier, G. J. (1996). Managing threatening behavior: The role of talk up and talk down. *Journal of Psychosocial Nursing and Mental Health Services, 34,* 25; Smith, P. (1981). Empirically based models for viewing the dynamics of violence. In K. Babich (Ed.), *Assessing patient violence in the health care setting.* Boulder, CO: Western Interstate Commission for Higher Education; Stevenson, S. (1991). Heading off violence with verbal de-escalation. *Journal of Psychosocial Nursing and Mental Health Services, 29,* 6.

Social Learning/Role Modeling/Operant Conditioning Risk Factors

- The family teaches and accepts violent behavior
- Violence is glorified in the media
- Parents who were abused as children are at risk for abusing their own children (Fig. 16.1)
    - The transmission of violence from one generation to the next is as much a component of subculture as any other learned behavior; some studies have shown that among adults who were abused as children, more than 20% later abuse their own children
    - Aggression as a learned (not instinctual) behavior
        - The correlation between earlier victimization and the later perpetration of physically and sexually violent crimes cannot be ignored; it has been postulated that males who were exposed to early victimization, including experiencing child physical or sexual abuse as well as witnessing domestic violence within the family, may be more prone to adapting to these negative experiences by using externalizing behaviors; these behaviors may include the increased acceptance and use of aggression, violence, and control within future relationships as well as other maladaptive behaviors, including lying, stealing, substance use, and truancy
- Sociologists have attempted to develop an integrated theory of several cultural and structural determinants and of social learning
    - Within this framework, growing up in a patriarchal society that emphasizes male dominance and aggression and female victimization, children are socialized into their respective sex roles; in addition, they learn through their experiences in the family or through exposure to the media; this learning becomes reinforced in the larger community, where male and female roles similarly rest on elements of macho culture

Biologic and Biochemical Factors

- Lesions in the brain, such as tumors, can produce changes that result in increased violence
- Neurotransmitters can be involved in anger; low serotonin levels have been correlated with aggression, and low dopamine levels with anger

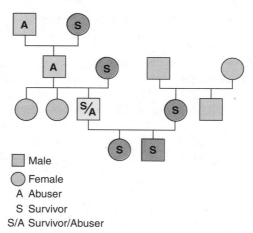

FIG. 16.1 Genogram demonstrates the multigenerational transmission of family violence. (From Stuart, G.W. [2013]. *Principles and practice of psychiatric nursing* [10 ed.]. St. Louis, MO: Mosby/Elsevier.)

Environmental and Socioeconomic Factors

- Environmental factors include stressful life events
- Socioeconomic factors include socioeconomic class, unemployment, poverty, crime, teenage pregnancy, and isolation
- The temporary placement of children in foster homes and informally with relatives exposes children to risks of violence from caretakers for whom the minimal moral constraints of the parenting role are less understood
- Social isolation
  - Social isolation has been identified as a characteristic of some families that are at high risk for physical and sexual abuse of a spouse or children; the isolation may be forced on the partner by the abuser; alternatively, shame may prompt the visibly battered spouse to withdraw even further; victims often become isolated from friends, the family of origin, neighbors, or anyone who could become acquainted with the events; some families isolate themselves in subtle ways by using unlisted telephone numbers or cell phones; they lack a means of transportation so that they cannot visit others, and their homes may be physically shuttered from the gaze of outsiders; they often lack community ties of any kind

INTIMATE PARTNER VIOLENCE/SEXUAL ASSAULT

Overview

- Sexual violence may include attempted or completed rape, sexual coercion and harassment, sexual contact with force or threat of force, and threat of rape
- More than half of all victims of sexual crimes, including rape and sexual assault, are women younger than 25 years old; often this violence occurs within the context of dating or acquaintance relationships, with the female partner the likely victim of violence and the male partner the likely perpetrator ; however, underage males can also be victims
- One in four girls and one in six boys will be sexually abused before they turn 18 years old
- Only approximately 33% of rapes are reported in the U.S.
- Sexual assaults may also include actions such as fondling or indecent exposure
- Previous victimization, including experiencing or witnessing violence during childhood, has also been linked with future victimization; sexual victimization during childhood is frequently a predictor of the experiencing of future sexual victimization; although past victimization does not guarantee future victimization, previous victimization—including a lack of control over one's body, sexuality, and choices—*may set relational norms that become acceptable in future intimate relationships;* furthermore, if childhood victimization went unrecognized or unreported—especially by someone charged with that child's care—the now adolescent victim may feel that his or her victimization is unimportant and that his or her abuse is of little consequence
- The way a cultural or ethnic group defines gender roles and the woman's place in society affects how rape will be perceived; in the U.S. multiple examples of male superiority and female subjugation exist in popular literature, media, fashion, art, and language; these cultural symbols help form attitudes and beliefs that are then further translated into laws, court proceedings, police behavior, educational curricula, and social service programs
- Myths that blame victims for rape and broad conceptualizations of sexual assault are influenced by ethnic-specific cultural values and norms

- Culturally sanctioned beliefs about the rights and privileges of husbands have historically legitimized a man's domination over his wife and warranted his use of violence to control her; however, women who have been forced into sex by an intimate partner may be at risk for the same results and consequences as if they had been raped by an unknown assailant (eg, sexually transmitted diseases, physical trauma, emotional issues)

Statutory Rape

- Although most adult women partner with slightly older males, the application of this social norm to adolescent females has been linked to an increased risk for victimization, including physical and sexual violence; furthermore, imbalances in power and control, financial resources, levels of life experience, and physical strength and stature may place younger females who are partnered with adult males at risk for experiencing unplanned and unprotected sex, unwanted pregnancy, and exposure to sexually transmitted infections, including human immunodeficiency virus (HIV) and acquired immunodeficiency syndrome (AIDS)
- Although partnering with an older male may be considered consensual in nature by the female, her peers, and possibly her family, sexual relationships with significantly older males may meet the legal definition of statutory rape; as such, teen advocacy and pregnancy prevention programs have called for the increased use of existing statutory rape laws to help with the prosecution and punishment of adult men who have sex with adolescent females
- Developmentally, adolescents must learn to control their newly gained independence from their parents as they master developmental milestones (eg, driving a car, dating) and learn to negotiate new relationships with peers and intimate partners; as such, youth—which is associated with limited knowledge and lack of experience in interpersonal relationships—is a significant risk factor for experiencing sexual victimization
- Adolescents are particularly vulnerable when their youth is coupled with early menarche, early dating, and early sexual activity, all of which have all been linked with an increased risk for the experiencing of victimization by an intimate partner
- Like adult victims, adolescent victims of sexual violence may experience negative physical health consequences after sexual victimization; although physical injuries do not always occur as a result of violence, victims may suffer physical trauma to the genital tract, including vaginal bleeding, bruises, lacerations, and contusions
- Trauma may be more extensive among younger females, especially those who have not yet reached menarche and who thus have less elastic and more easily damaged vaginal tissue; virginal adolescents may also be at increased risk for physical trauma, including hymeneal and perineal tears; this trauma increases the adolescent's risk of contracting sexually transmitted infections, including gonorrhea, chlamydia, herpes, and HIV
- Victims are at risk for sexually transmitted infections even without trauma
- They may also be at risk for unplanned pregnancy; among adult victims, almost 5% of pregnancies are the result of rape; the incidence of rape-related pregnancies among adolescent victims is likely higher because younger women may be unaware of or have limited access to postcoital contraceptives and may not be using any long-term contraceptive method (eg, birth control pills) at the time of the assault
- Several factors have been linked with an increased risk for either experiencing or perpetrating sexual victimization during adolescence, including age and developmental level, previous victimization, drug and alcohol use, and adherence to rigid social roles that dictate acceptable behaviors
- Minors and people with cognitive impairments are regarded as unable to give consent; sexual activity between a minor or a cognitively impaired adult and a competent adult is a form of sexual assault

Date Rape

- Although victims may be sexually assaulted after knowingly ingesting illegal drugs (eg, marijuana, heroin, cocaine), they may also be unknowingly drugged by so-called "date rape drugs"; two of the more common date rape drugs, γ-hydroxybutyrate and flunitrazepam, are central nervous system depressants that, when dissolved in both alcoholic and nonalcoholic beverages, become odorless and tasteless
  - After a person has ingested these drugs, he or she becomes disoriented and confused. Dissociation and unconsciousness for several hours may result
  - In an effort to reduce the incidence of drug-facilitated rape, pharmaceutical companies recently included a color additive in the drug flunitrazepam
  - In addition to similar preventative measures, the criminalization of drug-facilitated rape is also enforced under the Drug-Induced Rape Prevention and Punishment Act of 1996 and the Hillory J. Farias and Samantha Reid Date-Rape Drug Prohibition Act of 2000
  - Sources of date rape drugs remain plentiful in the U.S., internationally, and online
  - As with other substances that are knowingly or unknowingly ingested by victims, memory impairment, a common side effect of the medication, may make it difficult for victims to remember and identify the perpetrators of the crimes
- One in 5 women and one in 16 men are sexually assaulted while in college.
- Research has indicated that approximately 44% of acquaintance rape victims (compared with less than 1% of stranger rape victims) are likely to be sexually assaulted more than once by the same offender
  - About 50% of the victims do terminate the relationship
  - Victims of acquaintance rape are often in a state of denial during the aftermath of the rape, and they often present for treatment years after the assaultive incident
- Alcohol use and intoxication are significantly related to the perpetration of sexual violence; among male users, intoxication has been linked with the misinterpretation of sexual cues as well as the overestimation of a woman's sexual interest, which may ultimately result in increased aggression and forced or coerced sex

Rape

- Clinical work with offenders and victims reveals that rape serves nonsexual needs; it is the sexual expression of power and anger; rape is motivated more by retaliatory and compensatory motives than sexual ones; it is an act that is complex with multiple causes and that addresses issues of hostility and control; the defining issue in rape is the lack of consent on the part of the victim; sexual relations are achieved through physical force, threat, or intimidation; therefore rape is first and foremost an aggressive act, and, in any given instance of rape, multiple psychologic meanings may be expressed with regard to both the sexual and aggressive components of the act
- Rape is an interactional process that involves at least two people and a control issue; one person feels that he or she must gain control over the other person; it becomes clear when talking with rape victims that, from their point of view, rape is an act that is initiated by the assailant; it is not primarily a sexual act but rather an act of aggression, power, and violence
- Myths that the woman must have done something to provoke the rape often keep women from reporting rapes
- Myths that men cannot be raped prevent men from reporting rape
- Incarceration increases risk of sexual assault
- Military sexual assault is a growing problem

Effects of Rape on the Victim

- Victims suffer a significant degree of physical and emotional trauma during the rape, immediately after the assault, and for a considerable time period afterward; victims consistently describe certain symptoms over and over; a cluster of symptoms has been described as the *rape trauma syndrome,* which most victims experience; it includes physical, emotional, and behavioral stress reactions that result from the person being faced with an event that threatens one's life or integrity
- The acute reaction to rape is often shock, disbelief, and dissociation from the event
- Victims show two main styles of emotion: *Expressed* and *controlled*
  - In the expressed style, the victim demonstrates such feelings as anger, fear, and anxiety; the victims express these feelings by being restless during the interview, becoming tense when certain questions are asked, crying or sobbing when describing specific acts of the assailant, or smiling in an anxious manner when certain issues are stated
  - In the controlled style, the feelings of the victim are masked or hidden, and the interviewer notes a calm, composed, or subdued affect; it is not uncommon for victims to have a flat affect, to be stoic in demeanor, or to be highly emotional; it is frequently observed that people in prison will shut down and inhibit their feelings because they do not know who they can trust
- Victims express other feelings in conjunction with fear; these range from humiliation, degradation, guilt, shame, and embarrassment to self-blame, anger, and revenge; victims report feeling distressed by reminders or cues of the assault; seeing a man who looks like the assailant will evoke a strong emotional reaction; victims become cautious with all people; after a stranger rape, the victim expects the assailant to be everywhere
- Many symptoms develop after a rape or a sexual assault; the woman will feel numb, and she continually tries to block the thoughts of the assault from her mind; that reaction may be observed as a flat affect or indifference; she will say that she is trying to push it out of her mind, but the thought of the assault continually haunts her; there is a strong desire for the victim to try and think of how she could undo what has happened; she reports going over in her mind how she might have escaped from the assailant and how she might have handled the situation differently; however, she usually ends up believing that she would have been beaten or killed if she had not done what the assailant demanded; note that 91% of rape and assault victims are women, so this example uses a woman.
- Dreams and nightmares are also symptoms seen among rape victims

Trauma and the Limbic System

- The importance of psychologic trauma is how it affects the brain, particularly key regulatory processes that control memory, aggression, sexuality, attachment, emotion, sleep, and appetite; the affected location of the brain, the limbic system, is the alarm system that protects the individual in the face of danger; it is the beginning place where all sensory information enters the human system and is encoded; when trauma occurs, the neurohormonal system releases epinephrine, which helps prepare an individual to act during dangerous states
- When individuals are trapped and cannot remove themselves either through fleeing or fighting, there is a particular type of learning called *trauma learning* that occurs; it does not allow for a reduction of stress through the adaptive means of the fight-or-flight response; as a result of excesses and depletion of stress hormones in the brain structures responsible for interpreting and storing incoming stimuli, alterations occur in memory systems; the individual becomes immobilized, and, as the level of autonomic arousal increases, there is a move into a

numbing state as a result of the release of opiates in the brain; this numbing state accounts for the disconnection of the processing and encoding of information

- When the trauma is over, the alarm system remains somewhat stuck between the accelerated fight-or-flight response and the numbing state, which causes an alteration in the individual's adaptive capacity; this alteration is a cellular change that becomes fixed in its patterning and that is difficult to change or extinguish; of particular importance are various theories of modulating effects in the brain; this fight-or-flight response and numbing in the face of danger make sense; in addition, trauma can have a lasting effect on basic processes of adaptation and growth

- Because the neurologic responses of arousal and numbing are intricately related to information processing and memory, there is a distinctive type of memory in which experiences are recalled as if they were happening (eg, a flashback); thus when external events trigger an association with the abuse itself, the person is thrown into this panic memory and feels subjected to a hostile and exploitative environment even though nothing like that is currently present; internal events can also trigger a trauma-specific reaction called *night terrors;* these experiences are not typical dreams; rather, they involve a vivid and visceral response, and the individual feels as if the trauma is currently occurring

- Somatic problems, sleep disorders, phobias, social withdrawal, and depression may occur as later responses, especially if therapy is not sought and received

Nursing Care of Survivors of Sexual Assault

- Treat physical injuries, protect against sexually transmitted infections, offer pregnancy prevention and emotional support
- Create a safe environment in which the victim may express feelings and regain some sense of choice and control
- Provide support to family and friends of the victim and direct them how to support the victim appropriately
- Refer to rape counselors and/or rape counseling centers for immediate help and for longer-term support
- Focus on providing physical care and emotional support; assist with gathering evidence for criminal prosecution if needed

DOMESTIC/INTIMATE PARTNER VIOLENCE

Courtship Violence

- Although large-scale surveys have documented the prevalence of abuse in teen dating relationships, this type of violence often escapes attention or concern
  - Research indicates that a large number of college students experience physical aggression in their dating relationships
  - Estimates of the prevalence of dating aggression among college students range from 20% to 50%
- Dating violence appears to begin as early as the age of 15 or 16 years
  - Typical tactics include slapping, pushing, beating, and threatening with or using weapons
- Recurring and escalating episodes of violence in a relationship are quite common if the relationship is not terminated
  - Called the *Cycle of Violence,* it contains these predictable stages:
    - Tension building: batterer escalates and becomes more controlling; battered person tries to prevent angry outbursts of batterer

■ Battering: various triggers, with batterer minimizing the severity
■ Honeymoon: behavior of batterer changes to loving and begging for forgiveness; battered person tries to make up with batterer

Stalking

- With courtship violence, the aggressor may not want the relationship to end; there can be threats, stalking behavior (see later in this chapter), parking outside of the victim's house, and harassing phone calls; the harasser cannot tolerate separation; he or she feels abandoned, angry, and depressed, and he or she may become suicidal; rage is often behind the depression, as rejection is an attack on the ego; frequently, these individuals feel that they cannot manage on their own, and the limbic system is actually affected; these individuals may lack impulse control
- Stalking is part of the constellation of behaviors that are associated with partner violence, especially when there is a difficult breakup with an intimate partner; stalking takes various forms and has varying definitions across states; from a legal point of view, stalking is the willful, malicious, and repeated following and harassing of another person, with fear of violence resulting in the victim; stalking behaviors can vary from seemingly benign acts or efforts at being reasonable, to hidden, threatening, and frightening behaviors

Family Violence

- Spousal assault is the single most common cause of injury for which women seek emergency medical attention (Box 16.1)
  - In a study of the emergency treatment of women in a metropolitan hospital, battered women were 13 times more likely than other women who were receiving emergency care to be injured in the breast, chest, or abdomen, and they were three times as likely to be injured while pregnant
- According to the U.S. Bureau of Justice Statistics (U.S. Department of Justice), for nonfatal domestic violence in 2003 to 2012:
  - Current or former boyfriends or girlfriends committed most domestic violence
  - Domestic violence accounted for 21% of all violent crime
  - Females (76%) experienced more domestic violence victimizations than males (24%)

BOX 16.1 **Fact Sheet on Domestic Violence**

- Thirty-one percent of U.S. women report being physically or sexually abused by a husband, former spouse, or boyfriend at some point in their lives
- Domestic violence leads to long-term health problems, including chronic neck or back pain; migraine and other frequent headaches; visual and hearing loss; sexually transmitted diseases; chronic pelvic pain; and chronic gastrointestinal disorders
- Emotional health effects include: 56% of women in violent relationships are diagnosed with a psychiatric disorder; 29% of all women who attempt suicide are battered; 37% of battered women are depressed; 46% have anxiety disorders; and 45% experience PTSD
- Ninety-two percent of women who were battered did not discuss these incidents with their physicians; 57% did not discuss these incidents with anyone
- Eighty percent of clients report that they would like their health care providers to ask them privately about intimate partner violence

From Stuart, G. W. (2013). *Principles and practice of psychiatric nursing* (10 ed.). St. Louis, MO: Mosby/Elsevier.

- Several characteristics distinguish family violence from stranger violence; although there is a continuing relationship among its members that is similar to that of other relationships (eg, teacher and student, employer and employee, child and caretaker), daily interaction in a shared domicile increases the opportunities for violent encounters; because these individuals are bound together in a continuing relationship, it is quite likely there will be repeat violations by the offender
- An unequal power relationship makes one more vulnerable to the aggression and violence of the offender; moreover, the offender often threatens additional violence if the incidents of violence are disclosed; the victim may refrain from disclosure in anticipation of stigmatization and denigration; finally, episodes of violence often occur in private places, are invisible to others, and are less likely to be detected or reported to police
- Violence that began during dating can continue within marriage
- Family violence has been linked to mental illness and personality disorders, although the links have been established for clinical populations rather than with the use of case-control methods or general population surveys; studies of women's shelter populations report that depression is common among women who are chronic victims of domestic violence; there is also a high incidence of bipolar depression, anxiety disorders, PTSD, panic disorder, and suicide ideation among chronically abused women
- A large group of batterers have been diagnosed as having borderline personalities that include a constellation of behavioral shifts: Anger outbursts, rage, intense jealousy, blaming, recurring moods, trauma symptoms, haunting fear of isolation and loss, binge drinking, and repetitive self-destructive thoughts

Violence During Pregnancy

- As many as one in five teenagers are the victims of domestic violence during pregnancy
- Although domestic violence during pregnancy is often preceded by a history of abuse, pregnancy may act as a trigger that increases the frequency and severity of the violence; this increase may be related to the financial implications of the pregnancy and birth, the stress surrounding altered relational and sexual roles, and the increased attention on the growing pregnancy
- In addition, pregnancy disclosure, especially in cases of questionable paternity, may also potentiate a volatile situation
- Intimate partner violence during pregnancy is associated with low birth weight and preterm birth

Homicide of Female Victims

- According to Bureau of Justice Statistics, females made up 70% of victims killed by an intimate partner in 2007, a proportion that has changed very little since 1993; females were killed by an intimate partner at twice the rate of males

Nursing Care of Survivors in Relation to Domestic Violence

- Overview
  - Includes child abuse (see later in this chapter), partner abuse, and elder abuse (see later in this chapter)
  - Abuse can be physical, emotional, sexual, and/or financial
  - Neglect of a dependent child or elder is more common than abuse; neglect is the failure to provide basic care needs such as nutrition, shelter, and health care
  - The incidence of psychiatric illness and addiction disorders is higher in families in which there is domestic violence

- Families in which abuse occurs are often isolated, with few support systems, have a history of abusive behaviors, and experience stressors such as unemployment or illness
- The child who is most likely to be abused has a physical or mental handicap (see later in this chapter) or was born prematurely or at a difficult time in the family's history; such children become scapegoats and are blamed for the family's problems; an elder adult who is abused may have physical or cognitive disabilities that make them more vulnerable and require caregivers to take on more responsibility
- Societal influences of violence, sexual imagery, cultural norms about family roles, and the use of physical punishment to discipline may increase the tendency toward domestic violence

NURSING CARE OF SITUATIONS OF DOMESTIC VIOLENCE/NEGLECT

Assessment

- Assess the woman's potential danger in cases of domestic violence; information regarding the pattern of abuse and its severity and frequency is vital; other critical signs that indicate increased danger are that the abuser has a weapon, that he has been violent outside of the house, that he is a substance abuser, that he has been stalking the woman, and that he has threatened suicide or homicide; at times, the woman may contemplate suicide
- Identify signs of violence/neglect
  - Unexplained or frequent injuries or accidents, conflicting stories about injuries, delayed treatment for injuries, injuries in various stages of healing (Box 16.2)
  - Inadequate hygiene, inappropriate dress, and eating and sleeping disorders
  - Depression; assess risk for suicide
  - Sexually transmitted infections; inappropriate (premature) sexual knowledge
  - Be alert to the possibility of human trafficking
- Report suspicions of child and elder abuse to the appropriate governmental agency, which is a requirement for nursing licensure in most states; the nurse does not need to be absolutely certain and provide proof—there only needs to be a reasonable suspicion

---

BOX 16.2 Physical Indicators of Possible Adult Abuse

General Appearance
Anxious and frightened; depressed and passive; ashamed and embarrassed; poor eye contact; weight problems; looks to partner for answers and partner does all of the talking; partner exhibits smothering and extremely possessive behavior

Skin
Contusions, abrasions, minor lacerations, scars, and burns, particularly on the breasts, arms, abdomen, chest, neck, face, and genitals

Musculoskeletal
Fractures and sprains, especially of distal bones (eg, skull, facial bones, extremities) compared with proximal bones; dislocated shoulders; evidence of previous fractures

Genital and Rectal
Evidence of vaginal or anal rape such as bruising, edema, and bleeding; also evidence of direct kicks or punches in this area

Abdominal
Internal bleeding or other injuries; chronic pelvic pain

Neuropsychologic
Acute stress disorder; hyperactive reflexes; chronic headaches and backaches; paresthesias from previous injuries

From Fortinash, K. M., & Holoday, P. A. (2012). *Psychiatric mental health nursing* (5th ed.). St. Louis, MO: Mosby

---

Planning/implementation

- The plan of care for any survivor of violence focuses on addressing critical physical problems, collecting appropriate evidence, securing the immediate safety of the victim, examining the implications of the abuse on the woman and other family members, and discussing future plans for safety
- The nurse develops the care plan with the client and recognizes that any effort to impose personal beliefs on the battered woman will fail; instead, the client needs reassurance that she is capable of making appropriate decisions for herself, even if her decision is to return to her abuser; it is only through empowerment—and not through threats and intimidation—that the woman is most likely to develop the strength to make independent decisions that foster growth
- When the battered woman's physical condition has been stabilized, it is critical to assess her future safety and to collaboratively explore her fears, anxieties, and concerns (Box 16.3)
  - Despite the need to leave the abusive situation, the woman may strongly believe that she has no other option except to return to her abuser
  - If the woman chooses to return to the batterer, it is important to respect this decision; making a decision to leave the batterer is usually a gradual process
  - However, it is critical that the woman realizes that she has options; the nurse may serve as the key factor in a beginning awareness that other options do exist
- All states have laws that provide some level of protection for survivors of domestic violence; however, the reality is that there is a large gap between the actual laws and their implementation by the police and the criminal justice system; in some localities, police are mandated to arrest the abuser if there is evidence of probable violence; in many states, the police must provide the battered woman with information about local shelters, domestic violence crisis lines, and her legal rights; however, if the police do not provide the information, the nurse can advise the battered woman of her legal rights

---

BOX 16.3 Nursing Interventions for Battered Women

Report abuse to police.
Provide medications to relieve pain and anxiety.
Discuss the validity of the woman's anxiety.
Encourage the woman to discuss the events that led to past and present abuse.
Point out the increasingly violent nature of the relationship, and acknowledge concern for her safety.
Insist that no person has the right to abuse another.
Explore the effectiveness of her current coping skills, and suggest additional skills.
Focus on her strengths, endurance, and abilities.
Discuss the destructive societal expectations of women.
Discuss the frequency of woman abuse.

Explore family and friends as support possibilities.
Discuss the potential for using community resources (eg, shelters, hotlines, police).
Describe current laws regarding domestic violence.
Explore the implications of pressing charges against the batterer.
Explore the meaning of the potential relationship loss.
Explore the various options for the future.
Provide a fact sheet about domestic violence.
Provide referrals.
Develop a safety plan with critical papers, money, clothing, and other essentials to be set aside for emergency exits.
Offer to be available for further questions.

From Fortinash, K. M., & Holoday, P. A. (2012). *Psychiatric mental health nursing* (5th ed.). St. Louis, MO: Mosby.

- Some women's rights advocates and criminal justice experts have differing perspective regarding mandatory reporting laws for domestic violence; women's rights advocates claim that mandatory domestic violence reporting laws discourage battered women from seeking treatment for their injuries because the women fear that their situations will be reported to the police and that they will consequently be in even greater danger of abuse; because some women are not ready to deal with the police, being forced to do so could be nontherapeutic and disempowering and even increase their risk of abuse
  - If no mandatory reporting laws exist, then the police should not be notified unless the woman consents; although some professionals choose to maintain confidentiality if the battered woman requests it, the deciding factor with regard to reporting is the degree of danger that the woman faces and whether state law mandates reporting
- Interventions
  - Interventions for elder and child abuse include education about usual growth and development, methods of discipline of children, referral to support groups and social services, anger management, assertiveness training, and relaxation therapy
  - Removal of at-risk children; dependent adults may be removed from the home for their safety
  - The battered woman is at greatest risk of harm when she tries to leave her abuser; therefore the woman must become aware of this risk, and the nurse must assist her with the development of a safety plan; such a plan typically involves helping the victim create an emergency exit from the home and plan a time to escape as well as providing the phone numbers of nearby shelters, crisis lines, and community resources; the woman should also be referred to the local victim's assistance program

Levels of Prevention

- Primary prevention for domestic abuse begins with making nonviolence a priority; education about the societal acceptance of violence against women as portrayed in films, television, magazines, and music must be exposed
  - Nurses can become more knowledgeable about factors that increase the risk of domestic violence, and they can work with other members of the community to establish public policy and programs to address these issues
- Secondary prevention of domestic abuse involves early case finding and decisive intervention
  - Specific nursing interventions depend on the stage that the battered woman is in because a woman who is in denial about the abuse requires a different strategy from one who is determined not to return to the relationship
- Tertiary prevention is required when the woman has been repeatedly abused; in such instances, the focus is on assisting the abused woman to overcome the physical and psychologic effects of the abuse and to prevent future abuse; because the abuser frequently threatens and harasses the woman when she attempts to leave, it may be difficult for her to follow through
  - Frequently, these women seek assistance from local shelters that can provide safety and counseling; nurses are often in the position to provide support and counseling to battered women in shelters

Prognosis

- Victims of partner abuse usually require several attempts before successfully leaving an abusive situation; victims should be helped to develop strategies for exiting an abusive situation, which include identifying financial resources, safe houses, and support groups; nurses should guard against expressing frustration to victims who choose to remain in their current situations

5. A recently married 22-year-old woman is brought to the trauma center by the police. She had been robbed, beaten, and sexually assaulted. The client, although very anxious and tearful, appears in control. The health care provider prescribes alprazolam 0.25 mg for agitation. The nurse should administer this medication when the:
   1. Client's crying increases
   2. Client requests something to calm her
   3. Nurse determines a need to reduce her anxiety
   4. Health care provider is getting ready to do an examination
6. A nurse in the emergency department is assessing a client who was beaten and sexually assaulted. After physical and psychological safety, which is the nurse's next priority assessment?
   1. The family's feelings about the attack
   2. The client's feelings of social isolation
   3. Disturbance in the client's thought processes
   4. The client's ability to cope with the situation
7. A nurse is working with a married woman who has come to the emergency department several times with injuries that appear to be related to domestic violence. When talking with the nurse manager, a nurse expresses disgust that the woman returns to the same situation. What is the nurse manager's **best** response?
   1. "She must not have the financial resources to leave her husband."
   2. "Most woman attempt to leave about six times before they are able to do so."
   3. "There is nothing the staff can do because people are free to choose their own life"
   4. "These women should be told how foolish they are to remain in their current situation."

See Answers on pages 323-325.

ABUSE OF CHILDREN

Homicide of Infants and Small Children

- Family violence can escalate to homicide; several patterns are noteworthy: Newborns and children between the ages of 1 and 4 years are more vulnerable to homicide than are children between the ages of 5 and 9 years
- Infants and small children are more likely to be killed by their mothers than their fathers, perhaps in part as a result of differential risk exposure; the risk of homicide for children who are younger than 5 years old is greater for male than female children

Nonfatal Child Abuse

Types of nonfatal child abuse include physical abuse, psychological abuse, and sexual abuse

- Because bruises, fractures, and lacerations are easily observed and detected, physical abuse is the type that is most often reported
- Psychologic abuse is difficult to detect and treat, and it is more long lasting than physical injury
- Sexual assault is not rare, but it is often concealed by the victim and the family

Physical Abuse

- Physical child abuse is the intentional physical infliction of injury by a parent or caretaker; the spectrum of injuries is broad, and it may range from a few bruises to injuries that cause death

- Types of physical abuse
  - Bruising is observed in the form of finger and palm prints on the face or buttocks and as human teeth or bite marks; loop and lash marks on the skin are easily identified and indicative of a doubled-over cord or belt; in most true accidents, bruising occurs on only one body surface, except when a fall occurs down a flight of stairs
  - Burns are another source of physical abuse; a cigarette may cause circular areas of similar size on the soles, palms, or abdomen; hot water burns are noted with a clear water level on the buttocks, perineum, or legs, and they may be caused by dunking the child as a disciplinary measure for problems with toilet training; dry contact burns to the palms and soles may result from holding the child against a hot radiator
  - Fractures of the long bones, ribs, or skull are often detected in abused and neglected children
  - Children with neurologic injuries may present in a coma or with convulsions and be found to suffer subdural or retinal hemorrhage, especially in shaken baby syndrome

NURSING CARE OF CHILDREN WHO ARE PHYSICALLY ABUSED

Assessment/Analysis

- History of injury: Objective data from examination does not match story told by parents (eg, "Toddler fell off of chair" when examination reveals spiral fracture of femur, which would not result from this type of fall) (Box 16.4)
- Physical status: Evidence of past injuries (eg, skeletal, soft tissue); failure to thrive (Box 16.5)
- Parent-child interaction
- Developmental level

Planning/Implementation

- Monitor for clues that indicate neglect or abuse
- Child
  - Unexplained injuries, scars, bruises
  - Physical signs of neglect (eg, malnourished, dehydrated, unkempt)
  - Cringes when physically approached, seems unduly afraid

BOX 16.4 Interview Guidelines for Assessment of a Child

Do
- Conduct the interview in private.
- Sit next to the child, not across the table or desk.
- Tell the child that the interview is confidential.
- Use language the child understands.
- Ask the child to clarify words that you do not understand.
- Tell the child if any action will be required.

Ask open-ended questions. Possible questions include:
- How did this happen to you?
- Who takes care of you?
- What do you do after school?
- Who are your friends?
- What happens when you do something wrong?

Do Not
- Allow the child to feel "in trouble" or "at fault."
- Suggest answers to the child.
- Probe or press for answers the child is not willing to give.
- Display shock or disapproval of parent, child, or situation.
- Force the child to remove clothing.
- Conduct the interview with a group of interviewers.

Modified from Varcarolis, E. M., & Halter, M. J. (2010). *Psychiatric mental health nursing: A clinical approach* (6th ed.). St. Louis, MO: Saunders.

BOX 16.5 Physical Indicators of Possible Child Abuse and Neglect

General Appearance
Excessive fearfulness and watchfulness
Disheveled and malnourished
Failure to thrive
Multiple injuries
No history of significant trauma

Skin
Unexplained bruises, welts, and scratches in various stages of healing (ie, different colors)
Regular patterns of bruises and welts (eg, bite marks, marks from electrical cords)
Untreated infected wounds
Lacerations from rope burns, especially on the neck, wrists, ankles, and torso
Bruises on the buttocks, genitalia, thighs, side of the face, trunk, and upper arms

Burns
Small round cigarette burns (however, infected insect bites can resemble cigarette burns)
Immersion burns (these have even boundaries that are glove-like, sock-like, or symmetric; accidental burns are asymmetric with splash marks)
Patterned burn marks (eg, from an iron or grill)

Fractures
Fractures in infants that are younger than 1-year-old fractures of the femur, humerus, posterior ribs, skull, and long bones and any uncommon fractures

Head Injuries
Skull fractures and subdural hematomas (these are the leading cause of death among abused children)
Brain hemorrhages or contusions without external signs of injury (eg, shaken baby syndrome)
Alopecia caused by hair pulling

Abdominal Injuries
Ruptured liver or spleen
Ruptured blood vessels
Kidney, bladder, or pancreatic injuries
Injuries to the jejunum or duodenum
Injuries to the eyes, ears, nose, and mouth
A wide variety of injuries, including missing teeth, bruising, perforation of the tympanic membrane, epistaxis, nasal fractures, retinal hemorrhage, detachment, corneal abrasions, and periorbital hematomas

From Fortinash, K. M., & Holoday, P. A. (2012). *Psychiatric mental health nursing* (5th ed.). St. Louis, MO: Mosby.

- Responses indicate avoidance of punishment rather than gaining reward
- Has excessive interest in sexual matters; has sexually transmitted infection
- Nursing care depends on type of injuries sustained
- Parental behavior
  - Offers inconsistent stories explaining injuries
  - Emotional response is inconsistent with degree of injury
  - May resist or fail to be present for questioning
- Protect from further abuse (Box 16.6)
- Know child abuse laws; report *suspected* abuse/neglect to designated authority
- Provide consistent caregiver
- Monitor when parents or others visit
- Help parents:
  - Address their dependency needs
  - Learn to control frustration through other outlets
  - Learn about childhood growth and development, expected behavioral characteristics, realistic expectations
  - Appropriate modes of limit setting and discipline

BOX 16.6	Nursing Interventions for the Physically Abused Child

Develop a trusting relationship with the parents.
Be direct and open but supportive.
Obtain a holistic history, including the stresses and problems that the family is experiencing.
Explore how the events that led to the abuse might be altered in the future.
Explore alternative strategies for childcare problems.
Discuss basic child growth and development.
Provide the parents with basic materials about child growth and development.
Have the parents apply child development principles.
Discuss the need for parenting classes.
Discuss strategies for anger control.
Discuss reporting laws regarding child abuse.
Explain the child welfare function of protective services.
Take steps to inform protective services.
Observe parent–child interactions unobtrusively.

Involve parents in childcare during the child's hospitalization, when appropriate.
Discuss the physical effect of abuse with parents.
Discuss the short-term and long-term psychologic effects of child abuse.
Provide a referral to postdischarge public health child nursing.
The public health nurse will coordinate services and monitor parental progress.
The public health nurse will serve as a role model and assist the parents with applying principles learned in parenting classes to their own lives.
Have the parent discuss how s/he will maintain her/his anger skills.
Teach the nonviolent parent to intervene if the other parent exhibits negative parenting.
Assist the parents with the development of social support systems.
Explore community resources with the family.

Modified from Fortinash, K. M., & Holoday, P. A. (2012). *Psychiatric mental health nursing* (5th ed.). St. Louis, MO: Mosby.

- Use therapeutic play with child to help express feelings
- Provide emotional support and therapy; abused children may grow to be abusive parents
- Refer family for group therapy, home visits, foster grandparent visits

Evaluation/Outcomes

- Child remains free from injury or neglect
- Parents demonstrate effective parenting activities

Psychological Abuse of Children

- Defined as sustained, repetitive, and damaging behavior that substantially reduces the creative and developmental potential of crucially important mental abilities of a child
  - These faculties include intelligence, memory, recognition, perception, attention, imagination, and moral development; psychologic abuse impairs children's capacity to understand and manage their environment, confuses or frightens them, and renders them vulnerable; such abuse affects education, general welfare, and social life; the consequences of psychologic abuse are determined by the nature, intensity, and duration of the abuse; the damaged mental abilities and processes; the age and stage of development of the abused child; and the quality of life, treatment, and therapy after the abuse has ended
  - Often the psychologic abuse of a child is ignored until the child's formative years have been impaired by the threats and rejection that are integral parts of these families' day-to-day routines; the deprivation and misery that were parts of many neglecting parents' own childhoods may be perpetuated in their roles as parents or caregivers; they may not wish to harm their children, but they have little capacity to help them; as a result, the children are more frequently withdrawn rather than aggressive

- Abusive language and verbal expressions of hostility are present in a high percentage of severely abusing families; some parents state bluntly that they hate their children and never wanted them whereas others threaten to kill them; frequently, the children are yelled at and called derogatory names such as "idiot;" they are referred to as objects of ridicule; hopelessness, despair, and defeat are obvious in these children's attention-seeking and approval-seeking overtures for love; they trust no one, and they expect little except rejection

Sexual Abuse of Children

- A person may achieve sexual contact with another person in three basic ways: (1) through consent, which involves negotiation and mutual agreement; (2) through exploitation, which involves a person capitalizing on a position of dominance (eg, economic, social, vocational) to take sexual advantage of a person in a subordinate position; and (3) through assault, which involves the threat of personal injury or the use of physical force
  - The latter two methods constitute sexual victimization; only through negotiation and consent can sexual relations properly be achieved; however, such consent is precluded in sexual encounters between a child and an adult by virtue of the adult being mature and occupying a position of authority and dominance with regard to the child; a child is not legally able to give consent; a child, by definition, is an immature person, and most children have not developed sufficient knowledge, wisdom, or social skills to be able to negotiate such an encounter on an equal basis with an adult; even a physically mature child is not mature enough to emotionally cope with sexual demands from an adult; the child can easily be taken advantage of by an older person or adult, and, although the child may agree to and cooperate with the sexual activity, the child does so without an awareness or appreciation of the effect that such activity may have on his or her subsequent psychosocial development (eg, personality formation, attitudes, values, identity issues)
  - In general, children are not well informed about human sexuality or adequately prepared for this important area of human behavior, and the offender can exploit their innocence in self-serving ways to the physical, social, psychologic, and emotional detriment of the children
- The sexual abuse of children includes a wide range of sexual acts perpetrated by persons who are older than the victim; these acts include exhibitionism, the fondling or manipulation of the genitals, digital penetration, penile penetration of the vagina or rectum, genital contact, the insertion of foreign objects into the genitals or rectum, and the use of children in pornography and prostitution
- Sexual abuse also includes noncontact sexual activity such as sexually explicit language directed toward a child, obscene telephone calls, showing pornographic materials to a child, and voyeurism; most sexually abused children experience multiple types of sexually abusive acts; the legal definition of sexual abuse varies by state jurisdiction, and nurses need to familiarize themselves with the laws in their district
- Gaining access to the child
  - The child predator may gain access to the victim through deception or by directly approaching the child; in the majority of cases, the offender will use some type of psychologic pressure (eg, enticement, encouragement) to persuade the child to enter into sexual activity; in some cases, the offender may resort to force, either in the form of threats and intimidation or through brute physical strength
- Pressure situations
  - The most common approach used by a child predator is to initially establish a nonsexual relationship with the victim that has meaning to the child; the offender becomes a familiar

and trusted figure in the child's life; over time, sexual intimacy is introduced into the context of this involvement; the offender may deceive the child by misinterpreting social standards (eg, "All boys and girls do this, so it's okay"), by misidentifying the activity (eg, "We're going to wrestle"), by tricking the child (eg, "I'm going to give you a bath"), or by presenting the activity in the context of game (eg, "I've hidden some money in my clothes, and, if you find it, you can have it"), and then rewarding the child's cooperation with money, gifts, candy, or toys; children will exchange the sexual activity for these other nonsexual rewards, and one of the most prized rewards is attention; the offender will capitalize on the child's need for attention to lure the child into the sexual activity by making the child feel special or important

- Forced situations
  - Although less likely, the offender may directly confront the child with sexual demands in the content of verbal threats (eg, "Do what I say and you won't get hurt"), intimidation with a weapon (eg, brandishing a knife), or direct physical assault (eg, grabbing the child); these tactics are directed at overcoming any resistance on the part of the victim, although the intent is not to hurt the child; such sexual assaults constitute child rape, in which sexuality becomes the means for expressing power and anger; the offender's approach is either one of intimidation, by exploiting the child's helplessness, naïveté, and awe of adults, or one of physical aggression, attacking and overpowering his victim
- Offenders
  - Characteristics of offenders are primarily based on the research of those cases that have been examined within the criminal justice system and that represent situations in which the sexual abuse was disclosed; most cases of sexual abuse are never reported, so these criminal cases are not believed to be representative of all offenders
  - Experts recognize that child sexual offenders make up a diverse population that is difficult to classify; the offenders vary with regard to age, gender, occupation, income, marital status, and ethnic group
  - Juvenile offenders exist, ranging in age from 5 to 19 years, and they represent all ethnic, racial, and socioeconomic classes; however, 90% are male; the majority of adult offenders report beginning their deviant sexual behavior during adolescence
- Characteristics of the nonoffending parent
  - When the abuser is the father, the mother is sometimes blamed for failing to satisfy her husband's psychologic and sexual needs or for being rejecting or dominating; in addition, when the child discloses the abuse to the mother, it has been claimed that the mother commonly denies that the abuse occurred or blames the child for initiating or encouraging it; these mothers are in denial
  - By contrast, many nonoffending mothers are initially shocked and unable to believe their child's claim of being sexually abused by their partner; it is especially upsetting to the woman if she loves and trusts her partner because she must now cope with her partner's betrayal in addition to her child being violated and traumatized; it is much simpler and less painful to believe that it did not occur; nevertheless, many mothers who are initially in shock experience a process that involves a crisis of disbelief and ambivalence that is followed by gradual acceptance and eventual dedication to healing the child's trauma as well as their own
- Long-term consequences
  - Nurses realize that, when traumatized children become upset, it is difficult for them to calm down, because the shifts in integrative behavior are driven by biologic dysregulation; there is a progression of symptomatology and behaviors among victims of a traumatic event

- Integration of trauma: No PTSD
    - The optimal response pattern from a traumatic event is resolution of the posttrauma symptoms, with subsequent integration of the traumatic event in to the life experience of the victim; in the integrated pattern, the client is able to relate to the sexual abuse experience, but is not compelled to dwell on it or to avoid it with the use of maladaptive psychologic defenses
- PTSD with a classic PTSD response, a biphasic response is noted; the victim may suffer intrusive thoughts of the abuse or display avoidant behaviors; exposure to stimuli can induce a state of hyperarousal and numbing, which may cause the victim to experience highly emotional states
    - Symptoms may include hyperactivity, headaches, stomachaches, back pain, genitourinary distress, and nightmares; symptoms of interpersonal disruption include behaviors such as excessive fear of others and an inability to assert or protect oneself; aggressive behaviors include agitation, aggression toward peers, family members, or pets, and potentially sexualized behavior toward others
- Several patterns of PTSD symptoms are noted in traumatized children:
    - The anxious pattern is characterized by generalized fears and anxious recollection of the abuse situation if probed or asked; anxiety disorders, eating disorders, and phobic and obsessive-compulsive disorders have been linked with unresolved trauma
    - The avoidant pattern is characterized by denial or recanting that the abuse has occurred; these youths may develop a substance use disorder history, depression and suicidal thoughts, phobic behavior, adjustment problems, or conduct disorders
    - The aggressive pattern is characterized by sexual or aggressive behavior; minimal acknowledgment or frank denial of prior abuse is typical; there is the testing and breaking of rules, impulsivity, and fighting with peers; diagnostic labels of hyperactivity, learning disabilities, conduct disorders, and impulse disorders are sometimes used
    - The disorganized pattern is characterized by fragmented and sometimes bizarre behavior; dissociative states can occur; there may be denial or frank amnesia regarding prior sexual abuse
- Delayed PTSD: Some victims of trauma may not initially develop PTSD but rather progress to delayed PTSD and display no visible sequelae to the event; avoidant behaviors include low sexual involvement, passivity, substance use to reduce tension, somatic complaints, and depression; aggressive patterns include participating in high-risk behaviors and antisocial acts, substance use as a stimulant, and high sexual involvement

Nursing Care of Sexually Abused Children
- See also Nursing Care of Children who are Physically Abused and Table 16.2

Assessment
- Nurse's own assumptions
    - As with the assessment of other victims of violence, the nurse should begin with an assessment of his or her own assumptions, beliefs, and attitudes about childhood sexual abuse
        - Nurses who believe that the child is responsible in any way for the sexual abuse will find it difficult to be supportive of the child
        - The nurse must be comfortable when speaking with the child about the abuse so that an attitude of discomfort is not conveyed to the child

TABLE 16.2 Types of Child Abuse and Physical and Behavioral Indicators		
Type of Abuse	**Physical Indications**	**Behavioral Indications**
Physical Abuse		
Occurs when a caretaker allows or inflicts intentional physical injury that causes a substantial risk to the child's well-being and health	Bruises/wounds in differing stages of healing Unexplained burns, bruises, welts, broken bones, internal injuries, bite marks, etc. Bald patches on scalp Subdural hematoma (child younger than 2 years) Retinal hemorrhage	Excessive fear of parents or constant effort to please Wary of adult contact Posttrauma syndrome (eg, nightmares) Obvious attempts to hide bruises or injuries Withdrawn, depressed, or aggressive disruptive behavior Regressive behavior
Neglect		
Failure to provide for the child's basic needs	*Physical neglect:* Malnourished Underweight, poor growth pattern Inadequately supervised Poor hygiene Unattended physical problems Inappropriate dress *Educational neglect:* School problems or failure Not enrolled in *mandatory* school for age *of* child	Soiled clothing; poor hygiene Begging, stealing food Emaciated or have distended belly Extended stay at school (early arrival and/or late departure) Psychosomatic complaints Delinquency Alcohol or drug abuse Abandonment Chronic truancy Special educational needs not being attended
Sexual Abuse		
Sexual abuse perpetrated on nonfamily member Some types include: • Exhibitionism • Touching or manipulating the child's sexual organs • Oral, anal, or vaginal sex • Having child touch perpetrator • Masturbation in front of or with the child	Difficulty in walking or sitting Vulvovaginitis Urinary tract infections Torn, stained, or bloody underclothing Bruises or bleeding in external genitalia, vaginal or anal areas Venereal disease, especially in preteens In boys, pain on urination or penile swelling or discharge Foreign matter in rectum, vagina, or urethra	Mistrust of adults Abnormal or distorted view of sex Bizarre, sophisticated, or unusual sexual behavior or knowledge Phobias: Fear of the dark, men, strangers, leaving the house Delinquent or running away Self-injury or suicidal thoughts or behaviors Mental disorders may develop (eg, PTSD, depression, multiple personality disorder, eating disorders, conduct disorders, anxiety disorder)

Continued

TABLE 16.2 Types of Child Abuse and Physical and Behavioral Indicators—cont'd

Type of Abuse	Physical Indications	Behavioral Indications
Emotional or Psychological Abuse		
Behaviors that convey to the child that he or she is worthless, flawed, unloved, or unwanted: • Constant criticism • Insults • Harsh demands • Threats and yelling • Ignoring the child • Denying child opportunities to receive positive reinforcement	Speech disorders Lag in physical development	Difficulty in learning and living up to potential Lack of self-confidence Inappropriate adult-like behavior or infantile behavior Dramatic behavior changes (eg, aggressiveness, compulsive seeking of affection or approval)

From Varcarolis, E. (2013). *Essentials of psychiatric mental health nursing* (2nd ed.). St. Louis, MO: Saunders.

- ▪ Children are adept at recognizing nonverbal cues, and the nurse's discomfort may be interpreted by the child as a sign that he or she should not talk about the abuse with the nurse or that he or she is not believed
- A holistic approach is essential; because childhood sexual abuse trauma is highly complex and affected by multiple interacting factors, it is important to gain as much information as possible without subjecting the child to unnecessary and repeated probing and questioning
- Most often the nurse encounters the sexually abused child in the emergency department or an outpatient clinic; often, the mother or another caregiver brings the child to a medical facility to determine whether the child has been sexually abused
- Whenever there is a suspicion of childhood abuse, a complete physical examination must be conducted, including assessment for failure to thrive; delayed growth and development
  - The primary objective is to establish a trusting relationship with the child so that he or she can relate relevant events and cooperate with the physical examination
  - It is important to assess the relationship between the caregiver and the child to determine whether the child is more comfortable with or without that person
    - ▪ Usually younger children do not want to be separated from their caregiver, whereas older children may be too inhibited to disclose in front of the caregiver for a variety of reasons such as fear of being blamed by family members, disbelieved, or instrumental in the family break-up
    - ▪ Sometimes the child may retract the disclosure in an effort to protect the abuser with whom he or she may have an ambivalent relationship
    - ▪ Finally, the developmental age of the child is an important factor in his or her ability to successfully provide data about the abuse; the younger the child, the less able he or she may be to describe events and to understand the interviewer's questions
  - The majority of children who have been sexually abused do not display any physical signs of abuse if the disclosure has been delayed for weeks or if there has not been any vaginal or anal penetration; the occurrence of oral copulation or mock intercourse is also difficult to physically document unless the child is examined within a short time after the activity

- In addition to the lack of physical evidence, the sexually abused child may not display any observable signs of emotional trauma, and he or she may deny, retract, and be inconsistent with regard to the description of the abuse; caregivers often interpret this behavior to mean that the abuse did not occur and that the child is lying; the significance of absent physical or emotional signs must be clearly explained to the child's caregivers
- Conversely, multiple emotional and psychologic indicators may be present; however, because many of these signs can also reflect other problems, their presence alone is not a conclusive sign that sexual abuse has occurred; pinpointing that sexual abuse has occurred is difficult and challenging, because there is no single profile or set of symptoms that guarantees its presence; many signs and symptoms must be viewed only as potential indicators of sexual abuse, whereas others are highly probable indicators
- The meaning of any child's acting-out behavior needs to be explored; such behavior in abused children usually reflects the anger, confusion, and sense of betrayal that the child is experiencing and unable to discuss; although many abused children are able to act out their feelings through rebellious and delinquent behavior, others withdraw, blame themselves, become guilt ridden, and continuously try to be a "better" or "good" child; such children may function at a high level in school and even be praised and admired for what appears to be mature behavior because they often assume major responsibility for adult caregiver roles in their homes
- Some children with abusive histories do not exhibit signs of trauma during childhood but instead go on to exhibit them later in life; the presence of sexual abuse trauma depends on a wide variety of complex factors; in particular, the degree to which the child receives validation, protection, and support after disclosure is crucial to the resolution of the trauma
- Multiple sources of information are gathered, including interviews with the child and family members, outside information from sources such as teachers and babysitters, and psychologic tests if needed
- The interview with the child ideally should take place in an environment in which the child feels safe and comfortable; as with all sensitive topics, questions should begin with the least sensitive and most positive topics and progress to the most sensitive and direct ones; initial questions are meant to gain the trust of the child and to assist him or her to relax and to become more spontaneous; the developmental age of the child is a critical factor in the type and level of question that is used; therefore, all techniques must be modified according to the child's needs; small children may have difficulty with nondirective and open-ended questions; interviewers must be extremely cautious to not use leading questions (eg, "Daddy likes to tickle your bottom, doesn't he?")
- Eventually, the child must be asked directly about the possibility of sexual abuse; in a non-emergency situation, questions such as these could be used with a small child whose father, stepfather, or other male caregiver is suspected of the abuse:
  - Do you know why you have come to see me
  - What have you been told
  - What kinds of games do you and (the alleged abuser's name) play when your mom isn't around
  - Are there any games that you and (the alleged abuser's name) play that you don't like

Planning/Interventions

- The nurse's role is to provide comfort and safety for the child (Box 16.7)
- The immediate physical and psychologic needs of the child must be determined and addressed
- After immediate needs have been addressed, it is always critical for the nurse and other health care professionals to make a determination as to whether the child will be safe if returned to his or her home

| **BOX 16.7** | **Physical, Behavioral, and Psychosocial Indicators of Possible Childhood Sexual Abuse** |

General Appearance

Varies from normal to anxious, fearful, and depressed

Probable Physical Examination Indicators

Bruises, lacerations, or bite marks on the breasts, neck, buttocks, extremities, and oropharynx

Presence of sexually transmitted disease, including HIV

Presence of adult pubic hair and semen

Edema, abrasions, petechiae, and erythema of the genital area

Lacerations of the vagina or anus

Alterations in or enlargement of the hymenal orifice

Dysuria caused by periurethral trauma

Rectal fissures, chafing, erythema, bruising, lacerations, and perianal scarring

Semen in the oropharynx or the nasopharynx

Scar tissue of the labia minora, hymenal membrane, and anus

High-Risk Family History Indicators

Substance abuse in caregivers

History of abuse in parents

Domestic violence

Inadequate impulse control or mental illness in caregivers

Alleged offender with sexual dysfunction, poor coping skills, and poor social skills

Socially isolated family

Sexual abuse of sibling

Behavioral Indicators

Disclosure and spontaneous discussion of the abuse

Preoccupation with drawing genitals or anxious avoidance of anything to do with genitals or sex

Inappropriate sexual play behavior with dolls or other children, compulsive masturbation, inserting objects into the vagina or anus, sexualized kissing, fondling the genitals of others, and imitating intercourse

Dissociation

Avoidance of particular people

School and learning problems

Antisocial behavior, promiscuity, and substance abuse

Running away and other self-destructive behavior

Possible Psychosocial Indicators

Increased anxiety, fears, and depression; low self-esteem

Multiple somatic complaints

Signs of posttraumatic stress disorder

From Fortinash, K. M., & Holoday, P. A. (2012). *Psychiatric mental health nursing* (5th ed.). St. Louis, MO: Mosby.

- Types of long-term treatment depend on the child's developmental level and the mother's potential for supporting and protecting the child in the future
  - With a younger child, play therapy is often used, because the child often has difficulty verbalizing feelings about his or her abuse
  - Group therapy with other young children is also useful because common fears and misperceptions can be addressed; as the child becomes able to repeatedly address these fears and misperceptions, they will gradually be resolved; group therapy with other children is also a powerful modality for teaching the child self-assertive behavior and about how to self-protect in the future

Evaluation/Outcomes

- Child remains free from any abuse or neglect

ELDER ABUSE

Background

- Elder abuse is frequently compared with child abuse because neglect is common in both cases; however, with elder abuse, elders continue to have the rights of adults unless they are declared incompetent by a judge; therefore decisions cannot be legally forced on the elder as they can with children
- Elders have the right to choose to remain in a particular environment, even when it is obvious that they are being abused or neglected; the age that defines a person as an elder varies from 60 to 65 years
- Types of elder abuse
  - The physical abuse of an elder is defined as the use of physical force that may result in bodily injury, physical pain, or impairment; physical abuse may include striking (with or without an object), hitting, beating, pushing, shoving, shaking, slapping, kicking, pinching, and burning; in addition, the inappropriate use of drugs and physical restraints, force feeding, and physical punishment of any kind are also examples of physical abuse
    - Nurses can observe for signs and symptoms of bruises, black eyes, welts, lacerations, and rope marks; bone or skull fractures; open wounds, cuts, punctures, or untreated injuries in various stages of healing; sprains, dislocations; and internal injuries or bleeding
  - Sexual abuse of an elder is defined as nonconsensual sexual contact of any kind with an elderly person or sexual contact with a person who is incapable of giving consent; it includes all types of sexual assault or battery such as rape, sodomy, coerced nudity, and sexually explicit photographing
    - Nurses can observe for bruises around the breasts or genital area; unexplained sexually transmitted disease or genital infections; unexplained vaginal or anal bleeding; and torn, stained, or bloody underclothing
  - The emotional or psychologic abuse of an elder is defined as the infliction of anguish, pain, or distress through verbal or nonverbal acts; emotional and psychologic abuse includes but is not limited to verbal assaults, insults, threats, intimidation, humiliation, and harassment; other examples include treating an older person like an infant, giving an older person the "silent treatment," enforcing social isolation, and isolating an elderly person from his or her family, friends, or regular activities
    - Nurses can observe for an elder who is emotionally upset or agitated; who is extremely withdrawn, noncommunicative, or nonresponsive; or who is exhibiting unusual behavior that is usually attributed to dementia (eg, sucking, biting, rocking)
  - Neglect is defined as the refusal or failure to fulfill any part of a person's obligations or duties to an elder; neglect may also include the failure of a person who has fiduciary responsibilities to provide care for an elder (eg, failing to pay for necessary home care-services) or the failure on the part of an in-home service provider to provide necessary care; neglect typically means the refusal or failure to provide an elderly person with such life necessities as food, water, clothing, shelter, personal hygiene, medicine, comfort, personal safety, and other essentials that are included in an implied or agreed-upon responsibility to an elder
    - Nurses may observe dehydration, malnutrition, untreated bedsores, poor personal hygiene, and unattended or untreated health problems
  - Financial abuse of the elderly is another form of elder abuse

Risk Factors

- The psychopathology of the abuser
- External and situational stress

- Dependency and family relationships
- Social isolation
- Transgenerational violence

Lack of Reporting

- Patterns of assault of the elderly and disabled are often not reported (see Chapter 20)
- Perpetrators are most likely family members or caregivers
  - About 40 million individuals in the U.S. are age 65 or older; the U.S. Census Bureau projects that more than 62 million Americans will be age 65 years or older in 2025
  - Older women are more than twice as likely than men to suffer from abuse, and slightly more than half of the alleged perpetrators of elder abuse are female; because older victims usually have smaller support systems and fewer physical, psychologic, and economic reserves, the effect of abuse and neglect is magnified, and a single incident of mistreatment is more likely to trigger a downward spiral that leads to a loss of independence, a serious complicating illness, and even death

Elder Sexual Abuse

- Approximately 1 in 10 Americans aged 60 years and older have experienced some form of elder abuse; some estimates range as high as 5 million elders who are abused each year; one study estimated that only 1 in 14 cases of abuse are reported to authorities
- A National Institute of Justice report notes fear of the offender as the major reason for nonreporting; such underreporting of sexual abuse continues to occur in all age groups in a significant number of cases, with the extent of nondisclosure or nonreporting estimated to be as high as 68%; for elders, the typically inherent nature of dependence on others (eg, family members, caretakers, agency staff) in combination with physical frailty and alterations in mental status can result in an increased risk of abuse with subsequently low rates of reporting
- From a medical standpoint, bruises may be attributed to the aging process rather than to an assault; sometimes nursing procedures are blamed to explain genital bruising and bleeding in institutionalized elderly as either a "botched catheterization" or "rough perineal care;" bruising of the abdominal area may be attributed to tight restraints; clearly, there are multiple reasons to believe that the known cases of elder sexual assaults underestimate the true number of such cases

Difficulties with Recognizing Elder Trauma

- There is no prevalence data regarding PTSD among elders who have been victimized by others during a crime or as a result of other forms of elder abuse; however, the literature suggests that elderly victims may meet the diagnostic criteria for PTSD; the delayed onset of PTSD is an infrequently diagnosed variant of the disorder that is receiving attention among older combat veterans
- Another reality with older adults is comorbid disorders; there are many physical illnesses that are attributed to elders, including cardiac, respiratory, and cognitive problems; psychiatric conditions are present as well, including depression, substance misuse, and personality disorders, which many of which may mimic diagnoses on the anxiety continuum, including PTSD
- Older adults who reside in nursing homes are an especially vulnerable group; they often require assistance with basic activities of daily living (eg, bathing, dressing, feeding) as a result of physical and cognitive impairments; these disabilities make an individual dependent on others and an easy target for a sexual predator
- There are approximately 17,000 nursing homes in the United States, and these house 1.5 million older adult residents; nearly 1 in 3 U.S. nursing homes were cited for violations of federal

standards that had potential to cause harm or that had caused actual harm to a resident during the 2 years 1999 to 2001; nearly 1 out of 10 homes had violations that caused residents harm, serious injury, or placed them in jeopardy of death

- Reasons for the untimely reporting of allegations concern: (1) residents may fear retribution if they report the abuse; (2) family members are troubled with having to find a new place because the nursing home may ask the resident to leave; (3) staff do not report abuse promptly for fear of losing their jobs or of recrimination from coworkers and management; and (4) nursing homes want to avoid negative publicity and sanctions from the state

Elder Abuse Offenders

- Most sexual assaults of the elderly are not witnessed; however, when the victim is infirm as a result of cognitive deficits, the lack of an eyewitness is a complicating issue during the assessment and investigation of these cases; the challenge is to reconstruct the events that surrounded the possible sexual injury; a widely held myth regarding sexual abuse and assault is that offender motivations are sexual in nature; professional research suggests that sexual attacks are prompted by the offender's inherent need to dominate and oppress the victim; in cases of rape of the elderly, it has been contended that the victims are more likely to suffer more brutality and violence during their attacks than their younger counterparts; a theoretic explanation for this difference includes the idea that elderly victims are perceived by the offender as authoritative or even oppressive; the use of violence helps the perpetrator overcome this oppression by venting hostility and rage onto the victim
- In one review of elder abuse, the average age of the offender was 37 years; mental deficiencies or physical disabilities were noted to be sparse in this population; the use of alcohol and drugs was found in nearly half (44%) of these cases; elder victims were more likely to have an established relationship to the offender (59%)

NURSING CARE OF ABUSED ELDERS

Assessment

- It is critical to interview the elderly client apart from the caregiver; in a hospital setting, it is quite easy to simply assert that hospital policy mandates that clients be seen alone; if the nurse is conducting the interview at the client's home, it may be much more difficult to gain private access to the elder
    - This assessment must determine whether an abuser who lives with the elder is a substance abuser or if he or she has a history of mental illness or violence because these factors may further compromise the nurse's safety; it is possible sometimes to identify a family member who is trusted and who is able to provide the nurse with an opportunity to visit the elder as well as to ensure the safety of the nurse
    - Having another nurse present during a home visit is always an option, but at no time should nurses intentionally place themselves in dangerous home-visit situations
- It is not uncommon for both the abuser and the abused to maintain secrecy about the abuse; as with other types of family violence, abusers frequently threaten their victims with harm if they disclose the abuse; even without threats of retaliation, however, a great deal of time often lapses before the abused elder is comfortable disclosing the mistreatment; reluctance is usually a result of shame or self-blame or of fear of abandonment, institutionalization, or serious consequences for the abuser; physical indicators of actual or potential elder abuse are shown in Box 16.8; many of these symptoms are present with normal aging; therefore, as with other

BOX 16.8 Physical Indicators of Actual or Potential Elder Abuse and Neglect

General Appearance
Anxious, fearful, and passive
Poor eye contact
Looks to caregiver for answers
Poor hygiene and inappropriate dress
Underweight or malnourished
Physically handicapped
No glasses, false teeth, or hearing aid, despite need

Skin
Contusions, abrasions, burns, and scars in various stages of healing
Pressure ulcers and urine burns
Rope marks

Abdominal and Rectal
Distended abdomen
Bleeding
Fecal impactions

Musculoskeletal Fractures
Evidence of old healed fractures
Current fractures and sprains
Limited range of motion
Contractures

Genital and Urinary
Vaginal lacerations, bruises, and infections
Urinary tract infections

Neurologic
Slurred speech
Confusion

Modified from Fortinash, K. M., & Holoday, P. A. (2012). *Psychiatric mental health nursing* (5th ed.). St. Louis, MO: Mosby.

types of family violence, the nurse must perform a comprehensive assessment and consider the physical symptoms within the broader context of the client's life history
- Nursing assessment questions for the abused elder:
  - Are you happy living with (the name of the suspected abuser)
  - Please tell me about your financial assets and how they are managed
  - Whom do you turn to when you are feeling down
  - How are family disagreements handled in your household
  - Has anyone ever hurt you or touched you when you didn't want to be touched
- In addition to possible physical signs and symptoms of elder abuse and neglect, it is also necessary to assess the older adult for signs of exploitation and abandonment
  - Signs of exploitation include complaints by elders or evidence of the misuse of their money, the loss of control over their finances, material goods taken without consent or approval, and unmet financial needs that are inconsistent with their actual financial status
  - Signs of abandonment include reports by or evidence of elders being left alone and helpless for extended periods without adequate assistance

Planning

- As with other victims of family violence, securing safety is a major aspect of the plan of care for abused older adults; because most states have mandatory elder abuse reporting laws, it is critical that nurses and other health care professionals remain open to the possibility of elder abuse whenever there are potential indicators for it
- Because older adults may deny the existence of the abuse, it is necessary to establish a trusting relationship with older clients to facilitate disclosure; the nurse is often in the best position to assess and identify abused clients

- Thus the plan of care should include the nurse's taking time to communicate concern, compassion, and a desire to explore options and resources; this can determine whether clients disclose critical information or continue to suffer in silence

Implementation

- As with other cases of family violence, the nurse is often called on to function as the coordinator of care; the nurse may need to work closely with the social worker to develop and implement the plan of care; because the nurse has frequent opportunities to discuss. problems with the elder, he or she will be a key person in assisting the elder to identify feelings, recognize strengths, realistically assess the situation, and explore all possible options before making decisions
- Thus the nurse is in a position to address the total biopsychosocial, spiritual, and cultural needs of the client

Nursing Interventions

- The highest nursing priority is to balance the elder's safety and autonomy (Box 16.9); it is also important to assist with learning about the community resources that are available in terms of maximizing mental and physical health
  - A plan must be made with the family if the elder insists on remaining with the abuser(s), and this plan must clearly explain the family's obligations, the elder's rights, and the consequences of abusive or neglectful behavior in the future
  - Ongoing monitoring and evaluation are necessary; this is a role that is becoming more important for nurses as they provide ever-increasing amounts of care for older clients in their homes
- The home health care nurse must be prepared to provide counseling, referrals, support, and education to older clients and their families
  - Sometimes the caregiver may be in desperate need of stress management techniques, general information about the aging process, basic nursing care principles, and community agencies that provide assistance for older adults
  - Providing such support may dramatically ease the burden of caring for the older relative and prevent the occurrence of abuse and neglect

---

BOX 16.9 Nursing Interventions for the Abused Elderly

Monitor the client's response to decreased cardiac output.

Monitor the client's response to medications.

Provide reassurance and support.

Educate the client about medications and limitations.

Monitor the client for increased depression and suicide potential.

Explore with the client the reasons for feelings of helplessness and grief.

Discuss the client's capabilities and strengths.

Explore options that provide the client with increased control.

Explore ways for the client to increase self-care.

Explore the client's feelings related to family abuse.

Explore the client's options for remaining with family or making alternate living arrangements.

Coordinate referrals.

Show respect for the client's decisions.

Evaluate the caregiver's motivation for seeking and using assistance.

Evaluate the family's coping skills.

Evaluate possible substance abuse by the caregiver.

Evaluate the caregiver's willingness to acknowledge and work on family problems.

Evaluation

- Evaluating the effectiveness of the outcomes and nursing care plan for elders who have been abused is important, because the abuse may continue and even escalate if older clients choose to return to the abusive environment; however, nurses are often not in a position to follow up with clients after the clients leave the hospital
- Certain clues can be helpful for determining whether nursing interventions will be successful; these include the willingness of the older client to acknowledge the abuse and the willingness of the older client and the abusive family members to accept outside interventions or the removal of the elder from the abusive environment
- Although many resources for the older client exist in most communities, the family cannot be assisted if they deny the existence of the abuse; similar to battered women, older clients may experience multiple occasions of abuse before they gradually make the decision to leave their abusive environment

Assault of Disabled Persons

- From 2011 to 2015, for each age group measured except persons age 65 years or older, the rate of serious violent crime (rape or sexual assault, robbery, and aggravated assault) for persons with disabilities (12.7 per 1000) was *more than three times the rate* of that for persons without disabilities (4.0 per 1000); the rate for simple assault was more than twice the rate of that for persons without disabilities
- Among those with disabilities, persons ages 12 to 15 (144.1 per 1000 age 12 or older) had the highest rate of violent victimization among all age groups measured
- Sexual assault of a cognitively impaired person is rape because the victim is not considered able to give consent
- See also previous domestic abuse, abuse of children, and elder abuse sections

APPLICATION AND REVIEW

8. A parent who has been physically abusing a son is undergoing treatment for anger management. What statement by the client indicates the development of some insight into the abusive behavior?
   1. "I think the root of the problem is my partner's drinking."
   2. "I promise not to get so upset when my son causes trouble."
   3. "I'll be better able to control my behavior once my son gets better."
   4. "If I feel upset at my son, I'm going to go into the bedroom and punch a pillow."
9. An injured child is brought to the emergency department by the parents. When interviewing the parents, the nurse becomes suspicious of child abuse. Which parental behaviors might support this conclusion? **Select all that apply.**
   1. Demonstrating concern for the injured child
   2. Focusing on the child's role in sustaining the injury
   3. Changing the story of the way the child was injured
   4. Asking questions about the injury and the child's prognosis
   5. Explaining how the injury occurred, which is not consistent with the injury
10. A young child who is suspected of being sexually abused asks the nurse, "Did I do something bad?" What is the nurse's **most** therapeutic response?
    1. "Do you think you did something bad?"
    2. "Who said that you did something bad?"

3. "What do you mean by something bad?"
4. "Are you concerned that I think you did something bad?"
11. A nurse is caring for a preschool-age child with a history of physical and sexual abuse. What is the most advantageous therapy for this child?
   1. Play
   2. Group
   3. Family
   4. Psychodrama
12. People who abuse elders are most often:
   1. Strangers
   2. Physicians or caregivers
   3. Family members or caregivers
   4. Physicians or family members

See Answers on pages 323-325.

ANSWER KEY: REVIEW QUESTIONS

1. **4 Once the client is agitated, trying to teach any information is not effective and may increase the client's anxiety. Teaching relaxation techniques can be done when the client calms down.**
   1 Being assertive (not aggressive) shows the client the nurse is confident in handling the situation. This may help reduce the client's anxiety. **2** Responding before agitation escalates makes interventions more likely to be successful. **3** Providing choices may help the client feel less threatened and avoids a power struggle.
   Client Need: Psychosocial Integrity; **Cognitive level:** Analysis; **Integrated Process:** Communication/Documentation; **Nursing Process:** Planning/Implementation

2. **2 Before progress can be made in treating anger, clients need to take responsibility for their behavior. As long as they blame others, they will not be motivated to change.**
   1 Clients may express remorse but continue to blame others and not feel the need for change. **3** Developing alternative methods to release feelings is a worthwhile goal, but it is more appropriate later in therapy. It is not an initial goal. **4** These clients need to change their behavior, not teach others to change.
   Client Need: Psychosocial Integrity; **Cognitive Level:** Application; **Nursing Process:** Planning/Implementation

3. **3 "It annoys me when people call me 'Dearie,' so I told him not to do it anymore" is an assertive statement; it clearly states what the problem is and sets limits on undesired behavior without being demeaning.**
   1 "I know I should put the needs of others before mine" is a nonassertive or passive statement that denies the individual's own needs and desires. **2** "I won't stand for it, so I told my boss he's a jerk and to get off my back" is a destructive aggressive statement that sets limits but does so through demeaning. **4** "It is easier for me to agree up front and then just do enough so that no one notices" is a passive-aggressive response that avoids direct, honest confrontation for devious manipulation.
   Client Need: Psychosocial Integrity; **Cognitive Level:** Analysis; **Integrated Process:** Teaching/Learning; **Nursing Process:** Evaluation/Outcomes

4. **Answers: 2, 4, 1, 3, 5.**
   2 Increasing tension in facial expression indicates increasing anxiety, but the client still is maintaining self-control. **4** Impulsivity, as demonstrated by the inability to take turns with others, indicates that the client is having some difficulty setting limits on his or her own behavior. **1** When anxiety escalates to the point of hyperactivity and pacing behaviors, the client is attempting to cope with the anxiety and to discharge physical and psychic energy. **3** Engaging in verbal abuse may precipitate physical abuse and is a sign that the client is not able to maintain self-control. **5** The laying on of the hands in an offensive manner is a physical act of aggression.
   Client Need: Safety and Infection Control; **Cognitive Level:** Analysis; **Nursing Process:** Assessment/Analysis

5. **2 Because a sexual assault is a threat to the sense of control over one's life, some control should be given back to the client as soon as possible.**

   1 The client's crying is a typical way to ventilate emotions; the client should be told that medication is available if desired. **3** The nurse determining a need to reduce her anxiety takes control away from the client; the client may view this as an additional assault on the body, which increases feelings of vulnerability and anxiety and does not restore control. **4** That the provider is preparing to do an examination takes control away from the client; the client may view this examination, especially any internal examination, as an additional assault on the body, which increases feelings of vulnerability and anxiety and does not restore control.

   Client Need: Psychosocial Integrity; **Cognitive Level:** Application; **Nursing Process:** Planning/Implementation; **Integrated Process:** Caring

6. **4 The situation is so traumatic that the individual may be unable to use past coping behaviors to comprehend what occurred.**

   1 The family's feelings about the attack may be a later concern. The client should be the focus of care at this time. **2** Social isolation is not an immediate concern. **3** Coping skills, more than thought processes, are challenged at this time.

   Client Need: Psychosocial Integrity; **Cognitive Level:** Application; **Nursing Process:** Planning/Implementation; **Integrated Process:** Caring

7. **2 Nurses who work with clients who are victims of partner abuse need to be supportive and client. It takes time and several attempts for most victims to be able to leave abusive relationships.**

   1 This may or may not be true. There is not enough information to support this conclusion. **3** The staff can encourage the woman to make plans for addressing various potential events. Information about social services and telephone help lines can be beneficial. **4** The nurse should not resort to shaming women in this position because it will make them less likely to seek help.

   Client Need: Psychosocial Integrity; **Cognitive Level:** Comprehension; **Integrated Process:** Teaching/Learning; **Nursing Process:** Planning/Implementation

8. **4 Stating "If I feel upset at my son, I'm going to go into the bedroom and punch a pillow" demonstrates some insight. The client assumes responsibility for her behavior and devises a preliminary plan of action.**

   1 Saying "I think the root of the problem is my partner's drinking" does not show insight but, instead, denies responsibility for the abuse and places it on the partner. **2** Stating "I promise not to get so upset when my son causes trouble" does not show insight; it places blame on the son and promises behavior that probably is unrealistic. **3** Saying "I'll be better able to control my behavior once my son gets better" does not show insight; it places blame on the son and promises behavior that probably is unrealistic.

   Client Need: Psychosocial Integrity; **Cognitive Level:** Application; **Nursing Process:** Evaluation/Outcomes

9. **Answers: 2, 3, 5.**

   2 The child is made the scapegoat in the situation; the parents blame the child because they have unrealistic expectations of the child. **3** Discrepancies or inconsistencies in the history result from attempts to present a story that is not based on fact. **5** Discrepancies between the parental explanation for the child's injuries and the physical findings or discrepancies in the history that each parent gives are common because the information that is being provided is not based on fact.

   1 Abusive parents show little or no interest in their child's well-being. **4** Abusive parents usually do not ask questions about the injury or prognosis and demonstrate little or no interest in their child's well-being.

   Client Need: Psychosocial Integrity; **Cognitive Level:** Application; **Nursing Process:** Assessment/Analysis

---

Memory Aid: In Chil**D** abuse, there are **D**iscrepancies between the histories of injury and explanations told by caregivers and child and the physical findings.

---

10. **3 "What do you mean by something bad?" elicits further clarification of what the child means by "bad."**

    1 The nurse must determine what the child means by the word "bad" before reflecting the term back to the child. **2** Asking "Who said that you did something bad?" is not helpful; it will do nothing to clarify the child's idea of what "bad" means or the child's feelings about what happened. **4** Before the nurse can explore the child's concerns, the nurse must first understand the child's use of words and their meaning to the child.

    Client Need: Psychosocial Integrity; **Cognitive Level:** Application; **Nursing Process:** Planning/Implementation; **Integrated Process:** Communication/Documentation

11. **1 It is the most effective method for the child to play out feelings; when feelings are allowed to surface, the child can then learn to face them by controlling, accepting, or abandoning them.**

    2 Group therapy is not child-specific and generally is more suited for adolescents, young adults, and adults. **3** Family therapy is not child-specific and generally is more suited for adolescents, young adults, and adults. **4** Psychodrama is not child-specific and generally is more suited for adolescents, young adults, and adults.

    Client Need: Health Promotion and Maintenance; **Cognitive Level:** Application; **Integrated Process:** Caring; **Nursing Process:** Planning/Implementation

12. **3 People who abuse elders are most often family members or caregivers.**

    1 Strangers are not the most common abuser of elders. **2** Physicians are not the most common abusers of elders. **4** Physicians are not the most common abusers of elders.

    Client Need: Health Promotion and maintenance; **Cognitive Level:** Knowledge; **Integrated Process:** Caring; **Nursing Process:** Assessment/Analysis

OVERVIEW

- Eating behaviors and perceptions of body shape and weight are severely disturbed
- Anorexia nervosa and bulimia nervosa may be present in the same client or exist separately
- Binge-eating disorder is another maladaptive behavior involving eating

ETIOLOGY (FIG. 17.1)

Biologic Factors

- Up to 50% of the risk for eating disorders is possibly genetic
  - The additive effects of several genes for high-risk personality traits and neurobiological dysfunction is a significant theory; it is not just one gene
- New research shows oversensitivity in the serotonin system in those with eating disorders
- There is evidence for a biologic serotonin dysregulation that the person tries to modulate with eating disorder behaviors
- Research with clients who have recovered from *anorexia nervosa* shows overactive dopamine receptors related to excessive worry and a lack of positive response to common comforts and pleasures, such as food

Sociocultural Factors

- Diet and fashion industries encourage young people to strive for an idealized body and suggest that dieting and exercise will help them achieve it
- Unrealistic expectations of parents can influence teens
- Another risk factor is participation in sports that encourage low weight, such as cheerleading, wrestling, swimming, and running track
- Participation in intensely competitive sports that encourage perfectionism and excessive exercise also carries a high risk

Psychologic Factors

- Some high-risk personality traits are common to all eating disorders, whereas some personality traits are more specific to anorexia nervosa or bulimia nervosa (Box 17.1)
- Cognitive therapy literature describes certain distorted thinking patterns as characteristic:
  - Perfectionist
  - May have self-esteem and peer problems
  - Decision-making deficits
  - Rigidity of thinking

Familial Factors

- Stereotypic "eating disorder family": Caucasian, upper middle class, intact, enmeshed, rigid, and hostile
- However, eating disorders occur among all socioeconomic levels, races, and cultures, as well as with a range of interactive family styles

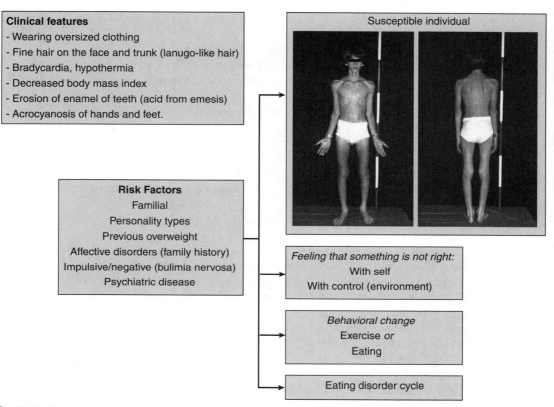

Clinical features
- Wearing oversized clothing
- Fine hair on the face and trunk (lanugo-like hair)
- Bradycardia, hypothermia
- Decreased body mass index
- Erosion of enamel of teeth (acid from emesis)
- Acrocyanosis of hands and feet.

Risk Factors
Familial
Personality types
Previous overweight
Affective disorders (family history)
Impulsive/negative (bulimia nervosa)
Psychiatric disease

Susceptible individual

Feeling that something is not right:
With self
With control (environment)

Behavioral change
Exercise *or*
Eating

Eating disorder cycle

FIG. 17.1 The slippery slope to eating disorders. (From Marcdante, K. J., & Kliegman, R. M. [2015]. *Nelson essentials of pediatrics* [7th ed.]. Philadelphia: Elsevier/Saunders.)

BOX 17.1 High-Risk Personality Traits for the Development of Eating Disorders

- Sense of ineffectiveness
- Low self-esteem
- Compliance and conflict avoidance
- Alexithymia (ie, difficulty naming and expressing emotions)
- Interoceptive deficits (ie, the inability to accurately identify and respond to bodily cues

Anorexia Nervosa
- Perfectionism
- Rigidity
- Risk and harm avoidance

Bulimia Nervosa
- Impulsivity
- Emotional dysregulation (ie, oversensitivity to and difficulty with modulating emotions and behavior)

From Fortinash, K. M., & Holoday, P. A. (2012). *Psychiatric mental health nursing* (5th ed.). St. Louis, MO: Mosby.

- *Enmeshed families* have poor boundaries, expect conformity, and discourage individuality and the direct expression of feelings
  - Parents are often controlling, critical, and demanding
  - Parents may demonstrate poor conflict resolution skills, displayed as the denial of disagreement, conflict avoidance, or constant and unproductive arguing; the result is tension and a fear of conflict
- Some theorize that influencing factors are the emphasis on body image, social acceptance, and achievement
  - Encouragement of dieting and avoidance of food may result from excessive concern with obesity
  - Attractiveness as way of receiving approval
- Parents may not encourage the child to be independent, to develop self-trust, or to have pride in one's individuality
  - If the child learns to avoid conflict to please others and to fear adult responsibilities, adolescence is a crisis
  - A sense of competence never fully develops; pressures to separate and be an individual are terrifying to both the child and the parents
  - Confronted with this crisis, the adolescent feels overwhelmed and out of control
- The myth of thinness as the key to confidence, success, and control is compelling; losing weight gives the adolescent a new sense of power and control, attention, and the ability to frustrate those who try to make her eat normally
- These secondary gains are often very rewarding, especially to a perfectionist, conflict-avoidant individual with low self-esteem
- Dieting can distract from actual conflicts and given her a sense of mastery
- Anxiety is reduced by control of food

Epidemiology

- Incidence of anorexia nervosa and bulimia is similar in all countries that have plentiful food supplies
- In the U.S. there is no difference in incidence of these disorders among racial, ethnic, or socioeconomic groups
- Mortality rate is reported at 4% to 20%, higher than that seen with any other psychiatric diagnoses
- Medical complications, substance-use–related death, and suicide are the main causes of death

Comorbidities

- Depression and anxiety are common in those diagnosed with eating disorders; depression is more common with bulimia nervosa than with anorexia nervosa
- Personality disorders, posttraumatic stress disorder (PTSD), social phobias, dissociative disorder, and substance use disorders are also common, as is a history of sexual abuse
- Careful diagnosis is necessary to separate the side effects of starvation and purging from the symptoms of coexisting mood disorders

Commanilities of Anorexia Nervosa and Bulimia

- Many underweight clients with anorexia nervosa binge and purge, and some clients diagnosed with bulimia nervosa use fasting or exercising, but not purging, to compensate for the binges
- There are eating disorders that may not fit the categories of Anorexia Nervosa, Bulimia Nervosa and Binge Eating Disorder that have been labeled Other Specified Feeding and Eating

Disorders. Half of those with eating disorders "migrate" from one diagnosis to another over time
- Other behaviors, such as stashing food and excessive exercise, are common to both eating disorders

General Assessment

- Involves sensitivity, thoroughness, and sharp observation skills
- First impressions set the tone for the entire treatment experience
- Clients diagnosed with eating disorders are sensitive to others and quick to judge whether others are trustworthy
- If the nurse forms a therapeutic alliance immediately, this can prevent many of the common power struggles
- Coexisting disorders must also be assessed
- Assess for suicide ideation and self-harm

Nursing Diagnosis

- Accuracy depends on thorough assessment
- Diagnoses are prioritized according to client needs from most urgent to least urgent

GENERAL NURSING CARE OF CLIENTS DIAGNOSED WITH EATING DISORDERS

Planning

- The nurse's *attitude toward the client* diagnosed with an eating disorder is as critical to the plan of care as any specific therapeutic intervention
- Clients appear fragile, and, although they are vulnerable, they are often quite rigid in their thinking and can be frustrating
- If the nurse does not form a good working alliance with a firm yet compassionate approach, client care can quickly turn into a series of power struggles, and the treatment will fail
- The plan of care has to include consistent and collaborative efforts by the client, the family, and the interdisciplinary staff

Client Needs

- Basic physiologic and safety needs to be met; safe, nonthreatening environment
- Acceptance
- Meaningful relationships
- Limit-setting of manipulative behavior
- Monitoring during and after mealtime
- Consultation with nutritionist to determine adequate dietary regimen

Usual Care

- Establish a relationship based on trust; promote self-worth
- Set limits that are realistic
- Create a structured and supportive environment with clear, consistent, and firm limits
- Support and encourage independence
- Teach more effective ways of coping
- Encourage participation in individual and family therapy
- Encourage the clients to express thoughts, feelings, and concerns about their body and body image

- Restore the client's minimum weight and nutritional balance through a behavioral program
- For underweight clients, coordinate with the dietitian to construct a behavioral plan for the client that includes weight-gain goals such as approximately 3 pounds per week, specific goals of eating 100% of meals, and reinforcements of increased privileges for compliance and goal achievement
- Continue to help the client improve understanding of own body image distortion
- Assume a caring yet matter-of-fact approach without being overly sympathetic or overly confrontational or authoritarian
- Normalize the client's lack of appetite and feelings of fullness as typical of the early refeeding process; normalize fears of obesity as part of the distorted thinking that is typical of eating disorders
- Intervene with the client's anxiety by helping the client increase tolerance for distress and to reframe anxiety as a signal of unrecognized feelings and needs
- Offer positive feedback when the client follows the treatment plan and works to maintain the goals of the individual contract
- Engage the client in therapeutic interactions and groups
- Assist the client with identifying issues of low self-esteem, separation and individuation, family dysfunction, and fear of maturity
- Discuss with the client how an obsession with food and weight may be a way to avoid more difficult life problems and challenges
- Collaborate with the dietitian to teach the client about adequate nutrition for the client's height and body type; educate the client about metabolic adaptations that are characteristic of starvation and refeeding such as the need to increase kilocalories as energy expenditure increases
- Collaborate with the social worker, family therapist, physician, occupational therapist, and other members of the interdisciplinary team
- Teach adaptive therapeutic strategies (eg, cognitive, communication, assertive)
- Educate the family about healthy eating behaviors as well as the importance of normal developmental separation and individuation
- Monitor for secretive vomiting and excessive exercise

Additional Care

- Treat comorbidities
- Treat side effects of eating disorders (hypokalemia, anemia, gastroparesis, laxative use)

Anorexia Nervosa

Onset: Usually during adolescence through young adulthood; less common in older adults but is increasing in perimenopausal women

Behavioral/Clinical Findings

- Subtypes
  - Restricting type: Weight loss is accomplished through dieting, fasting, or excessive exercise; may stay at the table or dining room for extended period (marathon meal) without ingesting much food
  - Binge eating/purging type: Weight loss is accomplished through purging (eg, use of self-induced vomiting and misuse of laxatives, diuretics, or enemas on a weekly basis)
- Weight less than 85% of expected weight; cachexia
- Distorted self-image; appear fat to themselves even when emaciated

- Intense fear of becoming fat, even though underweight
- May have history of compulsive traits such as rigidity, ritualistic behavior, and meticulousness; need to control or prove control
- Usually very manipulative
- Usually high achiever academically
- Frequent discord in family relationships; often chaotic
- Often interested in food and cooking in general; serves as a control strategy
- Cessation of menses for more than 3 months in females (amenorrhea)
- Inability to sustain self-starvation may result in bulimic episodes (binging of food followed by self-induced vomiting)
- Fatigue or hyperactivity
- Gastrointestinal (GI) disturbances (eg, feeling of fullness after small intake, nausea, and constipation)
- Hypotension; bradycardia
- Fluid and electrolyte disturbances that can lead to dysrhythmias; dependent edema; muscle cramping
- Low blood glucose level
- Anemia
- Sensitivity to cold
- Erosion of tooth enamel (if vomiting)
- Lanugo (fine, brittle body hair); dry skin

Outcome Identification

- The client will:
  - Participate in therapeutic contact with staff
  - Consume adequate calories for age, height, and metabolic needs
  - Achieve a minimum healthy weight
  - Maintain normal fluid and electrolyte levels
  - Resume a normal menstrual cycle
  - Demonstrate improvement in body image with a more realistic view of body shape and size
  - Demonstrate more effective coping skills to deal with conflicts
  - Manage family conflicts more effectively
  - Verbalize awareness of underlying psychologic issues
  - Achieve ideal body weight for age, height, and metabolic needs
  - Perceive body weight and shape as normal and acceptable
  - Resume sexual interest and age-appropriate sexual behavior
  - Demonstrate an absence of food rituals, preoccupation with food, or fears of food
  - Maintain appropriate levels of exercise for health maintenance

Therapeutic Interventions

- Unified team approach
- Behavior modification techniques that focus on client's responsibility for weight gain and reward positive behavior
- Regular weighing (may be daily) of patient under identical conditions (same time of day, same clothing, etc.)
- Time limit on meals; monitor client after meals to prevent purging
- Use of enteral feedings if weight loss is so great or fluid and electrolyte imbalance is so severe that it causes a threat to life

- Limit on excessive physical activity
- Psychotherapy focusing on self-image
- Group and cognitive therapy
- Family therapy with all members of family involved
- Gradual increase in calories and protein under guidance of nutritionist
- Antidepressants are helpful with comorbid depression
- Prevent edema, congestive heart failure, hypophosphatemia (ie, a low phosphate level), and other serious electrolyte imbalances with slow refeeding and careful monitoring

NURSING CARE OF CLIENTS DIAGNOSED WITH ANOREXIA NERVOSA

Assessment/Analysis

- Complete physical and dental examination to rule out associated medical complications of eating disorder; involved systems include central nervous system (CNS), renal, hematologic, GI, endocrine, cardiovascular, and integumentary
- Weight and height
- Signs of fluid and electrolyte imbalance
- History of amenorrhea
- Excessive exercise
- Behavior reflecting obsessiveness with food
- History of stringent control of food intake
- Depressive mood and level of anxiety
- Motivation to change maladaptive eating patterns
- Heart rate and rhythm
- Emergence of suicide or self-harm ideation or behaviors especially as patient gains weight

Planning/Implementation

- See General Nursing Care of Clients Diagnosed with Eating Disorders
- Develop a therapeutic relationship and environment
- Establish a behavior modification program
- Help client identify feelings
- Briefly discuss dietary modification in a nonthreatening manner
- Provide diet high in nutrient-dense foods
- Avoid focusing on eating or weight loss; focus on healthy coping

Evaluation/Outcomes

- Maintains dietary intake adequate to meet daily caloric requirements
- Reaches and maintains appropriate body weight; commonly, a goal of 3 lb/week is considered safe
- Develops realistic body image
- Identifies and verbalizes feelings
- Accepts age-appropriate role
- Resolves separation and individuation issues

Bulimia Nervosa

Onset: Most common in adolescent through 30-year-old population

Behavioral/Clinical Findings

- Engages in purging behaviors that occur at least weekly for a minimum of 3 months

- Eating binges characterized by rapid consumption of excessive amounts of high-caloric foods in brief periods, followed by induced purging (eg, vomiting, enemas, laxatives, diuretics) in the purging subtype
  - These clients feel a lack of control over their binge-eating
  - These clients often hide their purging, or perform it in secret
- Periods of severe dieting or fasting between binges
- Sporadic vigorous exercising between binges
- Weight may be within expected range with frequent fluctuations higher than or lower than expected range because of alternating binges and fasts
- A feeling of lack of control over eating during episode
- Depression and self-deprecating thoughts follow binges
- Extroverted
- Possible intermittent substance misuse
- Self-evaluation based on body image and appearance
- Repeated attempts to control or lose weight

Therapeutic Interventions

- Unified team approach
- Behavior modification techniques that focus on client's responsibility for weight gain if needed
- Time limit on meals; monitor client after meals to prevent purging
- Limit on excessive physical activity
- Psychotherapy focusing on self-image
- Group and cognitive therapy
- Family therapy with all members of family involved
- If appropriate, gradual increase in calories and protein under guidance of nutritionist
- SSRI medications—particularly fluoxetine—are effective for the treatment of bulimia nervosa
- Treatment of depression, which is the most frequently observed psychologic concomitant condition associated with bulimia

NURSING CARE OF CLIENTS DIAGNOSED WITH BULIMIA NERVOSA

Assessment/Analysis

- Behavior indicative of purging such as self-induced vomiting and use of enemas, laxatives, and/or diuretics
- Obsession with excessive exercise
- Pattern and duration of binging
- Undue concern with body weight and shape
- Physiologic changes such as dental caries, chipped teeth, enlarged parotid glands, calluses or scars on knuckles from induced vomiting
- Signs of fluid and electrolyte imbalances
- Weight and height
- History of consuming tremendous amounts of calories in a short period of time
- Symptoms of depression or obsessive-compulsive behaviors
- Bone mineral density screening for osteopenia and osteoporosis
- Assessment for amenorrhea
- Substance misuse (drugs, pattern, duration)

Outcome Identification

- The client will:
  - Participate in therapeutic contact with staff
  - Maintain normal fluid and electrolyte levels
  - Consume adequate calories for age, height, and metabolic needs
  - Cease binge/purge episodes when in the inpatient setting and cease dieting
  - Demonstrate more effective coping skills to deal with conflicts
  - Demonstrate age-appropriate boundaries with family
  - Verbalize an awareness of underlying psychologic issues
  - Demonstrate an improved awareness of body sensations and emotional states
  - Perceive body shape and weight as normal and acceptable

Implementation

- See General Nursing Care of Clients Diagnosed with Eating Disorders
- Provide a nonjudgmental, accepting environment
- Set realistic limits; keep under close observation to prevent purging
- Encourage verbalization of feelings
- Help identify feelings associated with binging and purging
- Shift focus from food, eating, and exercise to emotional issues
- Encourage journaling to identify situational and emotional triggers to binging

Evaluation

- Limits dietary intake to caloric requirements
- Reduces episodes of binging
- Reduces episodes of purging
- Identifies feelings
- Verbalizes emotions and needs
- Reports no depressive symptoms
- Develops a healthy lifestyle balancing eating and exercise

APPLICATION AND REVIEW

1. An adolescent is admitted to the psychiatric service with the diagnosis of anorexia nervosa. The adolescent has lost 20 pounds in 6 weeks and is very thin but is excessively concerned about being overweight. What is the **most** important initial nursing intervention?
   1. Compliment the physical appearance of the adolescent
   2. Explore the reasons why the adolescent does not want to eat
   3. Explain the value of adequate nutrition to the adolescent
   4. Attempt to establish a trusting relationship with the adolescent
2. What is an appropriate goal for a client with anorexia nervosa?
   1. Eat every meal for a week
   2. Gain 1 pound of weight a week
   3. Attend group therapy every day
   4. Talk about food for 1 hour a day
3. Evaluation of clients diagnosed with anorexia nervosa requires reassessment of behaviors after admission. Which finding indicates that the therapy is beginning to become effective?
   1. Food is hidden in pockets of clothing
   2. Statement that the hospitalization has been helpful
   3. Weight gain of 6 pounds since admission 3 weeks ago
   4. Remains in the dining room eating for 1 hour after others have left

4. A cachectic adolescent with the diagnoses of anorexia nervosa, dehydration, and electro-lyte imbalances is admitted to a mental health facility. The adolescent has been obsessed with weight, has exercised for hours every day, has taken enemas and laxatives several times a week, and has engaged in self-induced vomiting. Which is a **priority** when a nurse plans care for this client?
   1. Identifying personal strengths
   2. Controlling impulsive behaviors
   3. Correcting electrolyte imbalances
   4. Developing a contract for treatment goals

5. A nurse is working with clients with a variety of eating disorders. Which characteristic unique to bulimia nervosa differentiates this disorder from anorexia nervosa?
   1. Is obese and attempting to lose weight
   2. Has a distorted body image and sees the body as fat
   3. Has behaviors and an appearance that appear appropriate
   4. Is struggling with a conflict between dependence and independence

6. What characteristic of the environment is **most** therapeutic for clients with the diagnosis of bulimia nervosa?
   1. Controlling
   2. Empathetic
   3. Focused on food
   4. Based on realistic limits

7. A nurse admits an adolescent to the psychiatric unit with the diagnosis of anorexia ner-vosa. What is the **primary** gain a client with anorexia achieves from this disorder?
   1. Reduction of anxiety through control over food
   2. Separation from parents secondary to hospitalization
   3. Release from school responsibilities because of illness
   4. Increased parental attentiveness related to massive weight loss

8. A nurse is caring for a client with the diagnosis of bulimia nervosa. The nurse understands that individuals with bulimia use food to:
   1. Gain attention
   2. Control others
   3. Avoid growing up
   4. Meet emotional needs

9. A nurse is caring for an underweight adolescent girl who is diagnosed with anorexia ner-vosa. What are common characteristic of girls with this disorder that the nurse should identify when obtaining a health history and performing a physical assessment? **Select all that apply.**
   1. Fatigue
   2. Pyrexia
   3. Tachycardia
   4. Heat intolerance
   5. Secondary amenorrhea

10. Anorexia nervosa follows a cyclic pattern. List the following statements in order of pro-gression through this cycle. Number 1 is the first step and number 5 is the fifth step in the cycle.
    1. _____ Self-esteem increases as weight is lost
    2. _____ Dieting in an attempt to maintain control
    3. _____ Progressive deterioration in physical status
    4. _____ Secondary gains reinforce the anorectic client's behaviors
    5. _____ Sociocultural attitudes exert pressure for people to attain an idealized body

11. A nurse considers the cultural factors that may influence the development of eating disor-ders. The nurse considers that eating disorders exist more frequently in:
    1. Affluent families
    2. European countries
    3. Industrialized societies
    4. Men rather than women

12. A 17-year-old client is admitted to the hospital because of weight loss and malnutrition, and the health care provider diagnoses anorexia nervosa. After the client's physical condition is stabilized, the health care provider, in conjunction with the client and parents, decides to institute a behavior modification program. What component of behavior modification verbalized by one of the parents leads the nurse to conclude that the parent has an understanding of the therapy?
    1. Rewards positive behavior
    2. Deconditions fear of weight gain
    3. Decreases unnecessary restrictions
    4. Reduces anxiety-producing situations

13. An adolescent diagnosed with anorexia nervosa frequently telephones home just before mealtimes. The client uses the phone calls to avoid eating. What client behavior supports the nurse's conclusion that the nursing plan to set limits on this avoidance behavior is effective?
    1. Begins to clip recipes from magazines
    2. Arrives on time for meals without being told
    3. Organizes an aerobic exercise group for other clients
    4. Contacts the family frequently by telephone between meals

14. What should the nurse do when interacting with an adolescent client with the diagnosis of anorexia nervosa?
    1. Set limits
    2. Maintain control
    3. Demonstrate empathy
    4. Focus on dietary nutrition

15. The parents of an adolescent female are upset about their daughter's diagnosis of anorexia nervosa and the treatment plan proposed. What is the **best** response by the nurse when the client's parents ask to bring food in for the client?
    1. "For now, allow the staff to handle her food needs."
    2. "Your concerns about food contribute to her problem."
    3. "While in the hospital, she should eat the hospital food."
    4. "It is important that you bring in what you think she'll eat."

16. The nurse interviews a young female client diagnosed with anorexia nervosa to obtain information for the nursing history. What will the client's history **most** likely reveal? **Select all that apply.**
    1. Ritualistic behaviors
    2. Desire to improve her self-image
    3. Supportive family relationship
    4. Low achievement in school and little concern for grades
    5. Satisfaction with and a desire to maintain her present weight

17. When talking with one of the day nurses, a client with the diagnosis of anorexia nervosa states that the day nurses give better care and are nicer than the night nurses. The client also asks a question that the day nurse is aware was already answered by one of the night nurses. What conclusion should the nurse make about the client?
    1. Needs assistance in exploring and verbalizing feelings about the night nurses
    2. Is trying to develop a bond of trust with a staff member, which should be supported
    3. Is attempting to divide the staff, and the behavior should be reported to the other staff members
    4. Has negative feelings about the night nurses, and the nurses should be informed of these feelings

18. A 16-year-old high school student diagnosed with anorexia nervosa tells the school nurse that she thinks she is pregnant even though she had intercourse only once, over a year ago. What is the **most** appropriate inference for the nurse to make about the student?
    1. Using magical thinking
    2. Submitting to peer pressure
    3. Lying about the last time she had intercourse
    4. Lacking knowledge that anorexia can cause amenorrhea
19. Which nursing action is **most** important when providing counseling to an adolescent diagnosed with anorexia nervosa?
    1. Avoid talking about food
    2. Limit discussion of trivial topics
    3. Help the client express concerns about body image
    4. Identify the role the parents played in the development of the disorder
20. A nurse is caring for a client who was admitted recently to the psychiatric unit with the diagnosis of bulimia nervosa. Which clinical assessment must be present to meet the diagnostic criteria for bulimia nervosa?
    1. Amenorrhea in postmenarchal females
    2. Lack of control over binge eating episodes
    3. Body weight less than 85% of that expected
    4. Binge-eating episodes that occur at least once a week

See Answers on pages 337-340.

ANSWER KEY: REVIEW QUESTIONS

1. **4 The problem is psychologic. Therefore the nurse's initial approach should be directed toward establishing trust.**
   1 The client is convinced of being overweight; complimenting the adolescent will not change the adolescent's self-perception. **2** Exploring why the adolescent does not want to eat may be a provider intervention after trust has been established. **3** The client is not ready to learn the value of adequate nutrition.
   Client Need: Psychosocial Integrity; **Cognitive Level:** Application; **Integrated Process:** Caring; **Nursing Process:** Planning/Implementation

2. **2 A goal focuses on where the client should be after certain actions are taken; this client needs to gain weight.**
   1 Eating every meal for a week may set up a struggle between the client and the nurse; the focus of care should not be on the actual intake of food. **3** Behavior modification techniques work much better than group therapy; these clients lack insight and will focus on food, not eating. **4** These clients talk freely about food; talking about food for an hour is not therapeutic.
   Client Need: Psychosocial Integrity; **Cognitive Level:** Application; **Nursing Process:** Evaluation/Outcomes

3. **3 This is objective proof that eating behaviors have improved.**
   1 "Stashing" of food is an eating disorder characteristic, not a sign of improvement. **2** A statement about the hospital by the client is subjective information and may be manipulative. **4** "Marathon meals" with little actual food ingestion is a common behavior of people with anorexia.
   Client Need: Psychosocial Integrity; **Cognitive Level:** Application; **Nursing Process:** Evaluation/Outcomes

4. **3 Electrolyte imbalances can precipitate dysrhythmias that can be life-threatening.**
   1 Although clients with the diagnosis of anorexia nervosa have low self-esteem and identifying and supporting strengths promote the development of a positive self-regard, it is not the initial priority. **2** These clients are perfectionists who usually do not display impulsivity. **4** Developing a contract for treatment goals is difficult to accomplish initially, because these clients often deny the illness and evade therapeutic treatment.
   Client Need: Physiologic Adaptation; **Cognitive Level:** Application; **Nursing Process:** Planning/Implementation

5. **3 These clients hide much of their binging and purging behaviors and, unlike clients diagnosed with anorexia, may have near-ideal body weights.**
   1 Clients diagnosed with bulimia nervosa usually are not obese. **2** A distorted body image perceived as fat is associated with clients diagnosed with both anorexia and bulimia. **4** Struggling with a conflict between dependence and independence is associated with clients diagnosed with both anorexia and bulimia.
   Client Need: Psychosocial Integrity; **Cognitive Level:** Comprehension; **Nursing Process:** Assessment/Analysis

6. **4 Realistic guidelines reduce anxiety, increase feelings of security, and increase adherence to the therapeutic regimen.**
   1 A controlling environment sets up a power struggle between these clients and the nurse. **2** These clients need realistic rules and regulations that they identify as helpful, not empathy. **3** Focusing on food is not therapeutic and may result in a power struggle between these clients and the nurse.
   Client Need: Psychosocial Integrity; **Cognitive level:** Comprehension; **Nursing Process:** Planning/Implementation

7. **1 The client controls anxiety by maintaining a childlike body build and by demonstrating mastery over food intake.**
   2 Families of people with anorexia usually are fused, so separation from parents is not a desirable gain. **3** People with anorexia generally excel in academic areas and receive attention and praise as the perfect child; they will not gain from having this source of attention removed. **4** Maintenance of control, not the resulting overattention of parents, is the primary gain.
   Client Need: Psychosocial Integrity; **Cognitive Level:** Comprehension; **Nursing Process:** Assessment/Analysis

8. **4 Clients diagnosed with bulimia eat to blunt emotional pain because they frequently feel unloved, inadequate, and/or unworthy; purging is precipitated to relieve feelings of guilt for binging and/or to limit the fear of obesity.**
   1 The binging and purging usually are done alone and in secret. **2** Clients diagnosed with bulimia often feel out of control and perform their behaviors in secret. **3** This is one of the psychodynamic theories related to anorexia nervosa, not to bulimia nervosa.
   Client Need: Psychosocial Integrity; **Cognitive Level:** Comprehension; **Nursing Process:** Assessment/Analysis

---

 Memory Aid: Personality traits peculiar to **b**ulimia are a **b**omb—"IED":
I: impulsivity
ED: emotional **d**ysregulation

---

9. **Answers: 1, 5.**
   1 Fatigue occurs because inadequate nutritional intake results in electrolyte imbalances and decreased RBCs. 5 Amenorrhea occurs because of endocrine imbalances resulting from starvation; it is thought that severe starvation damages the hypothalamus.
   2 Many of these clients have lowered body temperature. **3** Anorexia nervosa clients have bradycardia. **4** Anorexia nervosa clients are cold intolerant.
   Client Need: Physiologic Adaptation; **Cognitive Level:** Comprehension; **Nursing Process:** Assessment/Analysis

10. **Answer: 5, 2, 1, 4, 3.**
    5 Sociocultural (eg, fashion, "superwoman" issues, and the diet and fitness industry), biologic, psychologic, and familial factors all influence the development of anorexia nervosa. **2** Dieting, exercise, purging, and laxatives are used to lose weight, with the resulting primary gain of a feeling of control over one's life. **1** As weight is lost, the individual feels a sense of accomplishment, and self-esteem increases. **4** Finally, secondary gains such as attention from parents and peers reinforce the behaviors associated with anorexia nervosa. **3** Continued dieting leads to multisystem dysfunction and a deterioration of physical status.
    Client Need: Psychosocial Integrity; **Cognitive Level:** Comprehension; **Nursing Process:** Assessment/Analysis

11. **3 Eating disorders are prevalent in industrialized societies that have an abundance of food; affected individuals likely equate food with pleasure, comfort, and love, and may have been nurtured, punished, or rewarded with food.**

    1 Eating disorders occur in all socioeconomic groups. **2** The incidence and prevalence of eating disorders around the world are similar in the U.S., European countries, Canada, Mexico, Japan, Australia, and other westernized countries with plentiful food supplies. **4** Studies indicate that 95% to 99% of persons with eating disorders are women not men.

    Client Needs: Psychosocial Integrity; **Cognitive level:** Comprehension; **Nursing Process:** Assessment/analysis

12. **1 In behavior modification, positive behavior is reinforced and negative behavior is punished or not reinforced.**

    2 Deconditioning the fear of weight gain may be a part of the program, but it is not a major component. **3** Decreasing unnecessary restrictions may be a part of the program, but it is not a major component. **4** Reducing anxiety-**producing** situations may be a part of the program, but it is not a major component.

    Client Need: Management of Care; **Cognitive Level:** Comprehension; **Integrated Process:** Communication/Documentation; **Nursing Process:** Planning/Implementation

13. **2 Arriving on time for meals without being told demonstrates a change in behavior, as well as a positive approach to meals.**

    1 The problem is not a lack of interest in food but a deliberate failure to ingest food. **3** Organizing an exercise group for other clients is a behavior typical of a client diagnosed with anorexia nervosa. **4** Contacting family by telephone between meals is unrelated to the behavior that needs to be changed.

    Client Need: Psychosocial Integrity; **Cognitive Level:** Analysis; **Nursing Process:** Evaluation/Outcomes

14. **1 The client's security is increased by limit setting; guidelines remove responsibility for behavior from the client and increase compliance with the regimen.**

    2 Simply maintaining control is not therapeutic and increases the power struggle. **3** The client needs structure not empathy. **4** Emphasis on dietary intake increases the power struggle between the client and the staff.

    Client Need: Psychosocial Integrity; **Cognitive Level: Comprehension**; **Integrated Process:** Caring; **Nursing Process:** Planning/Implementation

15. **1 It is most therapeutic for the staff to control food needs, thus removing the parents from the struggle.**

    2 Explaining that the parents' concerns about food may contribute to the daughter's problem may be interpreted as accusatory and increase the parents' guilt. **3** Saying that the daughter must eat hospital food when in the hospital is nontherapeutic; it cuts off the parents from future involvement. **4** Asking parents to bring in food they think the daughter will eat is nontherapeutic; it only continues the struggle between the parents and the client.

    Client Need: Psychosocial Integrity; **Cognitive Level:** Analysis; **Nursing Process:** Planning/Implementation; **Integrated Process:** Communication/Documentation

16. **Answers: 1, 2.**

    1 Clients diagnosed with anorexia nervosa frequently have a history of ritualistic behaviors, rigidity, and meticulousness; these reflect a need to control. **2** Clients diagnosed with anorexia nervosa have a disturbed self-image and always see themselves as fat and needing further reducing. **3** Family relationships often are not supportive, but conflicted. **4** Usually, there is high achievement and great concern about grades. **5** Usually, there is dissatisfaction with weight and a desire to lose weight.

    Client Need: Psychosocial Integrity; **Cognitive Level:** Comprehension; **Nursing Process:** Assessment/analysis

---

🔑 **Memory Aid:** Clients diagnosed with anorexia nervosa are not cats, but they are trying to be PuRRfect as seen in these personality traits:

P: perfectionism
R: rigidity
R: risk and harm avoidance

---

17. **3 Clients diagnosed with anorexia nervosa use manipulation to divide the nursing staff; sharing this knowledge alerts health team members.**

    1 Helping the client explore and verbalize feelings about the night nurses is counterproductive because it supports the client's manipulative behavior. **2** The client is attempting to manipulate the staff, which is not how trust is established. **4** Telling the night nurses about the clients feelings is counterproductive because it supports the client's manipulative behavior.

    Client Need: Management of Care; **Cognitive Level:** Application; **Nursing Process:** Planning/Implementation; **Integrated Process:** Communication/Documentation

18. **4 The loss of body fat due to anorexia can cause amenorrhea; the client needs information.**

    1 No data are available to support that the client is using magical thinking, which is characterized by the belief that thinking or wishing something can cause it to occur; in light of the client's diagnosis of anorexia, that is not the first conclusion. **2** Submitting to peer pressure is not a way that adolescents are expected to use to demonstrate peer pressure. **3** Although the nurse should question the time line again, the client's nutritional status should be explored first.

    Client Need: Psychosocial Integrity; **Cognitive Level:** Application; **Nursing Process:** Assessment/Analysis

19. **3 Expression of thoughts, feelings, and concerns helps the client clarify eventually the underlying factors of the disorder, which may be associated with issues such as identity, intimacy, sexuality, and/or adult responsibilities.**

    1 Food can be discussed through a matter-of-fact approach as long as it is not pervasive, authoritarian, or guilt-producing. **2** Limiting discussion of trivial topics may interfere with the nurse-client relationship; the nurse must listen, because what appears trivial or insignificant to the nurse may not be trivial or insignificant to the adolescent. **4** Blame for the disorder should not be placed on anyone.

    Client Need: Psychosocial Integrity; **Cognitive Level:** Application; **Nursing Process:** Planning/Implementation; **Integrated Process:** Communication/Documentation

20. **2 Ingestion of an excessive amount of food within a discrete time period (eg, a 2-hour period), accompanied by a feeling that one cannot stop eating or control what or how much one is eating, is a diagnostic criterion for bulimia nervosa.**

    1 Amenorrhea is a diagnostic criterion for anorexia nervosa. **3** Body weight less than 85% of expected is a diagnostic criterion for anorexia nervosa. **4** Binge-eating episodes accompanied by inappropriate compensatory behaviors must occur, on average, at least twice a week for at least 3 months.

    Client Need: Psychosocial Integrity; **Cognitive Level:** Comprehension; **Nursing Process:** Assessment/Analysis

Sexual Disorders $\quad$ 18

OVERVIEW

- Changing social and cultural mores have removed many of the sexual behaviors that were once considered deviations from the list of "abnormal practices"
- Today, sexual activities are considered abnormal only if they are directed toward anyone or anything other than consenting adults or are performed under unusual circumstances
- Sexual needs are basic human needs
- DSM-5 lists three categories of sexual disorders: Sexual dysfunctions, paraphilias, and gender dysphoria

GENERAL NURSING CARE OF CLIENTS WITH SEXUAL AND GENDER DYSPHORIA DISORDERS

- Reflect on own sexual values and customs
- Accept individual as a person in emotional pain
- Create a safe, nonjudgmental environment that permits open communication
- Begin with less sensitive topics and move gradually to more personal issues
- Avoid punitive or judgmental remarks or responses; maintain a matter-of-fact manner
- Provide for privacy and protect individual from others
- Set limits on sexual acting out behavior
- Report suspected child or elder abuse to appropriate protective service agencies

SEXUAL DYSFUNCTION

Overview

- Sexuality is essential to the well-being of individuals and of couples
- Inhibition or interference with the desire, excitement, orgasm, or resolution phases of the sexual response cycle is sexual dysfunction (Fig. 18.1)
- Can be lifelong or acquired
- Can be generalized or situational
- Often a combination of psychogenic and physiologic factors
- Nurses need to be aware that assisting their clients with the achievement of positive sexual expression is an important goal
- Nurses need to reflect on their own attitudes and values as well as their comfort with and knowledge of sexuality
- The goal of intervention is assisting the individual to achieve sexual satisfaction; the length of time that it takes to achieve varies among individual and couples

Etiologic Factors (Box 18.1)

- Physical/biologic factors
  - Testosterone stimulates sexual desire in males and females
  - Stress reduces sexual arousal and interest

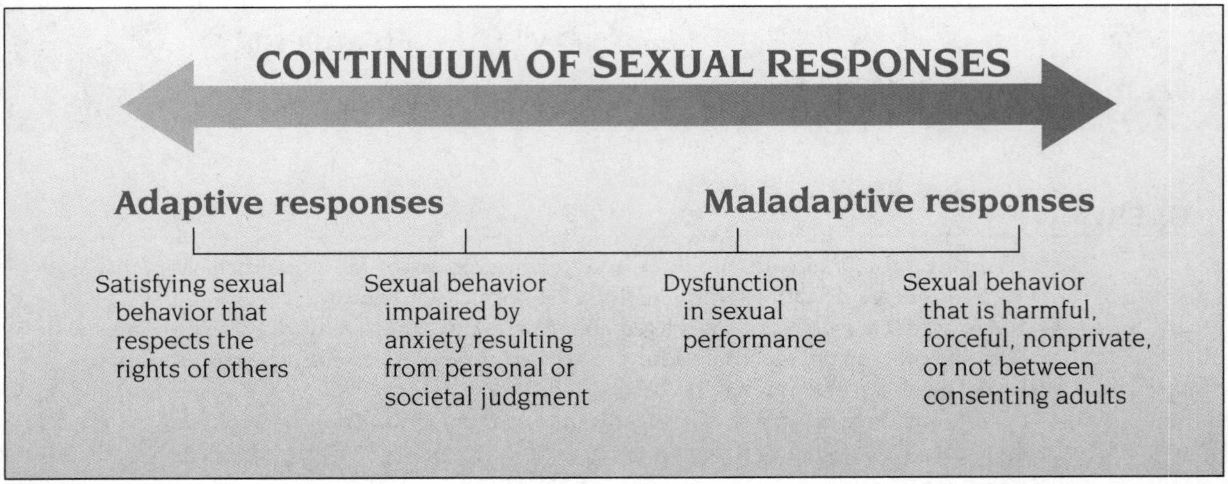

CONTINUUM OF SEXUAL RESPONSES

Adaptive responses

Maladaptive responses

Satisfying sexual behavior that respects the rights of others

Sexual behavior impaired by anxiety resulting from personal or societal judgment

Dysfunction in sexual performance

Sexual behavior that is harmful, forceful, nonprivate, or not between consenting adults

FIG. 18.1 Continuum of sexual responses. (From Stuart, G. W. [2013]. *Principles and practice of psychiatric nursing* [10th ed.]. St. Louis, MO: Mosby.)

BOX 18.1 Etiologic Factors for Sexual Dysfunctions

Physical/Biologic Factors
Vascular
- Cardiac disease
- Diseases of the blood vessels

Neurologic
- Stroke
- Head injuries
- Spinal cord disorders
- Epilepsy
- Parkinson's disease
- Peripheral nerve disorders

Endocrine
- Diabetes
- Altered hormonal levels (especially testosterone)

Pharmacologic
- Antidepressants
- Antihypertensives
- Hormonal therapy
- Mind-altering and mood-altering substances
- Alcohol

Other Causes
- Cancer
- Connective tissue disorders, including arthritis
- Pain disorders
- Depression
- Incontinence
- Sexually transmitted diseases

Psychologic/Emotional Factors
- Childhood experiences
- Body image
- Anxiety and stress
- Learned pattern for response

Cultural Factors
- Misinformation regarding sex
- Lack of sex education
- Different social standards for men and women
- Sexual myths and attitudes
- Religion

Relational Factors
- Differences in sexual desire or interests
- Lack of attraction
- Lack of communication
- Lack of trust

From Fortinash, K. M., & Holoday, P. A. (2012). *Psychiatric mental health nursing* (5th ed.). St. Louis, MO: Mosby.

- Vascular, neurologic, and endocrine disorders as well as a range of problems, including cancer, connective tissue and pain disorders, depression, incontinence, and sexually transmitted diseases, all contribute to the development of sexual dysfunctions
  - Medications—especially antidepressants, antihypertensives, and hormonal treatments—also affect sexual response
  - Substance use disorder is epidemic in U.S. society; these problems can seriously affect an individual's ability to function sexually
- Psychologic/emotional factors
  - Anxiety, stress, and depression also contribute to changes in sexuality
  - Positive and negative perceptions of one's body image affect sexual interest and function
- Cultural factors
  - Cultures vary distinctly with regard to the interpretations that they have for sexual behavior
  - Gender roles can be prescribed, and different social standards are set the behavior of men and women
  - Sexual myths influence attitudes toward sex
  - Many religions place restrictions on sexual behavior that is other than procreative; however, many religions advocate for a happy and vital sexual relationship, albeit generally within the context of marriage
- Relational factors
  - Problems within relationships, including financial and family stress, often pull a couple apart and disrupt their sexual satisfaction
  - Couples often have poor or ineffective communication regarding their sexual likes and dislikes
  - Couples often do not discuss what they do or do not enjoy sexually or share their feelings about the experience
  - Differences in sexual drives and interests further complicate the relationship

Types of Sexual Dysfunction and Behavioral/Clinical Findings (Box 18.2)

- Sexual desire disorders: Deficient, absent, or extreme aversion to and avoidance of sexual activity
  - Male hypoactive sexual desire disorder
  - Female sexual interest/arousal disorder

BOX 18.2 Sexual Dysfunctions

Male Hypoactive Sexual Desire Disorder
Erectile Disorder
Delayed Ejaculation
Premature (Early) Ejaculation
Female Sexual Interest/Arousal Disorder
Female Orgasmic Disorder
Genito-Pelvic Pain/Penetration Disorder
Substance/Medication-Induced Sexual Dysfunction
Refer to the DSM-5Manual for the Diagnostic Criteria for each disorder.

Modified from Fortinash, K. M., & Holoday, P. A. (2012). *Psychiatric mental health nursing* (5th ed.). St. Louis, MO: Mosby; Keltner, N. L., & Steele, D. (2015). *Psychiatric nursing* (7th ed.). St. Louis, MO: Mosby/Elsevier.

- Sexual arousal disorders: Partial or complete failure to achieve a physiologic or psychologic (subjective) response to sexual activity
  - Erectile disorder
  - Female sexual interest/arousal disorder
- Orgasm disorders: Delay in or absence of orgasm, premature ejaculation
  - Ejaculation disorders
  - Female orgasmic disorder
- Sexual pain disorders: recurrent or persistent genital pain before, during, or after sexual activity (dyspareunia)
  - Genito-pelvic pain/penetration disorder

Prognosis

- Drug companies provide statistics regarding the efficacy of products such as drugs for erectile dysfunction, which have been useful for men but much less so for women
- Most therapy for sexual dysfunction involves the use of cognitive-behavioral techniques
- The success of these techniques directly reflects the client's willingness and persistence in implementing them

Therapeutic Interventions

- First, treatment of underlying physiologic cause if present
- Psychologic-based interventions: Sexual counseling for client and partner
  - Sensate focus is a way of developing relaxation, learning to tune in to the body rather than the thoughts, and creating an atmosphere in which there is no demand for sexual pleasure or sexual release
  - To develop better arousal response and better orgasmic capacity, sex therapists may teach their clients masturbatory training exercises
  - Educational needs vary from specific ways to masturbate to theories about sexual response
  - Cognitive restructuring involves replacing negative or unpleasant thoughts about sexuality with more positive or realistic thoughts
- Relation-based interventions
  - Determination of whether there is a true sexual dysfunction, or whether the problem is within the relationship
  - Better communication can begin in the therapist's office, where both members of the couple are encouraged to talk and to listen
  - The most significant predictors of a couple's prognosis for healing their sexual intimacy issues are the respect, regard, and genuine liking for one another
- Vacuum constriction device for males for treatment of impotence
- Pharmacologic therapy:
  - Sildenafil, tadalafil, alprostadil for men for erectile dysfunction
  - Anxiolytics have been successful for the treatment of vaginismus (painful spasmodic contraction of the vagina)
  - Topical preparations of lidocaine as well as gabapentin are effective for treating genital pain disorders
- Hormonal treatments
  - Exogenous testosterone used in males improves sexual desire and possibly sexual function in general; a low level of the male hormone testosterone is called hypogonadal syndrome,

or andropause, and symptoms include abdominal weight gain and decreases in bone and lean muscle mass
- Lowered levels of testosterone lead to hypoactive sexual desire in women, and testosterone replacement improves sexual functioning; however, researchers do not fully understand the relationship between testosterone levels and sexual desire in females; lowered estrogen levels cause decreased lubrication, vaginal wall thinning, and vaginal pain; thus detecting levels of estradiol in the blood and estrogen replacement are sometimes necessary; localized estrogens are available that do not appear to increase circulating estrogens
- Surgical intervention: Semirigid or inflatable penile prosthesis

NURSING CARE OF CLIENTS WITH SEXUAL DYSFUNCTION

Assessment/Analysis (Box 18.3)
- Feelings about difficulties in functioning sexually
- Expectations regarding sexual ability
- Effect of sexual dysfunction on sexual relationship(s)
- A firm knowledge base, expert use of the nursing process, and a nonjudgmental attitude are necessary
- Nurses need a clear understanding of the complexity of the symptoms and the areas of dysfunction
- Sexual assessment is holistic and includes all assessment factors such as background, physical health, religious and cultural beliefs, education, occupation, significant relationships, and social relationships
- In addition to assessment of the specific complaint, the nurse also considers the individual's or couple's perspective of the problem and the associated desire to change

---

BOX 18.3 Principles of Sexual Assessment

- Before beginning a sexual assessment, examine your own feelings, attitudes, and level of comfort.
- Ensure a private and quiet space, ample time, and an unhurried attitude for the assessment.
- Do not ask questions about sexuality first. Begin with background information, and fit the sexual assessment into the overall assessment.
- Begin questioning about sexuality with the least sensitive areas, and then move to areas of greater sensitivity. For example, begin by asking, "Where did you first learn about sex?"
- Maintain appropriate eye contact and a relaxed and interested manner.
- Be professional and matter-of-fact about information that is asked or obtained. Avoid extreme reactions. The maintenance of an open and nonjudgmental attitude is essential.
- Use language that is professional but that will be understood by the client being interviewed. This is a good opportunity to teach the client about the words of sex.
- The nurse's tone of voice and manners reflect trust. If clients feel that they can trust the nurse, they will be more open.
- Sex is not something that most people are used to talking about, and this can make interviewing difficult. However, if the nurse has the right attitude, clients will generally be open, willing, and even eager to talk.

Modified from Fortinash, K. M., & Holoday, P. A. (2012). *Psychiatric mental health nursing* (5th ed.). St. Louis, MO: Mosby.

Planning/Implementation

- See General Nursing Care for Clients with Sexual and Gender Dysphoria Disorders
- Accept that the problem is real to client regardless of age
- Accept that desire to function sexually does not diminish with age
- Teach how to support/promote an erection (eg, avoid alcohol, recreational drug use, sedatives/hypnotics); use penile vacuum constrictive device
- Teach side effects of erectile agents (eg, sildenafil, tadalafil): Headache, flushing, dizziness, hypotension, diarrhea, dyspepsia, prolonged erection; avoid concurrent use with nitroglycerin because it can cause cardiovascular collapse
  - Men taking erectile agents need to contact their physicians immediately if they experience erections that last longer than 4 hours, painful erections, chest pain, a sudden loss of vision, fainting, rash, or urinary problems
  - Drugs are generally considered safe for erectile dysfunction as long as the client provides a complete medical and drug history
- When a client's individual beliefs prevent the implementation of a plan of care, treatment success depends on the further exploration of the problem or an alternative plan of care
- Implementation includes education, counseling, and assistance with identifying specific strategies, referrals, and support (Box 18.4)
- The nurse's role is to help the client express concerns about sexual functioning, express his or her feelings about the effect of these concerns, and to build client's knowledge base, self-esteem, and communication skills
- The nurse can recommend a physical examination, or suggest sex therapy, an advanced practice skill
- Nurses monitor client compliance and progress in treatment

BOX 18.4 **Client and Family Teaching Guidelines:** *Sexual Dysfunctions*

Teach Individual Clients
- Engage in breathing and relaxation techniques to reduce anxiety.
- Incorporate ways to increase comfort with and knowledge of one's body, using gradual and progressive touch. These exercises can be done in the shower or the bath or with the use of a mirror.
- Begin specific body image exercises that involve positive affirmations and mirror work.
- Practice the use of fantasy, erotica, self-stimulation, and toys to enhance sexuality.
- Provide information about human sexual response principles and current knowledge of the hormonal and biochemical control of sexual functioning.

Teach Couples
- Teach couples to schedule their sexual experiences for mutually agreed upon times.
- Help couples develop communication skills that enhance the ability to openly discuss sexuality, including ways to express likes and dislikes.
- Suggest that couples take turns planning a favorite sexual or sensual scenario that they will then act out together.
- Create a positive sexual atmosphere through the use of sexual humor, flirtation, touch, and the enjoyment of one another. Help couples have fun together.
- Inform couples about theories regarding the individuality and variance of sexual interest and levels of desire.
- Encourage couples to try something new, such as a full body or genital massage, sexual play at spontaneous moments, or variations in the time or location of sexual activity.

Modified from Fortinash, K. M., & Holoday, P. A. (2012). *Psychiatric mental health nursing* (5th ed.). St. Louis, MO: Mosby.

- Nurses need to stress to the client or couple that treatment success largely depends on following through with the plan of care
- These nursing interventions are prioritized according to client needs from most urgent to least urgent:
  - 1: Assist the client to better understand the human sexual response
  - 2: Teach the client about sexual dysfunctions, including possible etiologies, symptoms, and treatment options; include various methods of assessment, such as physical, urologic, gynecologic, and laboratory examinations as well as a psychosocial sexual assessment
  - 3: Educate the client about positive communication and relationship skills
  - 4: Help the client explore fears and anxieties related to sexuality; do this in a private, trusting, and open atmosphere; encourage the client to talk about what he or she learned about sexuality early in life and what his or her experiences were; teach breathing and relaxation techniques to facilitate ease when dealing with these issues
  - 5: Assist the client with enhancing self-esteem related to sexuality; encourage positive self-talk such as affirmations, cognitive therapy exercise, and body image exercises; discuss variations of sexual expression and treatment
  - 6: Refer the client to physical treatment modalities or sex therapy, as applicable
- The history of sex therapy involves the use of psychodynamic and cognitive-behavioral techniques, because originally theorists believed that the reasons for sexual problems were psychologic and relational in nature
- The current treatment emphasis is on physiologic causation (although often causes are unknown) and on combining biologic, psychologic, and couples-related approaches

Evaluation/Outcomes

- Determining the effectiveness of interventions is an ongoing process
- After intervention, the client will:
  - Develop a better understanding of the cause and symptoms of the disorder
  - Develop communication strategies to be able to express desires, likes, and dislikes to partner
  - Develop appropriate coping strategies to deal with frustrations and setbacks
  - Demonstrate use of appropriate intervention techniques that are designed to alleviate the specific disorder
  - Reports increased satisfaction with sexual functioning
  - Reports sexual ability approaches sexual expectations

APPLICATION AND REVIEW

1. A client in whom sexual dysfunction is diagnosed comments to the nurse, "Well, I guess my sex life is over." What is the **most** appropriate response by the nurse?
   1. "I'm sorry to hear that."
   2. "Oh, you have a lot of good years left."
   3. "You are concerned about your sex life?"
   4. "Have you asked your health care provider about that?"
2. Sildenafilis prescribed for a man experiencing erectile dysfunction. A nurse teaches the client about which common side effects of this drug? **Select all that apply.**
   1. Flushing
   2. Headache
   3. Dyspepsia
   4. Constipation
   5. Hypertension

3. During a routine yearly physical examination, an older adult says to a nurse, "I have not had sex lately because I can no longer get an erection!" What should be the nurse's initial response?
   1. "Let's discuss this concern a little more."
   2. "Be sure to tell your doctor about this problem."
   3. "There is medication available for erectile dysfunction."
   4. "This is an expected physiologic response to getting older."

4. What statement during a yearly physical examination indicates to a nurse that a male client may have a sexual arousal disorder?
   1. "I have no interest in sex."
   2. "It doesn't get hard during sex anymore."
   3. "I climax almost before we even get started."
   4. "It takes forever before I finally have an orgasm."

5. A 67-year-old man diagnosed with type 2 diabetes sadly confides in the nurse that he has been unable to have an erection for several years. What is the best response by the nurse?
   1. "At your age sex is not that important."
   2. "Sex is not what it is implied to be."
   3. "You sound upset about not being able to have an erection."
   4. "Maybe it is time that you speak to your health care provider about this."

6. Without knocking, a nurse enters the room of a young male client with the diagnosis of panic disorder and observes him masturbating. What should the nurse do?
   1. Say "Excuse me" and leave the room.
   2. Tactfully assess why he needs to masturbate.
   3. Pretend nothing was seen and carry out whatever task needs to be done.
   4. In a calm, quiet manner say, "This behavior is inappropriate in the hospital."

See Answers on pages 356-359.

PARAPHILIAS

Overview

- Paraphilias: Sexual urges or fantasies that are directed toward nonhuman objects or infliction of pain to self, partner, children, or other nonconsenting individuals
- To be considered a paraphilic disorder, a paraphilia must have negative consequences, such as distress or impaired functioning, or harm to client or others
- Concurrent overt or covert disorders include mood disorders, anxiety and impulse disorders, substance-related disorders, and antisocial and other personality disorders
- Recurrent intense behavior that continues for at least 6 months
- Usually begin in adolescence
- About half of clients seen clinically for paraphilic disorders are married

Etiologic Factors

- No one etiology is clear
- People do not voluntarily decide what types of sexual arousal patterns that they will have
- Contributing physical/biologic factors
  - In the biologic domain, two areas are addressed in research: Chromosomal functioning and hormonal levels
  - Klinefelter syndrome (extra X chromosome)

- Early life experiences are theorized to influence development of sexual disorders
- Some neuropsychiatric disorders have higher incidences of sexual disorders
- Evidence suggests that children who were sexually abused by adults during childhood were being environmentally influenced and therefore potentially predisposed to the development of a pedophilic disorder

Behavioral/Clinical Findings Based on Type of Paraphilia

- Exhibitionistic disorder: Sexual pleasure by exposing the genitals
- Fetishistic disorder: Sexual pleasure using nonliving objects
- Frotteuristic disorder: Sexual pleasure involving physical contact against a nonconsenting person
- Voyeuristic disorder: Sexual gratification by watching sexual play or nakedness of others
- Transvestic disorder: Sexual arousal from cross-dressing or dressing as the opposite sex
- Sexual masochism disorder: Sexual gratification obtained from self-suffering or humiliation
- Sexual sadism disorder: Sexual gratification through cruelty to others; acting on impulses may result in abuse of vulnerable person (eg, child, older adult, significant other)
- Pedophilic disorder: Attraction to children generally 13 years old or younger as sex objects; acting on impulses results in child abuse; person is at least 16 years old and at least 5 years older than the child

Therapeutic Interventions

- Successful only if there is motivation to change
- Cognitive and behavioral therapy may be effective if change is desired
- Treatment generally occurs on an outpatient basis

NURSING CARE OF CLIENTS DIAGNOSED WITH PARAPHILIAS

Assessment/Analysis

- History of sexual behavior
- Presence of other psychosocial difficulties
- Level of anxiety regarding sexual behavior (Box 18.5)
- Potential for violence toward others or self
- Reason for seeking treatment
- Pending criminal charges

BOX 18.5 Nursing Assessment Questions: Paraphilias

1. What brings you here for treatment? *To assess the client's level of insight*
2. Do you think that you have a sexual disorder? *To determine whether cognitive distortions are present*
3. Do you think that you have caused any physical or emotional harm to your victims? *To determine whether there are disturbances of feelings present*
4. How has this problem affected your lifestyle and relationships? *To determine the presence of disturbances in relationships*

Modified from Fortinash, K. M., &, Holoday, P. A. (2012). *Psychiatric mental health nursing* (5th ed.). St. Louis, MO: Mosby.

- Some untoward sexual practices, such as female genital mutilation, may be driven by cultural and religious beliefs or the customs of a specific country; it is important for the nurse to elicit and include client information about religious and cultural or customary beliefs during the initial evaluation before formulating a diagnosis

Planning/Implementation

- See General Nursing Care for Clients with Sexual and Gender Dysphoria Disorders
- The nurse should involve the client in the development of an individualized plan of care, with the expectation that the client will participate in the planning process
- The nurse should work with the client to develop an individualized plan of care that will help the client identify the presence of cognitive distortions (if appropriate), prevent reoffending by identifying triggers that provoke inappropriate sexual activity, and develop effective relapse-prevention strategies
- Relapse prevention strategies for paraphilias
  - Teach the client and significant others how to identify triggers that provoke inappropriate sexual thoughts and desires by listing the precursors to inappropriate sexual acting out
  - Be sure that the client understands that relapse prevention strategies are based on the identification of triggers; identifying triggers helps the client avoid reoffending behaviors
- In the population of clients with paraphilic disorders, it is not uncommon to find cognitive distortions; nurses must be aware of this possibility as they obtain client input into the development of the plan of care; for example, a client who is in denial of a paraphilic disorder may not be able to fully cooperate with the planning of care or to view client-centered outcomes as realistic
- The nurse should also explain the significance of treatment on recidivism and stress the importance of medication compliance and follow-up care with outpatient group psychotherapy
- Providing nursing care to clients diagnosed with paraphilias may be difficult because of the sensitive nature of these disorders; nurses must recognize this possibility and be aware of their own comfort level when discussing sexual issues with these clients; identifying the presence of a paraphilic disorder may have devastating effects on clients and their significant others; it is important for nurses to include significant others in the interventions to the extent that they can participate (Box 18.6)

Additional Treatment Modalities

- Sex drive depressants/antiandrogenic medications: Progestogens; luteinizing hormone–releasing hormone agonist; antiandrogen and progestogen (Box 18.7)
- SSRIs: Fewer side effects than antiandrogenic medications
  - Increased serotonin activity may decrease sexual appetite
- Individual and group psychotherapy and psychoeducation
  - Nurses may lead or colead psychotherapy and psychoeducation groups with the physician or with another member of the treatment team if he or she has the appropriate group psychotherapy credentials
  - Address cognitive distortions and provide education to this client population regarding the identification of triggers, relapse prevention strategies, the importance of treatment compliance, self-esteem issues, appropriate coping strategies, and problem-solving skills

BOX 18.6 Nursing Interventions for Paraphilic Disorders

- Help the client confront cognitive distortions through direct questioning methods that promote reality orientation regarding the client's offending behavior.
  - Open confrontation by the nurse may be needed, including an explanation of the effect of these distortions on treatment outcomes.
  - Journaling may assist with the breakdown of cognitive distortions and help the client track inappropriate sexual fantasies.
  - Client must be aware of the presence of a problem and willing to acknowledge its existence to potentiate treatment success.
- Educate the client and significant others about paraphilic disorders and aspects of treatment, such as identifying triggers that provoke inappropriate sexual activity and methods that help the client avoid relapse.
  - Encourage active participation in the educational process by compiling lists in a journal for review by the client and the nurse.
  - Copies of these lists should be placed in the client's medical record to inform other team members about the client's progress and provide a foundation for treatment.
- Enhance the client's compliance with treatment by openly discussing with him or her the effect that inappropriate sexual behaviors have on others. Provide research studies regarding the effects of treatment on recidivism rates and handouts about the scope of treatment and how compliance can assist the client with regaining control of sexual behaviors. Compliance with treatment may reduce the risk of relapse.
- Teach the client appropriate coping strategies, assertiveness skills, and problem-solving techniques to promote relapse prevention.
- Promote the client's development of appropriate social skills, and provide support and encouragement to the client for his or her efforts to control of the disorder.

Modified from Fortinash, K. M., & Holoday, P. A. (2012). *Psychiatric mental health nursing* (5th ed.). St. Louis, MO: Mosby.

- Recreational and occupational therapy may also be provided to assist the client with time structuring, which may be viewed as a relapse-prevention strategy
- Family and couples therapy may also be recommended, depending on the individual client care needs; usually provided by the social worker, but it may also be provided by a masters-prepared nurse or a physician

Evaluation/Outcomes

- Ceases socially unacceptable behavior
- Seeks and continues long-term therapy
- Limits paraphilic behavior to consenting adults
- Uses safer sex practices

Outcome Criteria

- The client will:
  - State the nature of the specific paraphilic disorder and its effect on the self and others (eg, if a breakdown occurs, if cognitive distortions are present)
  - Identify personal triggers (ie, stimuli that heighten unacceptable sexual cravings and that provoke inappropriate sexual behaviors)
  - Develop appropriate relapse prevention strategies
  - Communicate and problem-solve effectively

BOX 18.7 Sex Drive Depressants: Medication Key Facts

Sex Drive Depressants
Sex drive depressants are indicated for the reduction of sexual arousal and libido and for inappropriate or disruptive sexual behavior in clients with dementia.

Progestogens
Medroxyprogesterone
- This drug decreases sperm count and produces hot flashes, sweating, impotence, and insomnia.
- Smoking when taking this drug may increase the risk for deep vein thrombosis.

Luteinizing Hormone–Releasing Hormone Agonist
Leuprolide and goserelin
- Leuprolide decreases sperm count and produces hot flashes, anxiety, and insomnia.
- A serious side effect is a decrease in bone density with long-term use.
- Severe allergic reactions include rash, pruritus, urticaria, itching, flushing, and purpuric skin lesions.

Antiandrogen and Progestogen
Cyproterone
- This drug causes the atrophy of the seminiferous tubules and gynecomastia with chronic use.
- Dietary considerations: The use of this drug may impair carbohydrate metabolism and fasting blood glucose levels; hypercalcemia and changes in plasma lipids can also occur.

Modified from Fortinash, K. M., & Holoday, P. A. (2012). *Psychiatric mental health nursing* (5th ed.). St. Louis, MO: Mosby.

- Practice appropriate coping strategies
- Identify support systems

Prognosis

- The need to protect both the client and society from possible relapse or recidivism is critical
  - The minimal expected period for outpatient treatment is 2 years, although the length of treatment may be considerably longer, and it is sometimes geared to align with the length of the client's probationary sentence
- These clients need to be carefully monitored for any changes in their status that could lead to relapse; monitoring may occur through weekly outpatient group therapy or, if group treatment is not indicated, by periodic visits with the client's therapist
- A client is formally discharged from outpatient treatment on the basis of the level of progress and current status regarding the paraphilic behaviors; one should not be confused into thinking that because a client has been discharged from paraphilic treatment that this means the client is now "cured"; there is no proven cure for the paraphilic disorders client at this time
- After a client has committed a sexual crime and been diagnosed with a paraphilic disorder, the client will forever be considered a sexual offender and must register with that state's sex offender registry
- Nurses should be cautioned when attempting to predict sexual recidivism, which is the chronic and repetitive inappropriate acting out of sexual behaviors that are considered to be unacceptable that have or have not resulted in criminal conviction; clients who are currently undergoing treatment for a sexual disorder may have a lower level of sexual recidivism; treatment compliance is a therapeutic issue that nurses who are treating this population must address

- With continued treatment compliance and strict client monitoring, these clients *may* present as a lesser risk to society; it is important for nurses to also acknowledge that treatment efficacy cannot be proven at this time

LEGAL IMPLICATIONS

Forensic Psychiatry and Paraphilic Disorders

- Forensic psychiatry is the application of psychiatry for legal purposes to address issues related to criminal responsibility and competency to stand trial for various crimes that have been committed
- Formulating a forensic opinion about the paraphilic disorders is difficult; a person who has committed a sexual crime in response to psychotic processes, such as hallucinations or delusions, may be considered to not be criminally responsible (insanity plea)
- A paraphilic disorder may or may not include forensic issues
- An important aspect to explore during a forensic evaluation is the client's ability to appreciate the criminality of the behavior (sexual crime) and the ability to conform the behavior to the requirements of the law, which is not intended to address the client's ability to control himself or herself
- This understanding is a part of the forensic opinion, and, depending on the results of this assessment, the outcome may be a prison sentence or a sentencing to a maximum security forensic psychiatric facility until such time that the client is assessed as no longer being a danger to society

Sexually Violent Predators Act

- In 1990 the state of Washington's legislature enacted a bill known as the *Community Protection Act,* which provided for the civil commitment of sexually violent predators (SVPs)
  - After a term of incarceration, an SVP may be civilly committed against his or her will to a state psychiatric facility until such time that he or she is deemed to be safe to return to the community
  - This was the foundation and model legislation for the development of similar laws referred to as the *Sexually Violent Predator Act,* which has been passed into legislation in 20 states, the District of Columbia, and within the federal government
- The law in Texas provides for outpatient commitment only, whereas the other states provide for inpatient commitment; the realization of the costs of such programs may have influenced the rest of the states as far as deciding to even approach the possibility of SVP commitment laws
- The law established a civil commitment procedure for "any person who has been convicted or charged with a sexually violent offense and who suffers from a mental abnormality or personality disorder that makes the person likely to engage in the predatory acts of sexual violence" (Wash. Rev. Code Ann. §71.09.030, 1991); Washington state law defines a predatory act as "an act directed toward a stranger or an individual with whom a relationship has been established or promoted for the primary purpose of victimization" (Wash. Rev. Code Ann. §71.09.030, 1991); therefore it is conceivable that most sexually violent predators are either pedophiles or rapists
- In 2006 a federal law for the civil commitment of "sexually dangerous persons" was enacted as part of the Adam Walsh Child Protection and Safety Act; it applied to offenders who had completed their sentence in the federal system but who were not yet ready to be released into the community; *however, there are no federal commitment facilities;* hence, these offenders are

committed to the custody of the U.S. Attorney General, who then tries to convince state officials to civilly commit these clients to one of their state facilities

Sexting

- Continuing advances in technology have made it very easy for consumers to access and transmit any kind of information via the Internet and cell phones; the trend practiced primarily by young teens is called "sexting"
- Sexting occurs when someone transmits sexually explicit photos of themselves or others, other sexual images, or sexually graphic text messages via a cell phone or the Internet
- The prevalence of sexting is supported by surveys
- Negative outcomes of sexting include potentially becoming a serious criminal offender
- Nurses need to educate adolescents and their families about the ramifications of such behavior, including ramifications established by state law
- It is illegal to possess and distribute sexually explicit photos, objects, and text messages that involve a minor to anyone; in several cases, adolescents have actually received prison sentences for sending or receiving sexy photos of their 15-year-old girlfriends and then "accidentally" sending the photos to others; this may result in a child pornography conviction, and now these teenagers have to register themselves as sex offenders within their states
- As of February 2009, minors have been arrested in 10 states for sexting, resulting in the criminalization of children who are not child predators but who engaged in sexting (see Levine in Bibliography); teens should be reminded and cautioned that, after they hit "Send," the message is gone, and the damage is potentially done

GENDER DYSPHORIA

Etiologic Factors

- Feelings of incongruence between assigned or biologic sex and one's gender identity
- Origins are unknown
- Most children are firmly committed to gender role expectations as early as 18 months, but usually by 3 years

Behavioral/Clinical Findings

- Persistent discomfort with one's assigned gender and a feeling that it is inappropriate or inaccurate
- Strong desire to be of the other gender
- Persistent preference for cross-sex roles

Therapeutic Interventions

- Individual and/or group psychotherapy
- Surgical sex reassignment only after thorough assessment for presence of any psychiatric disorders that may be the primary disorder and these steps:
  - Psychotherapy for at least 6 months
  - Exploration of all issues: Surgical, financial, legal, etc.
  - Hormonal treatment and relationship changes over time
  - Individual's attitudes to reassignment may change, so surgery may not be chosen; for some individuals, hormonal treatment is sufficient.
  - Certainty before surgery is essential, because the surgery is not reversible.

NURSING CARE OF CLIENTS DIAGNOSED WITH GENDER DYSPHORIA DISORDERS

Assessment/Analysis

- Distress about assigned sex role
- Behaviors, social habits, and cross-dressing incongruent with sexual gender
- Preoccupation with becoming, being, or behaving like a person of the opposite sex
- History of sexual orientation (eg, asexual, homosexual, bisexual, heterosexual)
- Presence of depressive behaviors and suicidal ideation

Planning/Implementation

- See General Nursing Care for Clients with Sexual and Gender Dysphoria Disorders
- Accept own feelings about client's cross-dressing
- Accept client's discomfort with gender
- Encourage client to become involved with support groups
- Monitor risk for depression, self-mutilation, and suicide
- Assist to arrive at a solution (eg, acceptance, suppression, surgical sex reassignment)

Evaluation/Outcomes

- Verbalizes increased comfort with self
- Accepts assigned gender, lives as the opposite sex, and/or explores surgical options
- Participates in support group

APPLICATION AND REVIEW

7. A male client with the diagnosis of gender dysphoria disorder has been dressing and functioning in society as a woman for 2 years and has decided to have sex reassignment surgery. He tells a nurse that all his life he has considered himself to be female. Place these nursing interventions in order of priority.
    1. _____ Treat the client with respect.
    2. _____ Investigate own feelings about sexuality.
    3. _____ Encourage the client to explore feelings.
    4. _____ Accept the decision to have sex reassignment surgery.
    5. _____ Explore ways that the decision can be shared with significant others.
8. Which is a frequent finding in clients with paraphilic disorders?
    1. Other covert or overt emotional problems
    2. Gonadal and pituitary hormone deficiencies
    3. Over association with society's fringe groups
    4. Inadequate development of the sexual organs
9. An adult client charged with molesting a child is admitted for psychiatric evaluation. When a nurse suggests the client come to dinner, the client refuses and states, "I don't want anyone to see me. Leave me alone." What is the nurse's best response?
    1. "Certainly. I respect your wishes."
    2. "You sound upset; let's talk about it."
    3. "It will be easier to face other people right away."
    4. "Only the staff members know why you are here."

10. A child tells the school nurse, "My father has been getting into bed with me at night and touching me." What should the nurse do next?
    1. Ask the child to describe the touching.
    2. Tell the teacher to report any inappropriate behavior
    3. Contact the father to come to the school immediately.
    4. Report the child's conversation to child protective services.

11. A male client with the diagnosis of pedophilia is admitted to the psychiatric hospital because of repeated episodes of exhibitionism. In the recreation room the client exposes himself to a nurse and begins to masturbate. How should the nurse respond?
    1. Turn away from the client and ignore the behavior.
    2. Tell the client that the behavior is unacceptable and to stop.
    3. Remove the client from the recreation room and escort him to his own room.
    4. Recognize that the behavior is part of his illness and obtain a prescription for a libido-lowering medication.

12. An adult client confides to the nurse that she enjoys engaging in sex with multiple male adult sex partners simultaneously. What is the nurse's most appropriate response?
    1. "I recommend that you seek counseling for this problem."
    2. "Don't you think that having sex with multiple sex partners is immoral?"
    3. "These men are abusing you, and you should go to the police to report them."
    4. "What are you using for birth control and protection from sexually transmitted infections?"

13. A client is admitted to a long-term care facility and placed in a semiprivate room. After the second night on the unit the client's roommate reports that the client is masturbating at night and demands another room. What is the nurse's most appropriate initial intervention?
    1. Move the roommate who made the report to another room.
    2. Provide the client who was masturbating with periods of private time.
    3. Tell the roommate that this is acceptable behavior and the client has the right to engage in it.
    4. Inform the client who is masturbating that this behavior is inappropriate and should not continue.

14. An adult confides to a clinic nurse, "I have urges and fantasies to have sexual relations with children." What is the nurse's most appropriate response?
    1. Ask the client, "Have you ever acted on these thoughts?"
    2. Explain that these thoughts are unacceptable and intensive therapy is needed.
    3. Question the client, "Are you able to control your thoughts about sexual relations with children?"
    4. Inform the appropriate child protective services about the client and the thoughts the client has reported.

See Answers on pages 356-359.

ANSWER KEY: REVIEW QUESTIONS

1. **3 Asking whether the client is concerned about his or her sex life explores the meaning of the statement and allows further expression of concern.**
   1 Saying "I'm sorry to hear that" does not allow an explanation of feelings and cuts off communication. **2** The response, "Oh, you have a lot of good years left" lacks both empathy and understanding; it also cuts off communication. **4** Asking the client whether they have asked their health care provider about sex shirks responsibility; the client may be embarrassed to ask the health care provider and needs the nurse to act as facilitator.
   Client Need: Psychosocial Integrity; **Cognitive Level:** Application; **Nursing Process:** Assessment/Analysis

2. **Answers: 1, 2, 3.**

    1 Flushing is a common central nervous system response to sildenafil. **2** Headache is a common central nervous system response to sildenafil. **3** Dyspepsia is a common gastrointestinal response to sildenafil.

    4 Diarrhea, not constipation, is a common gastrointestinal response to sildenafil. **5** Hypotension, not hypertension, is a cardiovascular response to sildenafil. It should not be taken with antihypertensives and nitrates, because drug interactions can precipitate cardiovascular collapse.

    Client Need: Pharmacologic and Parenteral Therapies; **Cognitive Level:** Analysis; **Integrated Process:** Teaching/Learning; **Nursing Process:** Planning/Implementation

3. **1 The response "Let's discuss this concern a little more" communicates to the client that the nurse is willing and able to explore this concern. It is an open-ended statement that allows the client to control the direction of the conversation.**

    2 With the response, "Be sure to tell your doctor about this problem," the nurse abdicates responsibility to the health care provider. The nurse is capable and legally responsible to collect information and explore client feelings and concerns. **3** Telling the client there is a medication available for erectile dysfunction is premature; it moves immediately to a solution before adequate information has been collected. Also, the term *erectile dysfunction* is related to a medical diagnosis, and its use at this time may increase client anxiety. **4** Although sexual functioning diminishes as men age, there are many factors that influence sexual functioning (eg, physiologic problems, interpersonal conflicts, emotional stress).

    Client Need: Psychosocial Integrity; **Cognitive Level:** Application; **Integrated Process:** Caring; Communication/Documentation; **Nursing Process:** Planning/Implementation

4. **2 Referring to the ability for an erection is related to a sexual arousal disorder, which is a partial or complete failure to achieve a physiologic or psychologic response to sexual activity.**

    1 The statement, "I have no interest in sex" may indicate a sexual desire disorder in which the individual has deficient, absent, or extreme aversion to and avoidance of sexual activity. **3** The statement, "I climax almost before we even get started" is related to an orgasmic disorder, which is a delay in or absence of an orgasm or premature ejaculation. **4** The statement, "It takes forever before I finally have an orgasm" is related to an orgasmic disorder, which is a delay in or absence of an orgasm or premature ejaculation.

    Client Need: Psychosocial Integrity; **Cognitive Level:** Application; **Nursing Process:** Assessment/Analysis

> **Memory Aid:** To recall that the four stages of the sexual response cycle are *d*esire, *e*xcitement, *o*rgasm, and *r*esolution, use the first letters of each stage, D-E-O-R, to imagine a client opening the door, spelled "DEOR," to recovery from sexual dysfunction.

5. **3 When a client reveals something, it is important for the nurse to gather more information. This response promotes further communication. Assessment is the first step of the nursing process.**

    1 The statement, "At your age, sex is not that important" is a subjective, judgmental response by the nurse that reflects the nurse's view of sexuality in older adults. **2** The statement, "Sex isn't what it is cracked up to be" interjects the nurse's view and violates the concept of neutrality when counseling clients. **4** Having the client speak to health care provider may be indicated eventually, but first the nurse must obtain more information.

    Client Need: Psychosocial Integrity; **Cognitive Level:** Application; **Integrated Process:** Caring; Communication/Documentation; **Nursing Process:** Assessment/Analysis

6. **1 The client has the right to privacy; his behavior is acceptable in the privacy of his room.**

    2 Masturbation is a sexual outlet; assessment is unnecessary unless the act is practiced to excess. **3** Carrying out tasks while the client is masturbating can cause needless embarrassment to the client and may close off further communication. **4** His behavior is not inappropriate because he was in the privacy of his own room.

    Client Need: Psychosocial Integrity; **Cognitive Level:** Application; **Nursing Process:** Planning/Implementation; **Integrated Process:** Caring

7. **Answers: 2, 1, 3, 4, 5.**

   2 Because "the self" is the most important factor the nurse brings to the nurse-client therapeutic relationship, the nurse must understand personal feelings about issues surrounding this client's situation and needs; this is part of the preorientation phase of a therapeutic relationship. **1** In a therapeutic relationship the client is the focus of care, and the relationship should be based on respect. **3** In an atmosphere of respect, the client will then more likely express feelings. **4** The client considering sex reassignment surgery should explore all alternatives. However, once the decision is made, the nurse should support it. **5** After this important decision is made, the client may need assistance with how to inform significant others.

   Client Need: Psychosocial Integrity; **Cognitive Level:** Application; **Integrated Process:** Caring; **Nursing Process:** Planning/Implementation

8. **1 Clients with these sexual disorders usually have many other emotional problems that may be overt or covert in nature.**

   2 There is no proof of a deficiency of hormones. **3** Association with fringe groups has no basis in fact. **4** There is expected development of sexual organs in individuals with paraphilic disorders.

   Client Need: Psychosocial Integrity; **Cognitive Level:** Comprehension; **Nursing Process:** Assessment/Analysis

9. **2 Stating, "You sound upset; let's talk about it" identifies feelings and provides the client with an opportunity to talk.**

   1 Saying that you respect the client's wishes ignores feelings and does not help the client cope with the situation. **3** Whether it will be easier to face other people right away may or may not be true and may be false reassurance. **4** The nurse does not know for a fact that only staff members know why the client is there.

   Client Need: Psychosocial Integrity; **Cognitive Level:** Application; **Integrated Process:** Caring; Communication/ Documentation; **Nursing Process:** Planning/Implementation

10. **4 The nurse is legally responsible to report suspected child abuse to the appropriate child protection agency. The agency must assess the situation and intervene if necessary to protect the child.**

    1 Asking the child to describe the touching may cause more psychologic trauma; the nurse should listen and demonstrate concern. **2** The nurse does not need any more data to have a reasonable suspicion of child abuse. It must be reported. **3** Contacting the father may result in more abuse or in the child not reporting future abuse.

    Client Need: Management of Care; **Cognitive Level:** Application; **Integrated Process:** Communication/Documentation; **Nursing Process:** Planning/Implementation

11. **2 Exposing the genitals and masturbating in a public place are unacceptable behaviors. Unacceptable behavior should be pointed out to the client and the client instructed to stop. Exhibitionism usually is done for shock value rather than as a preamble to sexual assault or rape. If the client wishes to masturbate, this activity can be carried out in private.**

    1 Unacceptable behavior should never be ignored. The client needs limits set on this type of behavior. **3** Removing the client and escorting him to his room may eventually be done. However, the client must first be given the opportunity to change his behavior. **4** Although the nurse must recognize that the behavior is related to his illness, it is not the nurse's role to seek out or prescribe medication.

    Client Need: Psychosocial Integrity; **Cognitive Level:** Application; **Integrated Process:** Caring; Communication/ Documentation; **Nursing Process:** Planning/Implementation

12. **4 Adults may have consensual sex as desired, but the nurse should encourage the use of birth control and protection from sexually transmitted infections.**

    1 The nurse is interjecting personal values by stating the client should seek counseling for this behavior. **2** The nurse is interjecting personal values by implying that the client's behavior is immoral. **3** If the sex is consensual it is not abusive.

    Client Need: Psychosocial Integrity; **Cognitive Level:** Application; **Integrated Process:** Communication/Documentation; **Nursing Process:** Planning/Implementation

13. **2 Masturbating is a healthy human sexual behavior. The client should be provided with private time. The client has the right to meet physical needs while not imposing the behavior on others.**

    1 Moving the roommate to another room could be ineffective because this may happen with the client's future roommate. **3** Telling the roommate that this is acceptable behavior and the client has the right to engage in it does not address either client's needs. **4** Masturbating is an acceptable human behavior if practiced in private.

    Client Need: Psychosocial Integrity; **Cognitive Level:** Application; **Integrated Process:** Caring; **Nursing Process:** Planning/Implementation

14. **If a client reveals a predilection for pedophilia, it is most important to assess if the client has ever acted on these thoughts, because the best predictor of future behavior is past behavior.**

    2 No human thoughts are unacceptable; therapy is indicated if they are ego-dystonic. **3** Humans may have bizarre sexual fantasies, but it is their behavior about which they will be judged, not their thoughts. **4** This is premature; the nurse has not obtained information about whether he has acted on these thoughts.

    Client Need: Psychosocial Integrity; **Cognitive Level:** Analysis; **Integrated Process:** Communication/documentation; **Nursing Process:** Assessment/Analysis

19 Trauma-Related and Stress-Related Disorders

ETIOLOGY

- Trauma-related and stress-related disorders develop after identifiable traumatic event in which an individual is exposed to a traumatic or stressful event
- Psychologic distress due to exposure to a traumatic or stressful event varies among persons
- Some respond with anxiety or fear; others respond with depressive symptoms or anhedonia (loss of pleasure); some respond with dissociative symptoms; and others may exhibit a combination of symptoms

Epidemiology

- Traumatic events are prevalent worldwide, and trauma victims seek help in numerous clinical and emergency settings
- Between 5% and 10% of those experiencing trauma develop posttraumatic stress disorder (PTSD)
- Risk factors and prognosis depend on multiple factors including age, environment, genetic influences, culture, gender and previous trauma
- PTSD can occur at any age, with onset after the first year of life, and symptoms generally begin within 3 months after the trauma; symptoms may last from several months to many years
  - Comorbidity: Individuals diagnosed with PTSD are much more likely to have another mental disorder (eg, depressive, bipolar, anxiety, or substance-related disorder) than are persons without PTSD
  - PTSD and traumatic brain injury (TBI) among military personnel and combat veterans serving in wars in the Middle East is 48%
  - Children diagnosed with PTSD generally have at least one other diagnosis (eg, oppositional defiant disorder; separation anxiety disorder)
  - There is significant comorbidity between PTSD and neurocognitive disorder
- Types of stress-related disorders covered in this review include PTSD, acute stress disorder, adjustment disorders, and prolonged grief syndrome; dissociative disorders were reviewed in Chapter 15

POSTTRAUMATIC STRESS DISORDER

Overview

- Follows a devastating event that is outside the range of usual human experience (eg, rape, assault, military combat, hostage situations, natural or precipitated disasters)
  - The trauma can threaten bodily or psychologic harm, or death to self or others
  - Witnessing a trauma or death can also precipitate PTSD
- Not every traumatized person develops PTSD
- Neurobiology of PTSD does not follow the usual fight-or-flight stress response; studies indicate a complex interaction of neuroendocrinology, neuroanatomy, genetics, and traumatic stress
- Symptoms begin 1 month or more after the traumatic incident, but sometimes they begin years or even decades afterward

- Symptoms must last more than a month and be severe enough to interfere with relationships or work to be considered PTSD
  - Reactions shorter than a month in duration are categorized as acute stress disorder (see later in this chapter)
- The course of the illness varies; some people recover within 6 months, whereas in some the condition becomes chronic
- An adult's response involves intense fear, helplessness, or horror whereas a child's response involves disorganized or agitated behaviors
- To be diagnosed with PTSD, an adult must have all of these for at least 1 month:
  - At least one reexperiencing symptom
  - At least one avoidance symptom
  - At least two arousal and reactivity symptoms
  - At least two cognition and mood symptoms
- Reexperiencing symptoms may cause problems in a person's everyday routine; the symptoms can start from the person's own thoughts and feelings; words, objects, or situations that are reminders of the event can also trigger reexperiencing symptoms
- Reexperiencing symptoms include:
  - Flashbacks—reliving the trauma over and over, including physical symptoms such as a racing heart or sweating
  - Bad dreams
  - Frightening thoughts or sense of reliving the experience
- Prompts that remind a person of the traumatic event can trigger avoidance symptoms; these symptoms may cause a person to change their personal routine (eg, after a bad car accident, a person who usually drives may avoid driving or riding in a car)
- Avoidance symptoms include:
  - Staying away from places, events, objects, or situations (including anniversaries) that foster recall of the event or are reminders of the traumatic experience
  - Avoiding thoughts or feelings related to the traumatic event
- Arousal symptoms are usually constant, instead of being triggered by things that remind one of the traumatic events; these symptoms can make the person feel stressed and angry; they may make it difficult to perform daily tasks such as sleeping, eating, or concentrating
- Arousal and reactivity symptoms include:
  - Being easily startled
  - Feeling tense or "on edge"
  - Having difficulty sleeping
  - Having angry outbursts
- Cognition and mood symptoms can begin or worsen after the traumatic event but are not due to injury or substance use; these symptoms can make the person feel alienated or detached from friends or family members
- Cognition and mood symptoms include:
  - Trouble remembering key features of the traumatic event
  - Negative thoughts about oneself or the world
  - Distorted feelings like guilt or blame
  - Loss of interest in enjoyable activities
- Some individuals respond with anxiety, avoidance, denial, or delayed PTSD symptoms
- Some people diagnosed with PTSD do not show any symptoms for weeks or months
- PTSD is often accompanied by depression, substance use disorder, or one or more of the other anxiety disorders

- Children and teens can have extreme reactions to trauma, but their symptoms may not be the same as adults
- PTSD symptoms are also noted in traumatized children who often respond in an agitated or confused manner
- In very young children (less than 6 years of age), these symptoms can include:
  - Wetting the bed after having learned to use the toilet
  - Forgetting how to or being unable to talk
  - Acting out the scary event during playtime
  - Being unusually clingy with a parent or other adult
- Older children and teens are more likely to show symptoms similar to those seen in adults; they may also develop disruptive, disrespectful, or destructive behaviors; older children and teens may feel guilty for not preventing injury or deaths; they may also have thoughts of revenge

Behavioral/Clinical Findings

- Client responds to traumatic event with intense fear, confusion, helplessness, horror, and/or denial
- Hypervigilance; hyperarousal; exaggerated startle reflex
- Avoidance of situations that remind the person of the trauma (associated stimuli) is characteristic
- Impairments in memory or concentration
- Reliving or reexperiencing the event through memories, dreams, or flashbacks
- Feelings of isolation and detachment; depression
- Difficulty sleeping, disturbed sleep, and nightmares
- Violent outbursts of anger
- Risk-taking behaviors; substance misuse in attempt to control symptoms
- Additional symptoms may include hyperactivity, headaches, stomachaches, and back pain
- Impaired social relationships related to the symptoms

Therapeutic Interventions

- Complete diagnostic workup to rule out physical illness
- Psychotherapy, family therapy, group therapy, cognitive/behavioral therapies to provide controlled exposure to recall of event
- Psychotropic medications: Sedative/hypnotic and antianxiety agents are used short term when client is unable to cope or accomplish daily activities and until healthier coping emerges; antidepressants are used prophylactically in long-term therapy and to treat comorbid anxiety and depressive disorders; Prazosin to decrease nightmares
- Use of eye movement, desensitization, reprocessing techniques (EMDR)
- Imagery, relaxation, and meditation
- Cognitive restructuring and reframing
- Some resilience factors that may reduce the risk of PTSD include:
  - Seeking out support from other people such as friends and family
  - Finding a support group after a traumatic event
  - Learning to feel good about one's own actions in the face of danger
  - Having a positive coping strategy or a way of getting through the bad event and learning from it
  - Being able to act and respond effectively despite feeling fear

NURSING CARE OF CLIENTS DIAGNOSED WITH POSTTRAUMATIC STRESS DISORDER

Assessment/Analysis

- History of traumatic experience
- Sleep pattern disturbances, outbursts of anger, and decreased concentration
- Screening for symptoms of major depressive disorder, phobias, and substance use disorder, risk for self-harm and for suicide
- Behaviors associated with other anxiety disorders

Planning/Implementation

- Provide an environment that limits demands and permits attention to resolution of conflicts; establish a trusting relationship
- Identify precipitating stressors and limit them if possible
- Stay with client when memory of event returns to conscious level
- Intervene to protect from acting out violently with disregard for safety of self or others
- Accept symptoms as real to client; do not emphasize or call attention to them
- Attempt to limit client's use of negative defenses, but do not try to stop them until ready to give them up
- Help develop appropriate ways of managing situations through problem solving and cognitive/behavioral therapies; assist to expand supportive network; assist significant others to understand the client's situation
- Collect and document information to assist with determining presence of both PTSD and depression (comorbidity)

Evaluation/Outcomes

- Uses positive coping mechanisms to manage anxiety and reactions to the traumatic event and its flashbacks
- Verbalizes a decrease in dreams or flashbacks regarding the traumatic event
- Follows prescribed treatment regimen
- See Discharge Criteria (later in this chapter)

ACUTE STRESS DISORDER

Overview

- Symptoms similar to PTSD in response to a traumatic event
- However, symptoms develop during or right after (within 1 month) of the trauma; this is the distinguishing characteristic between acute stress disorder and PTSD
- The person demonstrates symptoms of dissociation (eg, a subjective sense of numbing or detachment); a reduced awareness of surroundings (being in a daze); derealization (unreal feeling); depersonalization (feeling alienated); and dissociative amnesia; the symptoms of dissociation occur during the traumatic experience or develop immediately afterward
  - At first, the person may feel confused or helpless, or be in denial about the event
- The person is unable to function in the usual social or occupational role (eg, the individual who has experienced the trauma is unable to perform some necessary task, such as obtaining medical or legal assistance or mobilizing personal resources, to cope with the incident)
- Early interventions are critical in preventing the development of PTSD

- Children experiencing inappropriate sexual behaviors may experience acute stress disorder, even without accompanying violence or injury
- The prevalence of acute stress disorder varies according to type of event and the context of the assessment
- Given the recent mass shootings in the U.S. and the traumatic events and disasters around the world, health care professionals can expect an increase in trauma-related and stressor-related disorders for years to come
- Risk factors include a history of a mental disorder, high levels of negative affect, avoidant coping style, hopelessness, or guilt related to the catastrophic event, and a history of previous trauma; there is often an exaggerated fear of future harm

Therapeutic Interventions and Nursing Care

- See Therapeutic Interventions for PTSD and Nursing Care of Clients with PTSD

APPLICATION AND REVIEW

1. A major feature of PTSD is:
    1. The presence of somatic symptoms that have no medical basis
    2. The reexperiencing of the stressor event
    3. Aggression and rage toward others
    4. Agoraphobia
2. People involved in a bioterrorism attack often exhibit immediate reactions to the traumatic event. Which responses can a nurse expect in survivors during the immediate period after a traumatic event? **Select all that apply.**
    1. Guilt
    2. Denial
    3. Altruism
    4. Confusion
    5. Helplessness
3. The parents of an adolescent who is experiencing PTSD have decided to care for their child at home. What is the **priority** intervention that the home health nurse must include in the plan of care?
    1. Encourage the parents to keep their child within the home environment
    2. Help the parents identify their child's problems that cause them to be fearful
    3. Assist the parents to understand that their child may avoid emotional attachments
    4. Discuss with the parents their feelings of ambivalence about what their child is enduring
4. The main difference between acute stress disorder and PTSD is:
    1. PTSD is milder
    2. PTSD resolves more quickly
    3. Symptoms develop faster after the event in PTSD
    4. Symptoms develop faster after the event in acute stress disorder

See Answers on pages 373-375.

ADJUSTMENT DISORDERS

Overview

- See also Chapter 11

- Adjustment disorders are characterized by emotional distress or short-term disturbance in mood or behavior with nonpsychotic manifestations resulting from identifiable stressor(s)
  - The main distinction of adjustment disorders is the identification of a specific psychosocial stressor, which may be a single event (eg, conflict with a coworker) or multiple events (eg, losing a job and going through a divorce)
  - A single stressor may also lead to other stressors (eg, conflict with a coworker can result in sleepless nights and calling in sick to work), so the initial stressor can have a "ripple effect"
  - Stressors may occur at any time in a person's life and in a number of situations; they include the stress of illness or injury and feeling "trapped" in a dissatisfying personal life or a difficult work environment
  - Adjustment disorders or reactions are not solely due to tragedy, loss, or change and can occur in anyone, regardless of age, religious or spiritual belief, culture, or socioeconomic status
- Symptoms are highly individualized and consist of marked distress and impairment in social, occupational, or academic functioning, sadness, tearfulness, withdrawal, mood disturbances, and preoccupation with the stressor
  - Symptoms are not severe enough for a diagnosis of PTSD
- Unlike depressive disorder, the adjustment disorder generally resolves or lessens once the stressor(s) is eliminated
- Suicide is always a risk factor in adjustment disorders and should be a primary consideration in all stress-related situations, especially in children or adolescents
  - Associated with increased suicidal risk, attempts, and completion
- Severity of the reaction is not proportionate to the severity of stressors
- Represent problematic response to life events, either developmental or situational
- Interaction of personality, crisis, developmental factors, and cultural influences
- Adjustment disorders may be diagnosed after the death of a loved one, when the grief response exceeds the typical pattern of grief and bereavement
- There is no apparent underlying mental disorder; however, there may be low self-esteem, and present behavior may be extremely disturbed
- Client exhibits capacity to adapt to overwhelming stress when given the time to do so
- Problems with distortions or interruptions in thinking processes and decision making tend to resolve themselves
- Adjustment disorders generally occur when the level of stress exceeds the person's usual expectations or coping abilities and typically occur within 3 months of the stressor
- Prevalence varies according to the population studied and the method of assessment
  - Although adjustment disorders are common, they have not yet received the attention of other major diagnoses
  - Nurses need to focus especially on children and adolescents who are experiencing death or loss of a significant person because their coping skills are not yet fully developed
- Suicide is the immediate concern, especially in adolescents, so nurses must be diligent in conducting a suicide assessment in all clients diagnosed with this disorder
- Persons living in poor neighborhoods, with fewer opportunities for a successful life, consistently experience a high rate of socioeconomic stressors that place them at an increased risk for adjustment disorders
- Comorbidity: Adjustment disorders may accompany a mental disorder or a medical disorder, but they are not considered to be an extension of a preexisting mental disorder

Behavioral/Clinical Findings

- Infancy: Extremely upset; demonstrating grief when separated from mother, a normal developmental stage
- Childhood: Regression to an earlier level of development when a new sibling arrives, although that may be a normal response; intense anxiety on entering school
- Adolescence: Struggle for independence; leads to hypersensitivity and frequent episodes of heightened anxiety
- Adult life: Heightened anxiety in response to stressors associated with events such as marriage, pregnancy, divorce, change of employment, purchase of a house
- Later life: Menopause and climacteric, "loss" of children to marriage, retirement, and death of a mate produce extreme stress
- Clinical Findings
  - Onset begins within 3 months of stressors and is out of proportion to the stressor
  - Significant impairment in social and occupational functioning
  - Duration of disorder lasts no longer than 6 months after stress ceases
  - Symptoms do not meet criteria of bereavement
  - Onset may occur at any age; commonly noted in children and adolescents
  - Anxiety may be related to a disturbance in self-esteem, and depression may be related to impaired social interaction
  - Not severe enough to meet criteria of acute stress response or PTSD

Therapeutic Interventions

- Complete diagnostic workup to rule out physical illness
- Psychotherapy, family therapy, group therapy, cognitive/behavioral therapies
- Psychotropic medications: Sedative/hypnotic and antianxiety agents are used short term when client is unable to cope or accomplish daily activities and until healthier coping emerges; antidepressants may be used prophylactically

NURSING CARE OF CLIENTS DIAGNOSED WITH ADJUSTMENT DISORDERS

Assessment/Analysis

- Individual's perception of problem
- Factors impinging on current situation
- Individual's personal strengths and support systems
- Level of anxiety
- Identification of type(s) of stressors and onset
- Risk for suicide

Planning/Implementation

- Help client and/or caregivers recognize and accept that a problem exists
- Maintain client safety
- Encourage identification and use of support systems
- Attempt to minimize environmental pressures
- Allow the client time to recover personal resources
- Treatment goals: To recognize relationship between stressor and emotions; then adjust to the new situation

Evaluation/Outcomes

- Reorganizes defenses
- Utilizes support systems
- Verbalizes a decrease in anxiety
- Develops more effective coping

COMPLICATED GRIEF

Overview

- Complicated grief (also called *prolonged grief syndrome*) presents similarly to depression (Table 19.1)
- Grief after loss of a loved one is a normal reaction and generally does not require professional mental health treatment
- Grief that is complicated and lasts for a very long time after a loss may require treatment
- Grief and depression coexisting makes the grief last longer

TABLE 19.1 Comparison of Grief, Depression, and Posttraumatic Stress Disorder

Aspect	Grief	Depression	Posttraumatic Stress Disorder
Process	Related to loss	Relatively static or cyclic affective disorder that is not necessarily related to loss	Relatively static anxiety disorder related to trauma; precipitating event is outside of the range of usual human experience
Manifestation of symptoms	Usually appear shortly after the loss	Sometimes associated with an identified loss	Often appear years after the trauma
Depressive symptoms	Dysphoric mood of sadness, hopelessness, and despair; anger and periods of agitation are common	Similar to but more intense than grief, except that the individual seldom expresses anger; psychomotor retardation, morbid guilt, and suicidal ideation are more common	Common; other symptoms include persistent reexperiencing of the trauma (rather than preoccupation with the image of the deceased, as with grief); increased arousal is common
Physical symptoms	Cover a wide spectrum; sometimes include heart disease and other chronic illnesses	Primarily neurovegetative	Sleep disturbances often resemble those of grief or depression; hypervigilance is common
Spiritual beliefs	Sometimes provide meaning or context	Seldom provide context or meaning	Seldom any relation

From Fortinash, K. M., & Holoday, P. A. (2012). *Psychiatric mental health nursing* (5th ed.). St. Louis, MO: Mosby.

Normal Grieving Process

- Loss is experienced when something of value (eg, object, person) is changed or gone
  - Actual: Can be validated by others (eg, death of spouse)
  - Perceived: Experienced internally; cannot be verified by others (eg, loss of youth)
  - Anticipatory: Occurs before loss is experienced (eg, scheduled amputation)
- Grief: Response to an actual or perceived loss
  - Bereavement: Emotional response to loss
  - Mourning: Behavioral response to loss; influenced by culture
- Theorists: Stages of grieving
  - Kübler-Ross: Denial, anger, bargaining, depression, acceptance
  - Lindemann: Somatic distress, preoccupation with image of the deceased, guilt, hostile reactions, loss of patterns of conduct
  - Engle: Shock/disbelief, developing awareness, and restitution/resolution

Behavioral/Clinical Findings

- Lasts longer than other types of grief
  - Up to some point, grief is normal; beyond that point, grief is considered pathologic or complicated; there is disagreement about a set amount of time when normal grief becomes complicated grief
  - Persons experiencing significant functional impairment for more than 6 months are likely experiencing a complicated grief reaction
- Characterized by greater disability or other more dysfunctional patterns than usual as defined by cultural values; associated with:
  - Unresolved issues in the relationship with the person who died
  - Inhibited expression of grief
  - Lack of social support
  - The "deritualization" of Western culture (eg, reduced mourning periods of 1 or 2 days)
  - Uncertain loss (eg, prisoners of war, kidnapping)
  - Traumatic loss (eg, by murder, in an accident)
  - Multiple losses (eg, war, natural disaster, mass murders)
  - Loss that is seldom discussed (eg, rape, abortion)
  - Undervalued loss such as that felt by some who experience miscarriages or other losses that may not be recognized by others as significant
  - The accumulated effects of current grief on past unresolved grief
- May suffer comorbid disorders such as anxiety, depression, or PTSD

Types of Complicated Grief

- *Traumatic grief* occurs when there is traumatic loss such as when a spouse is murdered, when a child dies suddenly and unexpectedly, or when rape or multiple deaths occur
  - PTSD is often a concurrent or complicating factor that is sometimes characterized by psychic numbing, intrusive thoughts, avoidance of stimuli, increased arousal, and other aspects of PTSD
  - For some clients, there is a distortion or exaggeration of one or more normative components of grief, with anger and guilt being the most common
- *Absent or inhibited grief* is characterized by the minimal emotional expression of grief, and it is sometimes related to trauma, as noted previously; absent grief sometimes converts to delayed grief, and the individual may experience it years after the loss

- *Conflicted grief* occurs when the relationship with the deceased individual or the lost object is characterized by ambivalence or conflict; initial responses to the loss are often minimal, and they then intensify rather than diminish over time; the survivor feels "haunted" by the deceased
  - An adult survivor of childhood sexual abuse whose abusing parent dies is an example of a person who is at risk for conflicted grief
- *Chronic Grief* is unending grief that occurs after a loss
  - Can be related to the survivor and the deceased having a highly codependent relationship
  - May result from a severe loss and a lack of resources or support to deal with the loss
  - Chronic grief is especially common in some cultural groups

Therapeutic Interventions

- Grief therapy provides guidance as one completes the tasks of successful mourning; its goal is to prevent unresolved and dysfunctional grief
- Several factors complicate grief work:
  - Grief work is extremely painful; many people are surprised at the intensity and depth of the pain, and they often make an attempt to avoid the distress by throwing themselves back into a busy schedule or by taking a vacation
  - The work is inherently contradictory; the pain demands expression, but many often fear that they will lose control over their feelings if they express the pain, saying, "I know that if I start crying, I will never stop"
  - Individuals need both emotion-based coping (eg, expressing deep, powerful feelings) and problem-solving coping (eg, developing strategies for going on with life) to successfully complete the work
  - In most of the Western world, cultural values support the avoidance of the expression of grief (eg, Western cultures value self-control highly, especially among men); there is a tendency to try to rush through grief and get back to work or get on with one's life; rituals that formerly helped with individual and community expressions of grief are now often brief "celebrations" of the deceased's life or other upbeat and usually brief events; after the burial or cremation, survivors are left alone with their pain and a long journey of healing ahead

Grieving Process and Nursing Care

- See Table 19.2

TREATMENT MODALITIES FOR TRAUMA-RELATED AND STRESS-RELATED DISORDERS

Individual and/or Group Therapy (see also Chapter 8)

- Some clients benefit from grief therapy (see above)
- Family therapy focuses on the family as a system rather than on just one individual's problem; the goals of family therapy are to foster self-worth of all members, promote clear and honest communication among members, create guidelines for interaction that are realistic and flexible, and link individuals and family with society in ways that are open and hopeful
- Psychoanalysis helps the individual become aware of repressed emotional conflicts, analyze their origin, and, through the process of insight, bring them into consciousness, so maladaptive behavior can be altered; it usually is not used to explore unresolved grief
- Psychoeducational therapy focuses on teaching clients and family members about disorders, treatments, and resources, with the goal of empowerment to participate in their own care once they have the knowledge

TABLE 19.2	Grieving Process and Nursing Care	
Stage of Grieving	**Client Response**	**Nursing Care**
Denial, disbelief	Disbelief, intellectualization	Accept response but do not reinforce denial
Anger, hostility	Verbally hostile	Do not become defensive, meet client needs
Bargaining	Seeks to avoid loss, may express feelings of guilt	Listen attentively, refer to spiritual counselor if appropriate
Depression, sadness	Grieves about what may never be, may be verbal or withdrawn	Listen attentively, sit quietly, use touch if appropriate
Acceptance, resolution	Comes to terms with loss, may make future plans, may have decreased interest in people and surroundings	Be quiet but available, help family to accept client's behavior

From Nugent, P. M., Green, J. S., Hellmer Saul, M. A., & Pelikan, P. K. (2012). *Mosby's comprehensive review of nursing for the NCLEX-RN examination* (20th ed.). St Louis, MO: Mosby.

Psychopharmacology (see also Chapter 8)

- Selective serotonin reuptake inhibitor (SSRI) (eg, paroxetine, fluoxetine, or sertraline) or a serotonin norepinephrine reuptake inhibitor (SNRI) (eg, venlafaxine) to reduce anxiety and stress level, as well as depressive symptoms
- Tricyclic antidepressants (TCAs) or mirtazapine may be prescribed if the client is unable to tolerate SSRIs and SNRIs, or if these drugs fail to reduce symptoms
- Clonidine and prazosin are used for panic and high arousal states; the most intolerable and troubling side effect of these medications is hypotension (low blood pressure); prazosin is used for nightmares specifically

General Nursing Care of Clients Diagnosed with Stress-Related Disorders

- Identifying the type of stress and stress pattern can lead to more effective interventions
  - There are many screening tools available for PTSD, and a more comprehensive assessment is conducted if the client tests positive (eg, a history is taken about the time of onset of the traumatic event; frequency of recurrence of the trauma; severity of the trauma; degree of distress; and functional impairment)
- Assessment for suicidal thoughts or behaviors or violence toward others is critical
- Assessment of self-injurious behaviors is also essential
- A family and social history is also conducted to determine whether the client has a support system and who in the client's life can be counted on to help him or her
- If the client is socially withdrawn, the nurse needs to ask further questions to determine the cause and nature of the withdrawn behavior
- There may be some underlying depressive symptoms or another disorder that needs to be examined
- Sleep habits and disorders, such as insomnia, need to be assessed, as well as the client's medical and psychiatric history and medication regimen
- See also specific assessment and behavioral/clinical findings for each disorder

Outcomes Identification

- General outcomes for clients diagnosed with trauma-related and stressor-related disorders include that the client will:
  - Verbalize concern for personal health and safety with absence of suicidality and self-injurious behaviors
  - Identify anxiety or stress-producing stimuli, circumstances, or events
  - Manage stress or anxiety through exercises such as mindfulness meditation and other stress-reducing techniques (see Chapter 8)
  - Demonstrate a decrease in physiologic, emotional, cognitive, and behavioral symptoms of stress or anxiety
  - Maintain the ability to function in mild stressful or anxiety states
  - Discuss the medicatios regimen and take medication as prescribed
  - Practice coping strategies (eg, deep breathing techniques; progressive relaxation exercises; thought; image and memory substitutions; and assertive [empowering] behaviors)
  - Utilize healthy, adaptive coping mechanisms
  - Report improved sleep patterns and ability to sleep through the night
  - Exhibit increased ability to problem-solve and make rational decisions
  - Demonstrate ability to perform activities of daily living
  - Verbalize feeling more hopeful and in control of life
  - Identify several friends and desire to socialize more
  - Recognize when to contact the therapist for more visits when a PTSD crisis occurs

Nursing Interventions

- Box 19.1 shows general nursing interventions for trauma-related and stress-related disorders
- See also specific interventions under each disorder

Discharge Criteria

- Persons with these disorders need close follow-up care (aftercare), specifically to prevent suicide and self-injurious behavior
- Follow-up care is especially critical in adolescents who do not have the ability to cope with their emotional and psychologic feelings of anger, rage, loneliness, and a general sense of being "different" and therefore unaccepted by peers
- A dysphoric or depressive mood state, in clients of all age groups, indicates that immediate evaluation is needed, and interventions, including medication, may need to be modified
- The client should always have a phone number of a contact person he or she can call in case of the sudden emergence of flashbacks, panic attack, or the reexperiencing of the traumatic stressor event, to protect the client from injury or suicide

APPLICATION AND REVIEW

5. A nurse is aware that a co-worker's mother died 16 months ago. The co-worker cries every time someone says the word "mother" or if the mother's name is mentioned. What does the nurse conclude about this behavior?
   1. It is an expected response
   2. Most people cry when their mother dies
   3. The co-worker may need help with grieving
   4. The co-worker was extremely attached to the mother

BOX 19.1	General Nursing Interventions for Trauma-Related and Stress-Related Disorders *(with rationale statements)*

1. Maintain safety for the client and the environment.
   A client's stress level or anxiety can escalate to a panic state, which can frighten and harm the client and others. The nurse's first priority is to protect the client and others in the environment.
2. Assess your own stress level and make a conscious effort to remain calm.
   Stress and anxiety are readily transferrable from one person to another.
3. Recognize the client's behaviors that may indicate PTSD and other stress-related disorders. Examples include: avoidance of questions asked; negative emotional state (fear, guilt, shame, sadness, confusion); withdrawn behavior; easily startled; problem with concentration.
   These behaviors may help the nurse implement a care plan that best fits the client's problems and symptomatology, which is the focus for nursing interventions.
4. Assist the client to manage their arousal level through stress-reducing activities, whenever they are threatened by images or flashback of the traumatic stressor event. Examples are: provide a safe and constant environment; teach stress- and anxiety-reducing exercises (eg, deep breathing, progressive relaxation, mindfulness meditation), and cognitive-behavioral strategies.
   Managing major symptoms and behaviors related to the traumatic event and the reexperiencing of the event helps reduce the stress level and affords the client some relief from the intensity of PTSD and related disorders.
5. Inform the client gently in the course of the nurse–client interaction that, although guilt is often a common outcome of trauma-related and stress-related disorders, the client is not responsible for the event and may recognize that in time.
   Sharing this important information counters the client's belief that he or she caused the event to happen, which helps the client put the event into a more realistic perspective and allows the healing process to begin. (Cognitive therapists state that guilt is not a feeling, but a belief held by an individual that is often erroneous, and needs to be gently challenged. Guilt, however, can invoke negative feelings that can be debilitating to the individual).
6. Connect the client and family with local support groups, in which the client and others can share their traumatic events in the presence of a professional group counselor.
   Describing the traumatizing event and listening to others' stories can help the client feel understood and supported, which reduces the stress level and adds to the healing process.

From Fortinash, K. M., & Holoday, P. A. (2012). *Psychiatric mental health nursing* (5th ed.). St. Louis, MO: Mosby.

6. A parent whose daughter is killed in a school bus accident tearfully tells the nurse, "My daughter was just getting over the chickenpox and did not want to go to school, but I insisted that she go. My child's death is my fault." How should the nurse anticipate that perceiving a death as preventable will likely influence the grieving process?
   1. Loss may be easier to understand and accept
   2. Mourner may experience a pathologic grief reaction
   3. Bereavement may be of greater intensity and duration
   4. Grieving process may progress to a psychiatric illness
7. Relatives of the victims of a home invasion attack in which several family members were killed received crisis intervention services. Which therapy is **most** beneficial after the immediate event has passed?
   1. Grief
   2. Family
   3. Psychoanalytic
   4. Psychoeducational

8. What is the most important observation a nurse makes with an adolescent diagnosed with an adjustment disorder?
   1. Depressive symptoms
   2. Manic symptoms
   3. Risk for suicide
   4. Anger and aggression
9. A client diagnosed with lung cancer says to the nurse, "If I could just be free of pain for a few days, I might be able to eat more and regain strength." Which stage of grieving does the nurse conclude the client is in?
   1. Bargaining
   2. Frustration
   3. Depression
   4. Rationalization
10. A client diagnosed with a terminal illness reaches the stage of acceptance. How can the nurse **best** help the client during this stage?
    1. Accept the client's crying
    2. Encourage unrestricted family visits
    3. Explain details of the care being given
    4. Stay nearby without initiating conversation

See Answers on pages 373-375.

ANSWER KEY: REVIEW QUESTIONS

1. **2 Reexperiencing of the stressor event is one of four hallmarks of PTSD.**
   1 The presence of somatic symptoms that have no medical basis is somatic symptom disorder. **3** Although it may occur, aggression and rage toward others is not a major feature of PTSD. **4** Agoraphobia is not a major feature of PTSD.
   Client Need: Psychosocial Integrity; **Cognitive Level:** Comprehensio; **Nursing Process:** Assessment/Analysis

   Memory Aid: Use "Re-AAC" for how to recall the four symptoms needed for the diagnosis of PTSD, as if the person is ***reaac***ting to the trauma: ***re***experiencing, ***a***voidance, ***a***rousal and reactivity symptoms, ***c***ognition and mood symptoms.

2. **Answers: 2, 4, 5.**
   2 Shock and disbelief are the initial responses to a traumatic experience; a situational crisis usually is unexpected, and its effect causes disequilibrium. **4** A crisis causes disequilibrium, and the individual experiences confusion, disorganization, and difficulty making decisions. **5** When a person is unable to cope, helplessness and regression often emerge; a crisis occurs when there is a painful, frightening event that is so overwhelming that an individual's usual coping mechanisms are inadequate.
   1 Feelings of guilt may emerge later when the individual moves from focusing on the self to an increased interaction with others. **3** Concern for others emerges later after the individual is able to set aside or resolve own needs.
   Client Need: Psychosocial Integrity; **Cognitive Level:** Comprehension; **Nursing Process:** Assessment/Analysis
3. **3 The client will tend to avoid emotional attachment to significant others because this is a common way to protect the self from the experience of potential future losses. The priority at this time is to have family members develop an understanding of what is happening to the client.**
   1 Although it is important to keep the client safe and secure when in the home, the family should not restrict the client to the home environment. **2** Although issues concerning the client's problems need to be resolved, it is not the priority. **4** Although a discussion with the parents their feelings of ambivalence may be necessary, it is not the priority.
   Client Need: Psychosocial Integrity; **Cognitive Level:** Application; **Integrated Process:** Caring; **Nursing Process:** Planning/Implementation

4. **4 Symptoms develop faster (within days to 1 month) after the event in acute stress disorder.**

1 PTSD is not milder or more severe; when the symptoms develop after the event is the distinguishing factor. **2** PTSD generally resolves more slowly than acute stress disorder. **3** Symptoms do not develop faster after the event in PTSD; they may be delayed by months, years or decades.

Client Need: Psychosocial Integrity; **Cognitive Level:** Comprehension; **Nursing Process:** Assessment/Analysis

5. **3 Crying is a release, but the individual should have developed effective coping mechanisms by this time. The co-worker may need help with the grieving process.**

1 Excessive crying 16 months after the death of a loved one is not considered an expected response. **2** People express grief in a variety of ways, not necessarily by crying. **4** That the co-worker was attached to the mother is an assumption and is not a valid conclusion.

Client Need: Psychosocial Integrity; **Cognitive Level:** Application; **Integrated Process:** Caring; **Nursing Process:** Planning/Implementation

6. **3 Deaths that are perceived as preventable cause greater guilt for mourners and therefore increase the intensity and length of the grieving process.**

1 It usually is more difficult to understand and accept a death perceived as preventable. **2** That the death may be perceived as preventable may prolong and intensify the mourning process but will not necessarily result in a pathologic reaction. **4** That the death is perceived as preventable may prolong and intensify the mourning process but will not necessarily result in a psychiatric illness.

Client Need: Psychosocial Integrity; **Cognitive Level:** Comprehension; **Nursing Process:** Assessment/Analysis

7. **1 Grief therapy provides guidance as one completes the tasks of successful mourning; its goal is to prevent unresolved and dysfunctional grief.**

2 Family therapy focuses on the family as a system rather than on just one individual's problem; the goals of family therapy are to foster self-worth of all members, promote clear and honest communication among members, create guidelines for interaction that are realistic and flexible, and link individuals and family with society in ways that are open and hopeful. No data indicate that the family became dysfunctional after the tragedy. **3** Psychoanalytic therapy usually is not used to explore unresolved grief. Psychoanalysis helps the individual become aware of repressed emotional conflicts, analyze their origin, and, through the process of insight, bring them into consciousness, so maladaptive behavior can be altered. **4** Psychoeducational therapy focuses on teaching clients and family members about disorders, treatments, and resources, with the goal of empowerment to participate in their own care once they have the knowledge. No evidence indicates that the families need this type of therapy.

Client Need: Management of Care; **Cognitive Level:** Application; **Nursing Process:** Planning/Implementation; **Integrated Process:** Caring

8. **3 Risk for suicide is the most important observation in clients with an adjustment disorder.**

1 Depressive symptoms, though common, are not the most important observation in clients with an adjustment disorder. **2** Manic symptoms are not the most important observation in clients with an adjustment disorder. **3** Anger and aggression, though important, are not the most important observation in clients with an adjustment disorder.

Client Need: Psychosocial Integrity; **Cognitive Level:** Application; **Nursing Process:** Assessment/Analysis

9. **1 Bargaining is one of the stages of grieving, in which the client promises some type of desirable behavior to postpone the inevitability of death.**

2 Frustration is a subjective experience, a feeling of being thwarted, but it is not one of the stages of grieving. **3** Classified as the fourth stage of grieving, depression represents the grief experienced as the individual recognizes the inescapability of fate. **4** Rationalization is a defense mechanism in which attempts are made to justify or explain an unacceptable action or feeling; it is not a stage of the grieving process.

Client Need: Psychosocial Integrity; **Cognitive Level:** Application; **Integrated Process:** Caring; **Nursing Process:** Assessment/Analysis

10. **4 The nurse's presence communicates concern and provides an opportunity for the client to initiate communication; silence is an effective interpersonal technique that permits the client to direct the content and extent of verbalizations without the nurse imposing on the client's privacy.**

      1 Crying, part of depression, usually ceases when the individual reaches acceptance. **2** During acceptance the client may decide not to have visitors, preferring time for reflection. **3** Detached from the environment, the client may find that the details of various procedures lose significance.

      Client Need: Psychosocial Integrity; **Cognitive Level:** Application; **Integrated Process:** Caring; **Nursing Process:** Planning/Implementation

CHILDREN AND ADOLESCENTS

Neurodevelopmental Disorders

- Arise during childhood and include autism spectrum disorders, attention deficit/hyperactivity disorder, oppositional defiant disorder, intermittent explosive disorder, and conduct disorder, as well as intellectual disabilities, learning disorders, and some movement and communication (language and speech) disorders
- These disorders may be characterized by physical as well as psychologic signs and symptoms and must be distinguished from expected variances in growth and development
- Psychiatric care of the child or adolescent is a subspecialty within psychiatric nursing; although there is a wide range of deficits with these disorders, there are fundamental principles that apply
- Care should be based on the child's developmental level and directed toward helping the child grow emotionally; all children, especially these children, require:
  - Protection from danger, including their own impulsive acts and self-destructive behavior
  - Love and acceptance
  - Basic physiologic needs to be met
  - Meaningful trusting relationships
  - Opportunities to explore the environment
- There is increasing awareness of mental illnesses in children and adolescents that were formerly believed to occur only in adults; these include bipolar disorder, schizophrenia, depression, and posttraumatic stress disorder (PTSD); manifestations of these illnesses in the younger population may differ from those in adults; treatments may be modified to meet the developmental level of the child and adolescent

Autism Spectrum Disorders

- Autism spectrum disorders (ASD) is the name for a group of neurodevelopmental disorders, "a spectrum" of symptoms, skills, and levels of disability
- ASD results in an alienation or withdrawal from social interaction; prognosis is guarded and depends on a multiplicity of factors
- People diagnosed with ASD often have these characteristics:
  - Ongoing social problems that include difficulty communicating and interacting with others; severe and pervasive impairment in reciprocal social interaction (eg, indifference or aversion to affection and physical contact) as well as severe and pervasive impairment of communication skills (verbal: eg, misuse of pronouns; nonverbal: eg, lack of eye contact)
  - Repetitive behaviors as well as limited interests or activities
  - Symptoms that typically are recognized in the first 2 years of life
  - Symptoms that impair the individual's ability to function socially, at school or work, or other areas of life
- The etiology of ASD is multifaceted but not precisely known
- Some people are mildly impaired by their symptoms, whereas others are severely disabled

- Treatments and services can improve a person's symptoms and ability to function, especially with early intervention; families with concerns should talk to their pediatrician about what they have observed and the possibility of ASD screening
- According to the Centers for Disease Control and Prevention (CDC), approximately 1 in 68 children has been identified with some form of ASD; males are diagnosed more often than females
- In the past, Asperger's syndrome and autistic disorder were separate disorders; they were listed as subcategories within the diagnosis of "Pervasive Developmental Disorders;" however, this separation has changed; the fifth edition from the American Psychiatric Association, the *Diagnostic and Statistical Manual of Mental Disorders* (DSM-5), does not highlight subcategories of a larger disorder; the manual includes the range of characteristics and severity within one category; people whose symptoms were previously diagnosed as Asperger's syndrome or autistic disorder are now included as part of ASD
- Behavioral/clinical findings
  - Not all people diagnosed with ASD will show all of these behaviors, but most will show several; the two main types of behaviors are "restricted/repetitive behaviors" and "social communication/interaction behaviors"
  - Restrictive/repetitive behaviors may include:
    - Repeating certain behaviors or having unusual behaviors (eg, motor activities, such as clapping or flapping of hands, spinning, rocking, swaying) and postures (eg, walking on tiptoes, odd postures, strange hand movements)
    - Having overly focused interests such as on moving objects or parts of objects (eg, a fan)
    - Having a lasting, intense interest in certain topics, such as numbers, details, or facts
  - Social communication/interaction behaviors may include:
    - Getting upset by a slight change in a routine or being placed in a new or overly stimulating setting
    - Making little or inconsistent eye contact
    - Having a tendency to look at and listen to other people less often
    - Rarely sharing enjoyment of objects or activities by pointing or showing things to others
    - Responding in an unusual way when others show anger, distress, or affection
    - Failing to or being slow to respond to someone calling their name or other verbal attempts to gain attention
    - Having difficulties with the back and forth of conversations
    - Often talking at length about a favorite subject without noticing that others are not interested or without giving others a chance to respond
    - Repeating words or phrases that they hear, a behavior called *echolalia*
    - Using words that seem odd, out of place, or have a special meaning known only to those familiar with that person's way of communicating
    - Having facial expressions, movements, and gestures that do not match what is being said
    - Having an unusual tone of voice that may sound sing-song or flat and robot-like
    - Having trouble understanding another person's point of view or being unable to predict or understand other people's actions
    - Not actively participating in simple social play or games
    - Preferring solitary activities
  - People with ASD may have other difficulties such as being very sensitive to light, noise, clothing, or temperature; they may also experience sleep problems, digestion problems, and irritability

- ASD is unique in that it is common for people with ASD to have many strengths and abilities in addition to challenges
  - Strengths and abilities may include:
    - Having higher than average intelligence—the CDC reports 46% of ASD children have higher than average intelligence
    - Being able to learn things in detail and remember information for long periods of time
    - Being strong visual and auditory learners
    - Exceling in math, science, music, or art
- Diagnosing ASD
  - The American Academy of Pediatrics recommends that all children between the ages of 18 and 24 months be screened for ASD; young children with ASD can usually be reliably diagnosed by age 2
  - Older children and adolescents should be evaluated for ASD when a parent or teacher raises concerns based on watching the child socialize, communicate, and play
  - Diagnosing ASD in adults is not easy; in adults, some ASD symptoms can overlap with symptoms of other mental health disorders, such as schizophrenia or ADHD; however, getting a correct diagnosis of ASD as an adult can help a person understand past difficulties, identify his or her strengths, and obtain the right kind of help
  - Diagnosis in young children is often a two-stage process
    - General developmental screening during well-child checkups
    - Every child should receive well-child checkups with a pediatrician or an early childhood health care provider; the Centers for Disease Control and Prevention (CDC) recommends specific ASD screening be done at the 18-month and 24-month visits
  - Earlier screening might be needed if a child is at high risk for ASD or developmental problems; those at high risk include children who:
    - Have a sister, brother, or other family member diagnosed with ASD
    - Have some ASD behaviors
    - Were born premature and at a low birth weight
  - Parents' experiences and concerns are very important in the screening process for young children; sometimes the health care provider will ask parents questions about the child's behaviors and combine this information with his or her observations of the child
  - Children who show some developmental problems during this screening process will be referred for another stage of evaluation
  - Additional evaluation: This evaluation is with a team of doctors and other health professionals with a wide range of specialties who are experienced in diagnosing ASD; this team may include:
    - A developmental pediatrician—a doctor who has special training in child development
    - A child psychologist and/or child psychiatrist—a doctor who knows about brain development and behavior
    - A speech-language pathologist—a health professional who has special training in communication difficulties
  - The evaluation may assess:
    - Cognitive level or thinking skills
    - Language abilities
    - Age-appropriate skills needed to complete daily activities independently such as eating, dressing, and toileting

- Because ASD is a complex disorder that sometimes occurs along with other illnesses or learning disorders, the comprehensive evaluation may include:
  - Laboratory blood tests
  - Hearing test
- The outcome of the evaluation will result in recommendations to help plan for treatment
- Diagnosis in older children and adolescents
  - Older children whose ASD symptoms are noticed after starting school are often first recognized and evaluated by the school's special education team; the school's team may refer these children to a health care professional
  - Parents may talk with a pediatrician about their child's social difficulties, including problems with subtle communication; these subtle communication issues may include understanding tone of voice, facial expressions, or body language; older children may have trouble understanding figures of speech, humor, or sarcasm; parents may also find that their child has trouble forming friendships with peers; the pediatrician can refer the child for further evaluation and treatment
- Nursing care of children diagnosed with ASD
  - See General Nursing Care Related to Disorders First Evident in Infancy, Childhood, or Adolescence for "Assessment/Analysis" and "Planning/Implementation" sections

Evaluation/Outcomes

- Remains safe from injury
- Decreases self-destructive behavior
- Uses fewer repetitive motor behaviors
- Increases use of first-person speech

Attention Deficit/Hyperactivity Disorder

- Attention deficit/hyperactivity disorder (ADHD) is a brain disorder marked by an ongoing pattern of inattention and/or hyperactivity-impulsivity that interferes with functioning or development
  - *Inattention* means a person wanders off task, lacks persistence, has difficulty sustaining focus, and is disorganized; also, these problems are not due to defiance or lack of comprehension
  - *Hyperactivity* means a person seems to move about constantly, including in situations in which it is not appropriate, or excessively fidgets, taps, or talks; in adults, it may be extreme restlessness or wearing others out with constant activity
  - *Impulsivity* means a person makes hasty actions that occur in the moment without first thinking about them and their high potential for harm or a desire for immediate rewards or inability to delay gratification; an impulsive person may be socially intrusive and excessively interrupt others or make important decisions without considering the long-term consequences
- Studies suggest an interaction between psychosocial and biologic factors; there is a strong correlation between genetic factors and ADHD; concordance is 51% in monozygotic twins and 33% in dizygotic twins; adoption studies also support genetics over environmental causes; ADHD occurs more often among the first-degree relatives of children diagnosed with ADHD
- ADHD occurs more frequently in males than females, with ratios from 2:1 up to 9:1; females with ADHD are more likely to have problems primarily with inattention
- Rates of ADHD among school-aged children are estimated at 3% to 7% of the population; as many as two-thirds of those diagnosed with ADHD also meet the criteria for another mental disorder

- Other conditions, such as learning disabilities, anxiety disorder, conduct disorder, depression, and substance use disorder, are common in people with ADHD
- Often diagnosed as child enters the school system
- For a person to receive a diagnosis of ADHD, the symptoms of inattention and/or hyperactivity-impulsivity must be chronic or long-lasting, must impair the person's functioning, and must cause the person to fall behind normal development for his or her age; the health care provider will also ensure that any ADHD symptoms are not due to another medical or psychiatric condition; most children diagnosed with ADHD receive a diagnosis during the elementary school years; for an adolescent or adult to receive a diagnosis of ADHD, the symptoms need to have been present before age 12
- ADHD symptoms can appear as early as between the ages of 3 and 6 and can continue through adolescence and adulthood; symptoms of ADHD can be mistaken for emotional or disciplinary problems or missed entirely in quiet, well-behaved children, leading to a delay in diagnosis; adults with undiagnosed ADHD may have a history of poor academic performance, problems at work, or difficult or failed relationships
- Symptoms persist in less severe form into adulthood
- ADHD symptoms can change over time as a person ages; in young children with ADHD, hyperactivity-impulsivity is the most predominant symptom; as a child reaches elementary school, the symptom of inattention may become more prominent and cause the child to struggle academically; in adolescence, hyperactivity seems to lessen and may show more often as feelings of restlessness or fidgeting, but inattention and impulsivity may remain; many adolescents with ADHD also struggle with relationships and antisocial behaviors; inattention, restlessness, and impulsivity tend to persist into adulthood
- Behavioral/clinical findings
  - Inappropriately inattentive; short attention span; easily distracted; learning disabilities
  - Excessive talking and impulsiveness (eg, cannot take turns, interrupts)
  - Difficulty organizing tasks and activities; does not complete tasks
  - Squirming and fidgeting; hyperactivity may or may not be present
  - Some people with ADHD only have problems with one of the behaviors, whereas others have both inattention and hyperactivity-impulsivity; most children have the combined type of ADHD
  - In preschool, the most common ADHD symptom is hyperactivity
  - It is normal to have some inattention, unfocused motor activity and impulsivity, but for people with ADHD these behaviors are more severe, occur more often, and interfere with or reduce the quality of how they functions socially, at school, or in a job
  - People with symptoms of inattention may often:
    - Overlook or miss details, make careless mistakes in schoolwork, at work, or during other activities
    - Have problems sustaining attention in tasks or play, including conversations, lectures, or lengthy reading
    - Not seem to listen when spoken to directly
    - Not follow through on instructions and fail to finish schoolwork, chores, or duties in the workplace, or start tasks but quickly lose focus and get easily sidetracked
    - Have problems organizing tasks and activities such as what to do in sequence, keeping materials and belongings in order, having messy work and poor time management, and failing to meet deadlines
    - Avoid or dislike tasks that require sustained mental effort, such as schoolwork or homework, or, for teens and older adults, preparing reports, completing forms, or reviewing lengthy papers

- Lose things necessary for tasks or activities such as school supplies, pencils, books, tools, wallets, keys, paperwork, eyeglasses, and cell phones
- Be easily distracted by unrelated thoughts or stimuli
- Be forgetful in daily activities, such as chores, errands, returning calls, and keeping appointments
  - People with symptoms of hyperactivity-impulsivity may often:
    - Fidget and squirm in their seats
    - Leave their seats in situations when staying seated is expected, such as in the classroom or office
    - Run or dash around or climb in situations in which it is inappropriate, or, in teens and adults, often feel restless
    - Be unable to play or engage in hobbies quietly
    - Be constantly in motion or "on the go," or act as if "driven by a motor"
    - Talk nonstop
    - Blurt out an answer before a question has been completed, finish other people's sentences, or speak without waiting for a turn in conversation
    - Have trouble waiting his or her turn
    - Interrupt or intrude on others, for example in conversations, games, or activities
- Therapeutic interventions
  - Although there is no cure for ADHD, currently available treatments can help reduce symptoms and improve functioning; treatments include medication, psychotherapy, education or training, or a combination of treatments
  - Note that people with autistic symptoms are at an increased risk for substance use disorder
  - Medications
    - For many people, ADHD medications reduce hyperactivity and impulsivity and improve their ability to focus, work, and learn; medication also may improve physical coordination
    - Stimulants: Although it may seem unusual to treat ADHD with a medication that is considered a stimulant, it works because it increases the brain chemicals dopamine and norepinephrine, which play essential roles in thinking and attention; the most commonly used is methylphenidate
      - Precautions: Stimulants can raise blood pressure and heart rate and increase anxiety; therefore a person with other health problems, including high blood pressure, seizures, heart disease, glaucoma, liver or kidney disease, or an anxiety disorder, should tell their health care provider before taking a stimulant
      - Side effects include decreased appetite with weight loss, sleep problems, tics (sudden, repetitive movements or sounds), personality changes, increased anxiety and irritability, stomachaches, and headaches
      - Restricting administration of stimulants to daytime hours (no later than 4 pm) may reduce the sleep disturbance side effects and giving the drug just after eating may reduce anorexia
    - Nonstimulants: These medications take longer to start working than stimulants but can also improve focus, attention, and impulsivity in a person with ADHD; used when a person has bothersome side effects from stimulants, when a stimulant was not effective, or in combination with a stimulant to increase effectiveness
    - Although not approved by the U.S. Food and Drug Administration (FDA) specifically for the treatment of ADHD, some antidepressants are sometimes used alone or in combination with a stimulant to treat ADHD; antidepressants may

help all of the symptoms of ADHD and can be prescribed if a client has bothersome side effects from stimulants; antidepressants can be helpful in combination with stimulants if a client also has another condition such as an anxiety disorder, depression, or another mood disorder; however, special caution is advised with the use of antidepressants in children and adolescents because increased suicide risk is a possibility

- Psychotherapy
  - Adding psychotherapy to treat ADHD can help clients and their families better cope with everyday problems
  - Behavioral therapy may involve practical assistance such as help organizing tasks or completing schoolwork or working through emotionally difficult events; it also teaches a person how to monitor his or her own behavior and give oneself praise or rewards for acting in a desired way such as controlling anger or thinking before acting
  - Giving positive or negative feedback for certain behaviors, establishing clear rules, chore lists, and other structured routines, help a person control his or her behavior; therapists may also teach children social skills such as how to wait their turn, share toys, ask for help, or respond to teasing
  - Cognitive behavioral therapy can also teach a person mindfulness techniques, or meditation; the therapist also encourages the person diagnosed with ADHD to adjust to the life changes that come with treatment such as thinking before acting or resisting the urge to take unnecessary risks
  - Family and marital therapy can help family members and spouses find better ways to handle disruptive behaviors, encourage behavior changes, and improve interactions with the client
- Education and training
  - Children and adults diagnosed with ADHD need guidance and understanding from their parents, families, and teachers to reach their full potential and to succeed; for school-age children, frustration, blame, and anger may have built up within a family before a child is diagnosed; parents and children may need special help to overcome negative feelings; mental health professionals can educate parents about ADHD and how it affects a family
  - Parenting skills training (behavioral parent management training) teaches parents the skills they need to encourage and reward positive behaviors in their children; it helps parents learn how to use a system of rewards and consequences to change a child's behavior; parents are taught to give immediate and positive feedback for behaviors they want to encourage and to ignore or redirect behaviors that they want to discourage; they may also learn to structure situations in ways that support desired behavior
  - Stress management techniques can benefit parents of children diagnosed with ADHD by increasing their ability to deal with frustration so that they can respond calmly to their child's behavior
  - Support groups can help parents and families connect with others who have similar problems and concerns; groups often meet regularly to share frustrations and successes, to exchange information about recommended specialists and strategies, and to talk with experts
- Nursing care of children diagnosed with ADHD
  - See General Nursing Care Related to Disorders First Evident in Infancy, Childhood, or Adolescence for "Assessment/Analysis" and "Planning/Implementation" sections

Evaluation/Outcomes

- Participates in home and school activities
- Completes tasks
- Follows directions

APPLICATION AND REVIEW

1. A 3-year-old child is diagnosed with autism spectrum disorder. Which behaviors should the nurse expect when assessing this child? **Select all that apply.**
   1. Imitates others
   2. Seeks physical contact
   3. Avoids eye-to-eye contact
   4. Engages in cooperative play
   5. Performs repetitive activities
   6. Displays interest in children rather than adults

2. What is the prognosis for a normal productive life for a child diagnosed with autism spectrum disorder?
   1. Dependent on an early diagnosis
   2. Often related to the child's overall temperament
   3. Ensured as long as the child attends a school tailored to meet needs
   4. Guarded because of interference with so many parameters of functioning

3. For what most common characteristic of autism spectrum disorder should a nurse assess a child suspected of having this disorder?
   1. Responds to any stimulus
   2. Responds to physical contact
   3. Seems unresponsive to the environment
   4. Interacts with children rather than adults

4. A nurse is assessing a child suspected of having ASD. At what age is ASD usually diagnosed?
   1. 2 years of age
   2. 6 years of age
   3. 6 months of age
   4. 1 to 3 months of age

5. For which clinical indication should a nurse observe a child suspected of having ASD?
   1. Lack of eye contact
   2. Crying for attention
   3. Catatonic-like rigidity
   4. Engaging in parallel play

6. A 6-year-old child diagnosed with autism spectrum disorder is nonverbal and has limited eye contact. What should a nurse do initially to promote social interaction?
   1. Encourage the child to sing songs with the nurse
   2. Engage in parallel play while sitting next to the child
   3. Provide opportunities for the child to play with other children
   4. Use therapeutic holding when the child does not respond to verbal interactions

7. A nurse is interviewing a child diagnosed with attention deficit disorder. For which major characteristic should the nurse assess this child?
   1. Overreaction to stimuli
   2. Continued use of rituals
   3. Delayed speech development
   4. Inability to use abstract thought

8. A hyperactive 9-year-old child with a history of ADHD is admitted for observation after a motor vehicle collision. What should be the focus of nursing actions when teaching about personal safety?
   1. Requesting that the child write at least three safety rules
   2. Asking the child to verbalize as many safety rules as possible

3. Talking with the child about the importance of using a seat belt

4. Encouraging the child to talk with other children about their opinions of safety rules

9. A 4-year-old child is diagnosed with ADHD. What information about the child's behavior should the nurse expect when obtaining a health history from the parents? **Select all that apply.**

1. Is impulsive
2. Talks excessively
3. Is spiteful and vindictive
4. Annoys others deliberately
5. Plays video games for hours
6. Does not follow through or finish tasks

10. A nurse anticipates that children diagnosed with ADHD may be learning-disabled. This means that these children:

1. Will probably not be self-directed learners
2. Have intellectual deficits that interfere with learning
3. Experience perceptual difficulties that interfere with learning
4. Are performing usually two grade levels lower than their age norm

11. A nurse is teaching the parents of a child diagnosed with ADHD about the prescribed medication methylphenidate. What time should the daily dose be administered?

1. Before breakfast
2. Just after breakfast
3. Immediately before lunch
4. As soon as the child awakens

12. A child is diagnosed with ADHD. What is a strategy that the nurse should teach the parents to assist in coping with this disorder?

1. Orient the child to reality
2. Reward appropriate conduct
3. Suppress feelings of frustration
4. Use restraints when behavior is out of control

See Answers on pages 403-407.

Oppositional Defiant Disorder

- Main features of oppositional defiant disorder (ODD): Disobedience, defiance, and hostility, mainly directed at adults or other authority figures in the child's life
  - The child often refuses to comply with normal rules or requests, deliberately irritates others, and blames others for his or her own mistakes and misbehaviors
  - Spitefulness and vindictiveness are also common
  - Manifestations of this disorder may exist in the home setting but not be present at school or elsewhere in the community; the child most often displays symptoms of this disorder with peers or adults he or she knows well
  - Children with this disorder generally do not consider themselves as oppositional, but instead view others as unreasonable or demanding
- Prevalence, risk factors, comorbidity
  - Higher prevalence in males than females and is consistent across cultures
  - Causative factors may be genetic or physiologic
  - Risk factors may be related to harsh or inconsistent discipline or neglect; moving from one foster care environment to another may also contribute to this behavior
  - Caregivers need to report suspected and actual child abuse to the appropriate authorities for further assessment and follow-up care
  - Coexisting conditions may be anxiety disorders, depressive disorders, and conduct disorders
  - The child may experience long-term problems in social and occupational functioning

Intermittent Explosive Disorder

- Characterized by recurrent episodes of impulsive, aggressive, hostile, or violent behaviors, or angry verbal outbursts
  - The individual often reacts in a way that is disproportionate to the situation; examples are road rage, domestic abuse, throwing or breaking objects without regard for their value, of other types of temper tantrums
  - The person may resort to attacking others or their possessions, which may result in bodily harm and/or destruction of property
  - The person may also injury himself or herself in the process
  - Persons with this disorder may be embarrassed or regretful after the fact
- Prevalence, risk factors, comorbidity
  - This disorder is seen in children and young adults as well as adults
  - Risk factors indicate that the neurotransmitter serotonin may play a role in its development, as well as a history of physical and emotional abuse and genetic and physiologic factors
  - Comorbidity includes the other conduct and disruptive disorders, as well as ASD
  - Anxiety disorders, depressive disorders, bipolar disorders, and substance use disorders may also be associated with this disorder

Conduct Disorder

- Characterized by disregard for society's rules/norms and rights of other people and animals and disregard and lack of empathy for the feelings of others
- Onset may occur as early as age 5 or 6, but usually is in late childhood or early adolescence; often diagnosed as having an antisocial personality disorder in adulthood; may be referred to by others as "bullies" because they abuse, intimidate, threaten, or aggressively harass others in order to gain power; they may initiate fights and use weapons for harm
- Behavior is repeated despite rational arguments and consequences; causes significant impairment in social, academic, or work performance
- Behavioral/clinical findings
  - Aggression toward people and animals; violent
  - Unfeeling toward others; are not concerned about hurting others
  - Destruction of property without remorse
  - Deceitfulness or theft
  - Serious violations of rules and laws such as theft and vandalism
- Prevalence, risk factors, comorbidity
  - Most begin in young children or teens
  - The disorders are more prevalent in males than in females
  - Risk factors are greater in children and teens who behave aggressively with both peers and adult figures; they are more likely to have similar problems as adults
  - Genetics, environmental factors, biologic parents with alcohol or substance use disorders, and mental illness all may have comorbid influence in the development of a conduct disorder
  - Poor parenting skills, harsh or inconsistent discipline, and poor living conditions may also contribute to this disorder
- Nursing care of children diagnosed with unspecified conduct disorder
  - See General Nursing Care Related to Disorders First Evident in Infancy, Childhood, or Adolescence for "Assessment/Analysis" and "Planning/Implementation" sections

- Evaluation/outcomes
  - Decreases destructive acts
  - Demonstrates increased ability to delay gratification

Separation Anxiety Disorder

- Etiology and epidemiology
  - May be experienced by infants age 6 to 30 months who are separated from their mothers; children who are entering school for the first time may also exhibit symptoms
  - Some degree of separation anxiety is developmentally appropriate between ages of 10 months to 2 years; the disorder is marked by excessive levels of anxiety or that occurs after age 2
  - More common among first-degree relatives, and it is possibly more common among children whose mothers have panic disorder or other anxiety disorders
  - Usually develops after a stressful event (eg, the death of a close and valued relative or pet, an illness in the child or parent, or a major change in the environment such as moving to a new neighborhood)
  - Occurs in approximately 4% of children and adolescents, and it is more common among females
- Clinical description
  - The child exhibits at least three symptoms: Excessive worry about being separated from the caregiver; significant distress when separated; and fear of being alone, which may include refusal to attend school, afterschool activities, and camps
  - Academic difficulties result from a refusal to attend school and thus increase the problem with social avoidance; school refusal occurs in about 5% of all school-aged children, primarily between the ages of 5 and 6 years and 10 and 11 years
  - Children with separation anxiety disorder demonstrate clinging behavior when in the presence of the caregiver, some to the point of following the caregiver to the bathroom
  - Bedtime is difficult, with the child or adolescent insisting that the parent remains with him or her until he or she falls asleep; during the night, these individuals often try to get into bed with parents or other significant figures; some will even sleep outside the parent's door if unable to enter the room; nightmares often contain elements of the child's fears such as family death as a result of fire, murder, or another catastrophe
  - Other symptoms of anxiety may also be present, including physical complaints such as stomachaches, headaches, nausea, and vomiting
  - Older children and adolescents may experience a racing or pounding heart, dizziness, and faintness; these somatic complaints may lead to numerous trips to physicians and subsequent medical procedures
  - Individuals with this disorder often experience recurrent and excessive distress when they are away from home or major attachment figures, and they are extremely fearful that imagined harm will happen to the significant others
  - Fears about danger to themselves or their families sometimes present as fears of animals, monsters, the dark, muggers, burglars, kidnappers, accidents, or plane or train travel; some fears also present as concerns about death and dying
  - These children show various moods, such as excessive worry that no one loves them and they therefore want to die, or unusual anger when someone tries to separate them from their parent or a significant other; at times the depressed mood justifies a diagnosis of major depressive disorder; when these clients reach adulthood, some will develop panic disorder with agoraphobia

- Comorbidities are not uncommon and include other anxiety disorders such as generalized anxiety disorder and social phobia, as well as major depressive disorder
- There may be periods of severity and periods of a reduction of symptoms; both the anxiety about possible separation and the avoidance of situations that involve separation may persist for many years
- Prognosis typically depends on the age of onset, the duration, and the coexistence of other disorders; children who attend school and afterschool activities and who have healthy peer and parental relationships do better than those who do not

Additional Anxiety Disorders of Infancy, Childhood, or Adolescence

- Some anxiety is expected in childhood and adolescence, because fears and worries are part of development
- Anxiety becomes a problem when there is a failure to move beyond the fears of a particular developmental stage
- Behavior interferes with daily functioning and educational and social achievement
- Behavioral/clinical findings (see Separation Anxiety Disorder)
  - School phobia: Severe anxiety about attending school
    - Overwhelming shyness and insecurity
    - Psychophysiologic (psychosomatic) symptoms used to justify nonattendance
    - Anxiety increases in response to attempts to force attendance
    - Nonattendance at school has emotional and legal implications
  - Selective mutism: Persistent failure to speak in specific social situations
    - Social involvement limited to family members or people who are familiar to the child
    - Excessive shyness or timidity with strangers
  - Reactive attachment disorder (a type of stressor-related disorder): Infant or young child does not develop healthy attachments with parents or caregivers; begins before age 5 years
    - Failure to initiate or respond to age-appropriate attempts at most social interactions
    - Child does not to seek out attachment figures
- Nursing care of children diagnosed with anxiety disorders of infancy, childhood, or adolescence
  - See General Nursing Care Related to Disorders First Evident in Infancy, Childhood, or Adolescence for "Assessment/analysis" and "Planning/implementation" sections

Evaluation/Outcomes

- States a decrease in anxiety and worry
- Demonstrates a decrease in physiologic symptoms
- Develops relationships outside of family members
- Attends school on a consistent basis

Mood Disorders in Childhood and Adolescence

- Depression and bipolar disorder can also begin in childhood or adolescence
- Bipolar disorder in children differs from adults in that children show more irritability; this behavioral difference decreases with development
- Bipolar disorder and ADHD can have similar presentations, so appropriate medication can be challenging
- See Chapter 11 for general information on mood disorders

GENERAL NURSING CARE RELATED TO DISORDERS FIRST EVIDENT IN INFANCY, CHILDHOOD, OR ADOLESCENCE

Assessment/Analysis (Box 20.1)

- Attainment or delay of developmental milestones (eg, motor, language, social, etc.)
- Parental behavior and attitude (eg, expectations, acceptance/rejection, encouragement/pressure)
- Personal and family health history (eg, vision, hearing, general health, perinatal history, familial disorders)
- Onset, characteristics, and pattern of speech; ability to communicate with others
- Level of anxiety, frustration, self-esteem
- Behavioral manifestations (eg, ability to perform activities of daily living [ADLs], hyperactivity, distractibility, attention span, impulsiveness, repetitive behaviors, tics, reports of somatic symptoms)
- Social abilities (eg, ability to connect with others/environment, aggressiveness, ability to follow directions/rules, respect for others and their belongings)

Planning/Implementation

- Develop a trusting relationship with the child and family
  - Be as truthful as possible
  - Provide consistent caregivers
  - Make explanations as clear as possible and at the appropriate cognitive level
- Help the child see self as worthwhile
  - Encourage verbalization of feelings
  - Accept child and focus on strengths to raise self-esteem
  - Foster independence by emphasizing abilities and achievements rather than limitations
  - Provide opportunities for the child to experience success and satisfaction
  - Use positive reinforcement for child's strengths and abilities
  - Teach and role model more adaptive coping behaviors
  - Increase sense of empathy through role modeling, role playing, group therapy
  - Support and encourage the child's movement toward independence but allow dependency when necessary
- Establish an environment in which the child can gain or regain a favorable equilibrium
  - Set realistic, attainable goals
  - Maintain routines based on the child's usual schedule; maintain safety
  - Manage hyperactivity and aggressive behaviors: Progress from avoiding situations that precipitate unacceptable behavior to monitoring behavior for increasing anxiety, signaling child to use self-control, and finally to placing child in "timeout" when appropriate
  - Set limits that are as realistic as possible but as firm as necessary, avoiding manipulation
  - Provide for consistency both in approach and in rules/regulations
  - Use a firm system of rewards and punishments within set limits
  - Point out reality, but accept the child's views of it
  - Recognize that the maladaptive behavior has meaning for the child or may be beyond the child's control (eg, tic disorder)
  - Plan activities to provide a balance between energy expenditure and quiet time
  - Introduce new situations gradually; permit child to have a familiar, comforting object
  - Engage in parallel play to connect with a withdrawn child in a nonthreatening manner

BOX 20.1 Nursing Interventions for Children and Adolescents *(with rationales)*

1. Conduct a thorough assessment with the parents or guardians and the client *to observe interactions,* and then assess them separately if appropriate.
2. Assess for the presence of suicidal ideation and for past aggressive behaviors including triggers of aggressive behavior *to ensure the client's safety and to prevent harm to others.*
3. Maintain a safe environment by continually assessing for contraband (eg, objects that are sharp, alcohol, illicit drugs) and being aware of any behavioral changes or signals that may indicate increasing anger or aggression *to prevent violence and to maintain a safe environment.*
4. Establish a therapeutic alliance and maintain appropriate boundaries *to ensure consistency and security.*
5. Help the client identify strengths and positive qualities *to foster self-esteem, self-assurance, and self-confidence.*
6. Demonstrate, teach, and reinforce cooperative, respectful, and positive behaviors *to assist the client with developing and redefining successful and positive relationships.*
7. Set clear and consistent limits in a calm and nonjudgmental manner *to promote a safe environment and to develop trust.*
8. Redirect disruptive behavior with recreational activities *to channel excess energy and to prevent escalation.*
9. Inform the client of the consequences of not adhering to the limits *to allow the client to have the opportunity to respond, to express feelings, and to cognitively process his or her options.*
10. Use timeouts or quiet time when the client does not respond to limits *to give the client time to deescalate in a quiet environment and to process the event.*
11. Role-play situations that trigger aggressiveness or self-mutilation or that encourage alcohol or illicit drug use *to explore and reinforce alternative methods of coping.*
12. Teach anger management techniques *to lessen the client's feelings of powerlessness and to prevent future escalation.*
13. For the younger child, initiate therapeutic play *to encourage the client to express thoughts and feelings in alternative ways in the absence of adequate language and to reestablish healthy boundaries.*
14. Establish a behavior modification program for the preschool-aged child and the school-aged child that rewards the client for expressing the self safely *to reinforce positive behaviors, to enhance self-esteem, and to foster a sense of accomplishment.*
15. Involve the adolescent client in developing a behavioral contract by identifying expected behaviors and privileges *to reinforce positive behaviors and to enhance self-esteem and independence.*
16. Engage the client in group therapy and recreational activities *to assist the client with developing positive peer communication and to improve social skills and motor skills.*
17. Provide positive feedback and recognition when the client adheres to the behavioral program and treatment plan *to promote self-esteem and to reinforce positive behaviors.*
18. Teach the parents and guardians about the client's disorder, the importance of consistency and structure, and the significance of medication compliance, if indicated, *to minimize guilt, to increase their knowledge base regarding the disorder, to help them develop realistic expectations, and to reinforce the consequences of medication noncompliance.*
19. Assess the parents and guardians for available support systems and refer them to support groups and individual and family therapy as needed *to increase their ability to cope and to minimize feelings of isolation and guilt.*

From Fortinash, K. M., & Holoday, P. A. (2012). *Psychiatric mental health nursing* (5th ed.). St. Louis, MO: Mosby.

- Involve family in parenting education and management training
  - Assist parents to:
    - Gain an accurate understanding of their child's strengths and weaknesses
    - Cope with feelings such as guilt, failure, or anger
    - Provide firm and consistent discipline and ignore temper tantrums
  - Help parents and child identify triggers to maladaptive behaviors
  - Involve family in multifamily therapy to work through problems of daily life and to gain new information and more adaptive coping skills
  - Provide parents with a list of available community resources
  - Assist family with placement of child when home care can no longer be provided because of changes in child or ability of caregivers
- Administer prescribed medications
  - Autism spectrum disorder: Antipsychotics (to treat irritability), stimulants for comorbid ADHD
  - ADHD: Amphetamine-like drugs (eg, methylphenidate); give after breakfast to ensure dietary intake; a second dose should be administered before 6 PM to limit insomnia
  - Tic disorders: Amphetamine-like drugs (eg, methylphenidate); atypical antipsychotics (eg, aripiprazole)
  - Enuresis: Desmopressin; tricyclic antidepressants for children older than 5 years of age
  - Anxiety disorders: Clonidine; some antidepressants are approved for use in children; S antianxiety agents (anxiolytics) not usually used in children
- Minimize long-term consequences
  - Identify and ensure that deficits are treated early
  - Support attendance at school, therapeutic nursery program, day treatment program, or special education program depending on age and degree of disability
  - Provide ongoing assistance to promote social and academic success
  - Provide activities appropriate for age and disorder (eg, play, games, sports)
  - Allow child time to verbalize, without completing words or sentences for child; use picture boards; use sign language; avoid nonverbal behavior that implies impatience
  - Support child and parents receiving treatment
    - Physical therapy
    - Occupational therapy
    - Speech therapy
    - Stimulation therapy
    - Early intervention programs
    - Psychotherapy (eg, play, group, or individual)

APPLICATION AND REVIEW

13. An 8-year-old child is diagnosed with oppositional defiant disorder. What behavior should the nurse identify that supports this diagnosis?
    1. Is easily distracted
    2. Argues with adults
    3. Lies to obtain favors
    4. Initiates physical fights
14. An adolescent with the diagnosis of conduct disorder since the age of 9 is placed in a residential facility. The adolescent has a history of fighting, stealing, vandalizing property, and running away from home. The adolescent is aggressive, has no friends, and has been

suspended from school repeatedly. What is the nurse's priority when developing a plan of care?
1. Preventing violence
2. Encouraging insight
3. Supporting self-esteem
4. Promoting social interaction

15. A nurse works with school-age children who have a conduct disorder, childhood-onset type. The nurse considers that these children are at risk for progressing to an additional disorder during adolescence, although technically the potential diagnosis is not used until age 18. For signs of which disorder should the nurse assess their present behavior?
1. Oppositional defiant
2. Antisocial personality
3. Pervasive developmental
4. Attention deficit hyperactivity

16. A nurse is planning care for a group of hospitalized children. Which age group does the nurse anticipate will have the most problem with separation anxiety?
1. 12 to 18 years
2. 5 to 11.5 years
3. 6 to 30 months
4. 36 to 59 months

17. A nurse is counseling the family of a child diagnosed with school phobia. What should the parents be taught to do?
1. Accompany the child to the classroom
2. Facilitate the child's return to school as soon as possible
3. Instruct the child as to why school attendance is necessary
4. Allow the child to enter the classroom before other children

18. What childhood problem has legal as well as emotional aspects and cannot be ignored?
1. School phobias
2. Fear of animals
3. Fear of monsters
4. Sleep disturbances

See Answers on pages 403–407.

Aging Individuals

- According to the U.S. Census Bureau, the number of adults age 65 years and older is expected to nearly double from 2012 (43 million) to 2050 (approximately 84 million)
- The U.S. Census Bureau projects that more than 62 million Americans will be age 65 years and older in 2025

Theories of Aging

- Theories of aging include biologic theories—genetic, immunologic, cross-linkage and free radical theories; psychosocial theories—disengagement, continuity, and activity theories

Biologic Theories of Aging

- Most biologic theories view the process of aging as either a normal, gradual wearing down of all systems or an abnormal series of cellular damages or mutations that eventually lead to the body's inability to make repairs
- Intrinsic or genetic theories focus on the process of aging as internal to the organism; researchers estimate that genetic factors account for about 30% of variance in life expectancy, with lifestyle and environmental influences having more profound effects on aging than was previously thought
- Extrinsic or nongenetic theories propose that aging occurs as a result of environmental factors that act on the organism, such as radiation, ozone, drugs, and toxic substances, which, researchers have theorized, damage cellular structures, thereby leading to aging and death
- A combination of genetic and environmental factors best explains why individuals age differently

- Four biologic theories of aging are genetic theory, immunologic theory, cross-linkage theory, and free radical theory
  - The *genetic theory* of aging represents a group of basic aging theories, all of which focus on an internal genetic code driving the aging process; genetic theory suggests that life span is determined primarily by inherited genes
    - An additional genetic theory is the biologic clock theory, which suggests the existence of a programmed internal genetic clock that regulates an organism's development and subsequent decline; this internal clock runs down over a predetermined length of time
    - Another genetic theory, known as *error theory,* explains the development of harmful genes that interfere with biologic processes such as protein synthesis; damage to biologic synthesis results in the development of damaged cells that interfere with normal biologic functions
  - *In the* immunologic theory, *i*mmune function significantly declines with aging; most biologists agree that changes in the immunologic system after puberty influence the process of aging; antibody production declines and autoimmune responses change in response to the decline; the body's ability to differentiate normal tissue from abnormal or foreign substances fails
  - *In the* cross-linkage theory, collagen tissue, which is an important component of connective tissue that maintains the structure of cells, tissues, and organs, changes with aging; with age, the combination of chemical changes and external stimuli causes the formation of molecular bonds in collagen—known as *cross-links*—that tend to stabilize the collagen fibers, thereby resulting in rigid and fragile tissue; scientists do not understand the mechanism that triggers the formation of cross-links, but they believe that the most active period of cross-link development is between 30 and 50 years of age
  - *In the* free radical theory, biologists theorize that some environmental stimuli interfere with cellular activity, thereby resulting in the production of free radicals; they sometimes interact with various cellular structures and cause damage to normal cellular function; free radicals are also formed during the normal process of cellular oxygenation when the cell removes waste products; although the cell is capable of neutralizing and removing such by-products, researchers theorize that, over time, the cell loses its capacity to eliminate waste and repair itself

Psychosocial Theories

- Sociologists have observed that an individual's role, relationships, and social experiences change as he or she ages; sociologic theories of aging attempt to explain the social aspects of the aging process; these three theories—*disengagement, continuity,* and *activity*—all take a different approach to the social aspects of aging; common to the three theories is the focus on action and adaptation by the individual (ie, the aging person needs to change or adjust to new situations)
- The disengagement theory suggests that a process of mutual withdrawal naturally occurs between the aging individual and society that is inevitable and universal in its occurrence; the retirement process is an example of this disengagement; society identifies the age of 65 years as the time for retirement; identifying a retirement marker or target is also a mechanism for society to open the opportunity for a young person to enter the workforce
  - Most criticism of this theory focuses on its presumed universality and that it does not allow for biologic, personality, or cultural differences; in addition, it presumes that the individual will see disengagement as an obligation to society; how ready and accepting older persons are to change roles determines their ability to adjust and, subsequently, their life satisfaction

- Another perspective is that individual personality traits and past experiences influence how an individual in society adapts to aging; a person who is withdrawn early in life will probably continue to withdraw and adapt if his or her social ties also support withdrawal behaviors; it is a combination of one's personal preferences and the needs of society rather than personal preference or societal needs alone that determine the degree and pattern of disengagement
- *The* continuity theory is based on the idea that people adapt best when they are allowed to be who they are; with aging, people become "more like themselves" in that they attempt to maintain the continuity of habits, beliefs, norms, values, and other aspects of the personality; the continuity theory allows for individual differences in the aging process and theorizes that each individual's personality contains a self-maintaining component, which means that the individual's long-standing behavior patterns affect coping and adjustment to new situations as they age
- *The* activity theory proposes that maintaining an active lifestyle and social roles offsets the negative effects of aging; activity theorists postulate that by retaining a high level of participation in his or her social environment, the older individual will report a higher level of overall life satisfaction and a more positive self-concept
  - The greater the loss in social roles (both formal and informal), the less the activity participation
  - The more activity maintained, the greater the social role support for the older person
  - Maintaining the stability of social roles supports a person's positive self-concept
  - The more positive a person's self-concept, the greater the degree of life satisfaction experienced
  - The importance, type, and availability of a particular activity as perceived by the older person is an essential consideration that affects self-concept and life satisfaction

Normal Aging Process

- The process of aging incorporates physiologic and psychosocial changes within the individual (see Summary: Aging Individuals for more details)
- Because the changes that characterize normal physiologic aging reflect pathologic changes, health care providers often confuse normal and abnormal aging processes; although aging is ultimately irreversible, people are still able to significantly delay disease and disability, even into very old age
- Psychosocial changes during aging in the areas of cognition, personality, social interactions, sexuality, and roles are even less distinct; personality and socioenvironmental factors play a huge role in determining psychosocial aging changes; particular aspects of such processes as cognition and memory decline with aging, whereas other aspects remain the same or are even enhanced with advanced age
- The physiologic aging changes that are considered part of normal aging affect all body systems, but not necessarily at the same rates; it is important to have an understanding of the common physiologic aging changes, because some of these changes indicate the development of pathologic conditions; many of these changes begin as early as the fourth and fifth decades of life; there are also individual differences in the rates of aging of some biologic systems as a result of factors such as heredity, environment, lifestyle, and nutrition

Psychological Aspect of Aging

- Psychosocial aging changes typically focus on an individual's responses to particular events across the life span; past coping mechanisms are not always effective for adjusting to stressful events in later life; because the life events of old age differ from those of younger ages, adaptation is sometimes more difficult for older adults

- Preparing for some life events will facilitate adjustment during old age; for instance, some employers offer preretirement counseling for older employees; psychosocial aging changes are reflected in several areas, including cognition, memory, personality, social support, sexuality, and role status; from a developmental perspective, the meaningfulness of life events is important for determining patterns of psychosocial aging in these particular areas
- *Cognition and memory*
  - Cognitive behaviors are divided into several interrelated processes that include intelligence, memory, attention, reaction time, and problem-solving
  - Many factors—health status, genetic profile, socioeconomic status, education, and lifestyle behaviors—contribute to the variability in cognitive functioning observed among older adults; in turn, cognitive losses often result in functional impairment and physical disabilities, which cause a spiraling decline for the older person
- *Intelligence and aging*
  - Crystallized intelligence develops from knowledge gained through the accumulation of experience and education; crystallized intelligence declines slightly, remains the same, or even increases with aging, depending on one's life experiences
  - Neurophysiologic processes across the life span affect fluid intelligence; declines in the nervous system with aging that affect one's attention span or reaction time reflect a loss of fluid intelligence
  - Some older adults have demonstrated an increased time needed to complete intelligence performance tests because they are more cautious and take additional time to make correct choices
- *Memory processes and aging*
  - Certain types of memory decline as a part of normal aging
  - Explicit memory, which is the ability to recall a specific name or place, tends to decline with aging
  - Working memory, which is the type of memory that is needed to perform daily activities, does not show an aging decline; because older adults often take longer to process information (which is also normal with aging) and have some specific recall problems, they often fear that this is an indicator of Alzheimer's disease; it is important to explain to them that this is not the case and to encourage older adults to seek ways to improve cognitive functioning through training and practice
  - Information that the brain processes in a more complex manner (eg, algebraic equations) is stored in a deeper area of memory and will last longer; information that the brain easily recognizes requires less attention; researchers believe that the automatic processing of information does not change with aging; offering cues to older adults will help them recall information that is stored in deeper areas of memory
- *Other cognitive functions*
  - The term *attention span* refers to one's ability to concentrate throughout the performance of some task; with aging, the ability to maintain the attention span through the completion of complex tasks diminishes, because complex tasks require dividing one's attention among several tasks at the same time
  - Two other segments of attention also show some decrements with aging; vigilance, which is the ability to sustain attention over longer periods of time, and selective attention, which is the ability to discriminate and focus on relevant information, are less acute among older adults

- Increased reaction time that results in decreased speed of performance on intelligence tests is one of the most obvious changes that occurs with normal aging, but researchers still do not fully understand why this happens; anxiety caused by unfamiliarity with performance or the fear of failure may affect the reaction time of older adults
- Problem-solving ability is a higher cognitive function; the complexity of the problem, past experiences, the amount of information that is irrelevant to the situation, and the individual's level of education are factors that influence problem-solving; there is little knowledge regarding normal changes in higher cognitive functioning during aging

- *Personality*
  - In general, most personality traits remain stable during the aging process; personality influences how an individual interacts and reacts within the social environment; personality traits develop over the life span, and they are influenced by internal and external environmental factors; an individual's ability to cope with stress and to adapt to change molds an individual's personality; self-concept reflects their personality
  - The individual's ability to adapt to change determines successful aging more than a particular category of personality traits
  - Some traits intensify with aging, including cautiousness, which is often an effective safety mechanism for older adults
  - The locus of control is another aspect of personality that remains stable over time; individuals with an internal locus of control perceive that they actively control their own destiny; alternatively, individuals with an external locus of control believe that they have no control over their destinies and that their behaviors have no effect on any outcomes; another phenomenon, the secondary locus of control, describes individuals with an external locus of control who learn to adapt to their beliefs; this has also been called *learned helplessness;* these individuals learn dependency and prefer that others make decisions for them

Sociocultural Aspects of Aging

- The quality of social support is a key area for interventions in the training of health care providers; social support is part of a communication process in which the facilitation of communication skills improves the quality of support
- Social networks are generally the web of social ties that surround a person and include several characteristics that are important in the study of the health and well-being of older adults; these include:
  - The size of the social network
  - The frequency of social contacts
  - The quality of the interactions
  - The degree of intimacy or closeness among members
  - The strength of the relationships
  - The geographic location of the members
  - The reciprocity of assistance
- Social networks and social supports are different concepts; the social network is the web or structure of the group and the social support is the emotional or tangible assistance that is obtained from the social network; not all social ties are supportive, and not all social supports come from the closest social network, such as a son or daughter living near older parents

Long-Term Care

- Long-term care options are continuing to increase for aging individuals

- Skilled nursing facilities, residential facilities, assisted living, day treatment, partial hospitalization, home health care, and community-based programs (see later in this chapter) are some of the options
- Long-term care can include a range of services and supports that may needed to meet an individual's personal care needs; most long-term care is not medical care, but rather assistance with the basic personal tasks of everyday life (ADLs) (Box 20.2). Other common long-term care services and supports are assistance with everyday tasks, sometimes called instrumental activities of daily living (IADLs)

Elder Abuse

- Little is known about the occurrence of domestic violence against elders in families for several reasons; most studies do not distinguish between elder abuse and elder neglect; families are unlikely to report the abuse because the responsible person may be a son or daughter; and many elderly people are homebound with no one available to see what is happening
- Older women are more than twice as likely as men to suffer from abuse, and slightly more than half of the alleged perpetrators of elder abuse are female
- Because older victims usually have smaller support systems and fewer physical, psychologic, and economic reserves, the effect of abuse and neglect is magnified, and a single incident of mistreatment is more likely to trigger a downward spiral that leads to a loss of independence, a serious complicating illness, and even death; nurses have a responsibility to be aware of the possibility of elder abuse and to recognize possible signs

Suicide

- Elderly individuals who are 80-years-old and older have much higher rates of death by suicide than other age groups (see also Chapter 6)
- Older individuals, especially men, usually choose a more lethal method of suicide, particularly firearms
- Of persons who complete a suicide, 90% have a psychiatric diagnosis (including substance use disorders), with affective disorders involved in 50% of completed suicides

Summary: Aging Individuals

- For all aging individuals, keep in mind that depression can look like dementia
- Note also that substance use disorders in the elderly have a complicated withdrawal secondary to other medical conditions

BOX 20.2 ADL and IADL Functional Assessment Categories	
ADL Categories	**IADL Categories**
Bathing	Shopping
Dressing	Meal preparation
Hair care	Transportation
Mouth care	Use of telephone
Nutrition/assist with feeding	Medication usage
Ambulation/mobility	Housekeeping
Mental status	Laundry
Elimination	Financial management

From Fortinash, K. M., & Holoday, P. A. (2012). *Psychiatric mental health nursing* (5th ed.). St. Louis, MO: Mosby.

- Assess fall risk in all older adults
- The young-older adult (age 60 to 74 years)
  - Physiologic development
    - Slowing of reaction time
    - Decrease in sensory acuity
    - Diminished muscle tone, strength
    - Problems associated with dental caries, ill-fitting dentures, or no teeth/dentures
    - Increased diversity in health status/function resulting from earlier lifestyle
    - Development of chronic health problems
  - Psychosocial development
    - Cognitive abilities may be affected by cardiovascular disease
    - Adjusting to retirement; some individuals experience loss of self-esteem; others enjoy freedom to explore other interests
    - Coping with altered economic status; adjusting to fixed income
    - Resolving death of parents and possibly spouse
    - Accepting separation from children and their families
    - Resolving developmental crisis between ego integrity and despair
    - May experience depression
  - Health problems: Cardiovascular disease, cancer, presbyopia, accidents, respiratory disease, osteoporosis/osteoarthritis, hearing loss (especially for high-pitched sounds), unbalanced/inadequate diet, depression
  - General nursing care of young-older adults

Assessment/Analysis

- Assess cardiovascular status (eg, vital signs, peripheral pulses, peripheral edema, shortness of breath, history of chest pain, changes in sensation)
- Measure visual/auditory acuities
- Obtain history relative to warning signs of cancer
- Assess coping skills, support systems

Planning/Implementation

- Encourage to maintain schedule of regular medical, dental, visual examinations to prevent or control health problems
- Assess living conditions for hazards that may cause accidents
- Refer widows/widowers to appropriate self-help groups as necessary
- Encourage to anticipate/plan for retirement and to develop new interests/support systems
- Encourage nutritional assessment/consultation to prevent nutrient deficiencies and to provide for diet modifications appropriate for aging

Evaluation/Outcomes

- Participates in exercise program
- Verbalizes fears to health care providers
- Remains free from injury
- Maintains satisfying interpersonal relationships
- Consumes nutritionally adequate diet
- Maintains therapeutic regimen
- The middle-older adult (age 75 to 84 years) and old-older adult (age 85 years and older)

- Physiologic development
  - Diminished sensation (eg, visual, auditory), diminished reaction time
  - Increased sensitivity to cold because of decreased subcutaneous tissue, decreased thyroid functioning, impaired circulation
  - Decreased enzyme secretion/motility of gastrointestinal (GI) tract
  - Decreased glomerular filtration rate
  - Decreased cardiac output
  - Arteriosclerotic changes with diminished elasticity of blood vessels
  - Decreased lung capacity
  - Demineralization and other degenerative skeletal changes, particularly in weight-bearing bones
  - Muscle atrophy
  - Decreased metabolic rate and declining function of organs (eg, liver, kidneys); increased risk of adverse reaction or toxicity when taking medications
- Psychosocial development
  - Cognitive abilities not necessarily affected by age but may be impaired as result of disease, leading to diminished awareness and increased safety risk
  - Resolving developmental crisis of ego integrity versus despair; depends on previous resolution of task of generativity versus stagnation
  - Adjusting to death of significant others
  - Adapting to decreased physical capacity, changes in body image
  - Adjusting to economic burden of fixed income
  - Recognizing inevitability of death
  - Reminiscing increasingly about past
- Health problems: Cardiovascular disease, cancer, accidents (eg, falls, automobile collisions), respiratory disease, cerebral vascular insufficiency, malnutrition, problems with perception (eg, cataracts, glaucoma, hearing loss)
- General nursing care of middle-older and old-older adults

Assessment/Analysis

- Assess cardiovascular status: Vital signs, peripheral pulses, peripheral edema, shortness of breath, history of chest pain, changes in sensation
- Identify neurologic deficits: Level of consciousness, orientation, motor function, sensory function
- Identify deteriorating musculoskeletal functioning, effect on quality of life
- Assess respiratory function: Respiratory rate, rhythm, depth; use of accessory muscles; breath sounds; pulmonary function tests; oxygen saturation level
- Review nutritional status (eg, dietary history, height/weight, skin condition, serum protein and albumin levels)
- Ascertain medications taken routinely (chronic health problems and use of over-the-counter medications leads to polypharmacy)
- Assess coping abilities
- Assess resources/support systems

Planning/Implementation

- Encourage to maintain schedule of regular medical supervision and exercise
- Promote maximal degree of independence
- Initiate appropriate referrals for those requiring assistance with ADLs

- Open channels of communication for reality orientation, reminiscing, emotional support; explain procedures/expectations; reinforce as necessary
- Refer to social services and other resources that can provide economic assistance
- Ensure appropriate fit of prosthetic devices (eg, dentures, contact lenses, eye prosthetics, hearing aids, braces, limbs); teach proper care of such devices
- Encourage to follow USDA dietary recommendations/reduced caloric intake

Evaluation/Outcomes

- Performs or assists with self-care activities
- Remains free from injury
- Uses community resources to maximize independence
- Maintains nutritionally adequate diet
- Maintains social relationships
- Adjusts to changes in functional abilities
- Maintains therapeutic regimen

SERIOUS AND PERSISTENT MENTAL ILLNESS

Populations at Risk

- Populations at risk include mentally ill persons who are homeless, who are in jail, who have substance use disorders, or who have AIDS

Community Mental Health Centers

- Provide outpatient services for children, the elderly, individuals who are chronically mentally ill, and those who have been discharged from an inpatient psychiatric facility; the services must include 24-hour emergency service as well as day treatment that may include partial hospitalization or psychosocial services; programs are specifically designed to manage the special needs of each group; services may also provide screening for persons to determine whether they are appropriate for admission to a state mental hospital
- Two separate philosophies that currently dominate the mental health care provider systems for persons with severe and persistent mental illness are freedom of choice versus continuity of care
  - *Freedom-of-choice* advocates argue that all people, regardless of their disabilities, should be able to choose from a variety of treatments; with this method, clients select from different treatments and treatment providers and receive care at a variety of agencies
  - *Continuity-of-care* advocates argue that persons with severe and persistent mental illness need to have one stable treatment provider throughout all phases of their illness; the assumption is that some symptoms of mental illness disrupt a person's care, so the symptoms also need to be treated; in this type of system, a central care provider or case manager is responsible for assessment, securing treatment, and referral to appropriate services
- Some systems—whether they offer freedom of choice or continuity of care—operate on the concept of *episodes of care*, which follows the medical model in which the client uses the system only when his or her symptoms require care; the advantage of this model is that it has the potential to serve increased numbers of clients because not all clients will require services at the same time; the disadvantage is that it does not make use of primary prevention
- Community mental health nurses have the challenge of identifying the diverse cultural populations within their community service areas and adapting or developing programs to meet the needs of these populations; a primary goal of hospitals, community health nurses, and

nurse educators is to demonstrate approaches to care that are culturally sensitive and competent for persons of all cultures and ethnic groups; community involvement, the development of trust, and cultural sensitivity training are all necessary components to accomplish this goal, and are essential for client and family compliance with treatment and medication regimens

- *Community mental health programs,* such as day-treatment programs, are outpatient programs that are staffed by interdisciplinary teams
- *Partial hospitalization* programs provide the most intensive treatment of the therapeutic models; they offer short-term care that is similar to that provided in an inpatient setting, except the client is able to return home each day
- Psychiatric *home visits* vary with regard to focus, time spent, intensity, and outcome; it is crucial that the nurse who is planning a home visit evaluate the potential risks of that visit before beginning the actual interventions; risk evaluation always includes the client's history, relationship with the nurse, current mental status, and living situation; visiting nurse programs and community mental health programs have specific guidelines that are designed to protect nurses
- *The Recovery Model* focuses on a client's competencies, not just treatment of symptoms.

Revolving-Door Syndrome

- Revolving-door syndrome refers to clients who are frequently rehospitalized
- Policies that have included deinstitutionalizing individuals have contributed to this situation
- Discharge from the hospital, often against medical advice, without follow-up is a contributing factor; however, those with long-term, pervasive mental illness are more likely to be committed and therefore unable to leave against medical advice
- The CDC summarizes this syndrome as:
  - There is a vicious cycle that sometimes links workplace violence, psychiatric treatment, and the "revolving door":
    - Stage 1: The intensive psychiatric hospital treatment for some mentally ill clients may be cut short because of insurance pressures for early discharge
    - Stage 2: Community-based follow-up treatment and medication monitoring are inadequately staffed and supervised
    - Stage 3: Client enters general hospital emergency department when in crisis
    - Stage 4: Deescalation and/or chemical restraint is applied
    - Stage 5: Client is discharged with minimal or no psychiatric follow-up
    - Stage 6: Client experiences a repeat crisis episode and admission to the emergency department—and the "revolving door" continues
- For those with severe and persistent mental illness, lack of follow-up care can lead to treatment and medication noncompliance, a return of acute symptoms, and frequent re-hospitalizations

Mentally Ill Persons in the Criminal Justice System

- Persons diagnosed with mental illnesses make up 15% of the total prison population compared with 5% of the general population; inmates with diagnoses of schizophrenia, major depressive disorders, bipolar disorder, and nonpsychotic disorders were most likely to have recurrent disorders
- As many as 70% of persons who are in prison for nonviolent offenses have a cooccurring substance use problem
- There are more nonwhites than whites in the prison system
- Persons diagnosed with mental illnesses are sometimes arrested because no treatment facilities are available; they are often arrested for minor offenses such as vagrancy, trespassing, disorderly conduct, or failure to pay for a meal; jails are inadequately prepared to care for the severely

mentally ill offender who is able to refuse to take psychotropic medications; the suicide rate among mentally ill offenders is higher than it is for any other group of offenders

- Family members often find it necessary to have a relative with severe and persistent mental illness arrested for violent or threatening behavior; in some situations, emergency involuntary admissions require that the person who is making the arrest or signing the commitment orders also has to witness the violent behavior; if that does not happen, the individual is jailed for his or her mental illness rather than admitted to a psychiatric facility; many persons diagnosed with severe mental illness serve long-term prison sentences with a minimal amount of psychiatric treatment; there is a concern that prison facilities are becoming like the asylums of the past; factors involved in the incarceration of mentally ill persons include:
  - Homelessness
  - Attitude of the community
  - Attitude of the police force
  - More strict commitment criteria
  - Lack of adequate community support
- Prisons usually direct the treatment of prisoners diagnosed with mental illnesses toward symptom management rather than illness management, which results in disciplinary treatment; severely mentally ill inmates are likely to remain in prison for longer periods of time than other prisoners with similar offenses; when they are finally released into an unstructured life with no prospect of rehabilitation, they are often unable to control their behavior, and they are likely to return to prison
- Nursing responsibilities in correctional institutions vary and include:
  - Assessing suicide risk and risk for self-harm
  - Evaluating mental status
  - Monitoring the effectiveness of medications
  - Providing a link between prisoners and community caregivers
  - Generating care when needed
  - Providing general mental health treatment
  - Educating prisoners and prison staff about mental illness
- Laws concerning the administration of psychotropic medications often frustrate nurses who are working with mentally ill prisoners; the medications are often necessary to contain clients' aggressive or violent behaviors; however, the law protects a prisoner's right to refuse psychotropic medication; unfortunately, when persons who are unable to think clearly because of mental illness refuse psychotropic medication, the result is both dangerous and tragic

Psychiatric Home Care

- Many home health agencies provide psychiatric home health care; home health nurses assess clients, their responses to treatment, and the safety of their living arrangements; the nurses also assess potential risk for emotional or physical harm from other household members
- Some studies estimate that 70% of mentally ill individuals live in the community
- To be eligible for home care, clients are unable to leave their homes, they need to demonstrate a medical necessity, and they require occasional care
- A broad range of psychiatric home visits are reimbursed by third-party payers, with each payer having specific criteria for reimbursement

Homelessness

- Homelessness is a major problem throughout the country as a result of poverty, unemployment, underemployment, substance abuse, and mental illness; men are more likely to be homeless, as are the racial and ethnic populations in specific areas of the country

- There have been numerous studies to determine the number of homeless persons in each state and major city
- It has been reported that 20% to 25% of the homeless population has a severe mental illness that interferes with an individual's ability to form relationships with family or care providers; persons diagnosed with severe mental illness are more likely to be noncompliant with medication as a result of a lack of finances, a lack of stability, and the inability to trust others to help them; in addition to uncontrolled mental illness, the homeless mentally ill population has poor hygiene and multiple health problems
- Racial and ethnic differences play a significant role in the family's response to members diagnosed with mental illness; some cultural groups are protective of the ill individual, whereas others soon become exhausted and emotionally drained with the care, dependency needs, and symptoms of the ill person
- Persons diagnosed with severe, persistent mental illness may move in and out of homelessness because of their symptoms or because they have stopped taking their medications; attempting to live a homeless existence and struggling to acquire food, shelter, and protection every day is difficult even for a healthy person; some clients seek shelter in places that they believe to be safe such as in tunnels, caves, secluded parks, or under bridges; if they were to become ill or injured, they would be unable to help themselves and might even die without being found for days or weeks
- The more disengaged these individuals are from society, the more difficult it is to offer them the services that they need

APPLICATION AND REVIEW

19. What principle of teaching specific to an older adult should the nurse consider when providing instruction to such a client recently diagnosed with diabetes mellitus?
    1. Knowledge reduces general anxiety
    2. Capacity to learn decreases with age
    3. Continued reinforcement is advantageous
    4. Readiness of the learner precedes instruction
20. A 76-year-old male client asks the nurse about the chances of getting osteoporosis like his wife. Which is the **best** response by the nurse?
    1. "This is only a problem for women."
    2. "Exercise is a good way to prevent this problem."
    3. "You are not at risk because of your small frame."
    4. "You might think about having a bone density test."
21. Which factor does the nurse consider **most** likely to contribute to the increased incidence of hip fractures in older adults?
    1. Carelessness
    2. Fragility of bone
    3. Sedentary existence
    4. Rheumatoid diseases
22. Which age-related change should the nurse consider when formulating a plan of care for an older adult? **Select all that apply.**
    1. Difficulty in swallowing
    2. Increased sensitivity to heat
    3. Increased sensitivity to glare
    4. Diminished sensation of pain
    5. Heightened response to stimuli

23. A nurse is caring for an older adult with a hearing loss secondary to aging. What can the nurse expect to identify when assessing this client? **Select all that apply.**
    1. Dry cerumen
    2. Tears in the tympanic membrane
    3. Difficulty hearing women's voices
    4. Decrease of hair in the auditory canal
    5. Overgrowth of the epithelial auditory lining

24. A 93-year-old client in a nursing home has been eating less food during mealtimes. What is the **priority** nursing intervention?
    1. Substitute a supplemental drink for the meal
    2. Spoon-feed the client until the food is completely eaten
    3. Allow the client a longer period of time to complete the meal
    4. Arrange a consultation for the placement of a gastrostomy tube

25. A 78-year-old client who has hypertension is beginning treatment with furosemide. Considering the client's age, what should the nurse teach the client to do?
    1. Limit fluids at bedtime
    2. Change positions slowly
    3. Take the medication between meals
    4. Assess the skin for breakdown daily

See Answers on pages 403-407.

ANSWER KEY: REVIEW QUESTIONS

1. **Answers: 3, 5.**

   3 Impairments in social interaction are manifested by a lack of eye contact, a lack of facial responses, and a lack of responsiveness to and interest in others. **5** Children diagnosed with autism spectrum disorder display obsessive ritualistic behaviors, such as rocking, spinning, dipping, swaying, walking on toes, head banging, or hand biting, because of their self-absorption and need to stimulate themselves.

   1 Impairments in communication and imaginative activity result in a failure to imitate others. **2** Children diagnosed with ASD are indifferent to or have an aversion to affection and physical contact. **4** Impairments in social interaction and imaginative activity are manifested by failure to engage in cooperative or imaginative play with others. **6** Children diagnosed with ASD are unable to establish meaningful relationships with adults or children because of their lack of responsiveness to others.

   Client Need: Psychosocial Integrity; **Cognitive Level:** Comprehension; **Nursing Process:** Assessment/Analysis

2. **4 Research studies have shown that the prognosis for normal productive functioning in people diagnosed with ASD is guarded, particularly if there are delays in language development.**

   1 Accurate diagnosis and early interventions have not been shown to promote a normal productive life; however, early interventions may help individuals to maximize their abilities. **2** Although temperament may affect the child's response to treatment, it does not affect prognosis to any extent. **3** Suggesting that a normal productive life is ensured by attending a school tailored to meet the child's needs is false reassurance and is not helpful.

   Client Need: Psychosocial Integrity; **Cognitive Level:** Knowledge; **Nursing Process:** Assessment/Analysis

3. **3 Poor interpersonal relationships, inappropriate behavior, and learning disabilities prevent these children from emotionally adapting or responding to the environment despite a possible high level of intelligence.**

   1 It is the lack of response to stimuli that is the clue to the possibility that the child may have ASD. **2** They have an aversion to physical contact. **4** They have impaired interpersonal relationships regardless of the age of the other person.

   Client Need: Psychosocial Integrity; **Cognitive Level:** Knowledge; **Nursing Process:** Assessment/Analysis

4. **1 By 2 years of age the child should demonstrate an interest in others, communicate verbally, and possess the ability to learn from the environment. Before these skills develop, ASD is difficult to diagnose. Usually, the signs of ASD become more profound by 3 years of age.**

   2 ASD can be diagnosed long before age 6. 3 Infantile ASD can occur at age 6 months but is difficult to diagnose. 4 Infantile ASD can occur at age 1 to 3 months but is difficult to diagnose.
   Client Need: Psychosocial Integrity; **Cognitive Level:** Comprehension; **Nursing Process:** Assessment/Analysis

5. **1 Children diagnosed with ASD usually have a pervasive impairment in reciprocal social interaction. Lack of eye contact is a typical behavior associated with ASD.**

   2 Crying for attention is not indicative of ASD in a child. 3 Catatonic-like rigidity is not indicative of ASD in a child. 4 Engaging in parallel play is not indicative of ASD in a child.
   Client Need: Psychosocial Integrity; **Cognitive Level:** Knowledge; **Nursing Process:** Assessment/Analysis

6. **2 Entering the child's world in a nonthreatening way helps promote trust and eventual interaction with the nurse.**

   1 Encourage the child to sing songs is unrealistic at this time; it is a long-term objective. 3 Expecting the child to play with other children is unrealistic at this time; it is a long-term objective. 4 The use of therapeutic holding may be necessary when the child initiates self-mutilating behaviors.
   Client Need: Psychosocial Integrity; Cognitive **Level:** Application; **Nursing Process:** Planning/Implementation

7. **1 A universal characteristic of these children is distractibility. They are highly reactive to any extraneous stimuli, such as noise and movement, and are unable to inhibit their responses to such stimuli.**

   2 Rituals are uncommon, although they do use repetition in language or movement. 3 Delayed development of language skills is not the major problem, but children diagnosed with attention deficit disorder may exhibit dyslexia (reading difficulty), speaking difficulty, dysgraphia (writing difficulty), or delayed talking. 4 Loss of abstract thought is not a universal characteristic associated with children diagnosed with attention deficit disorder.
   Client Need: Psychosocial Integrity; **Cognitive Level:** Knowledge; **Nursing Process:** Assessment/Analysis

> 🔑 **Memory Aid:** To recall that distractibility is a component of ADHD: for the ***AD*** of ADHD, think ***a***ttention ***d***istractibility.

8. **3 Focusing on specifics is important for children who are easily distracted.**

   1 Focusing on more than one item at a time might be difficult for an easily distracted child. 2 Hyperactive children respond best to concrete tasks; verbalizing safety rules is not a concrete task. 4 A child who is easily distracted has difficulty talking to a group of children regarding a particular topic.
   Client Need: Health Promotion and Maintenance; **Cognitive Level:** Application; **Integrated Process:** Teaching/Learning; **Nursing Process:** Planning/Implementation

9. **Answers: 1, 2, 5, 6.**

   1 Impulsivity, the inability to limit or control words or actions, results in spontaneous, irresponsible verbalizations or behaviors. 2 Hyperactivity occurs with both words and actions. 5 Games that are fun, engaging, and interactive often maintain the focus of children diagnosed with attention deficit hyperactivity disorder. 6 Inattention and distractibility result in an inability to focus long enough to complete tasks.

   3 Spitefulness and vindictiveness is associated with oppositional defiant disorder and is reflective of negativistic, hostile, defiant behavior toward others. 4 Annoying others deliberately is associated with oppositional defiant disorder and is reflective of insubordinate, hostile behavior toward authority; children diagnosed with attention deficit hyperactivity can be annoying, but the behavior is not deliberate.
   Client Need: Psychosocial Integrity; **Cognitive Level:** Knowledge; **Nursing Process:** Assessment/Analysis

10. **3 ADHD interferes with the ability to perceive and respond to sensory stimuli, which causes a deficit in interpreting new sensory data. This makes learning difficult and results in learning disabilities.**

1 That these children will probably not be self-directed learners is not necessarily true. **2** That these children have intellectual deficits that interfere with learning is not true. **4** That these children usually perform two grade levels lower than their age norm is not necessarily true.

Client Need: Psychosocial Integrity; **Cognitive Level:** Knowledge; **Nursing Process:** Assessment/Analysis

11. **2 Methylphenidate is an appetite suppressant; it should be given after meals.**

1 Methylphenidate at this time may suppress the child's appetite. **3** Methylphenidate at this time may suppress the child's appetite. **4** Methylphenidate at this time may suppress the child's appetite.

Client Need: Pharmacologic and Parenteral Therapies; **Cognitive Level:** Application; **Integrated Process:** Teaching/Learning; **Nursing Process:** Planning/Implementation

12. **2 External rewards can motivate as well as increase self-esteem.**

1 Orienting the child to reality is unnecessary because children diagnosed with attention deficit hyperactivity disorder are alert and oriented. **3** Feelings of frustration should not be suppressed, but rather the child should learn how to cope with these feelings in an acceptable manner. **4** The use of restraints is contraindicated because they are restrictive and punitive.

Client Need: Psychosocial Integrity; **Cognitive Level:** Application; **Integrated Process:** Teaching/Learning; **Nursing Process:** Planning/Implementation

13. **2 Oppositional defiant disorder is a repeated pattern of negativistic, disobedient, hostile, defiant behavior toward authority figures usually exhibited before 8 years of age.**

1 Being easily distracted is associated with ADHD and reflects an inability to sustain focus on a task. **3** Lying to obtain favors is associated with conduct disorder and reflects a violation of a societal norm. **4** Initiating physical fights is associated with conduct disorder and reflects a violation of the rights of another.

Client Need: Psychosocial Integrity; **Cognitive Level:** Knowledge; **Nursing Process:** Assessment/Analysis

14. **1 Clients with conduct disorder are at risk for physically, emotionally, or sexually harming themselves or others; safety of the client and others is the priority.**

2 Although encouraging insight is important, it is not the priority; these children have difficulty being insightful. **3** Although supporting self-esteem is important, it is not the priority. **4** Although promoting social interaction is important, it is not the priority.

Client Need: Safety and Infection Control; **Cognitive Level:** Application; **Nursing Process:** Planning/Implementation

15. **2 Children who exhibit behaviors associated with conduct disorder before the age of 10 rather than during adolescence, have a higher incidence of developing antisocial personality disorder during adolescence.**

1 If an oppositional defiant disorder persists for at least 6 months, it may be a precursor of a conduct disorder. **3** Pervasive developmental disorders are characterized by impairments in reciprocal social interaction and communication skills; types include autistic, Asperger, Rett, and childhood disintegrative disorders; they are not preceded by conduct disorder. **4** ADHD is often dually diagnosed with oppositional defiant disorder or conduct disorder and may precede the development of Tourette syndrome.

Client Need: Health Promotion and Maintenance; **Cognitive Level:** Comprehension; **Nursing Process:** Assessment/Analysis

16. **3 Infants and toddlers 6 to 30 months of age experience separation anxiety; it is this age group's major stressor and is most traumatic to the child and parent.**

1 Adolescents are often ambivalent about whether they want their parents with them when hospitalized. Peer group separation may pose more anxiety for the adolescent. **2** The school-age child is more accustomed to periods of separation from parents. **4** Separation anxiety occurs in this age group (36 to 59 months), but it is less obvious and less serious than in the toddler.

Client Need: Health Promotion and Maintenance; **Cognitive Level:** Comprehension; **Nursing Process:** Assessment/Analysis

17. **2 The longer these children stay out, the more difficult it is to get them to return to school because more fantasies and fears develop.**

1 Accompanying the child to the classroom feeds into the child's fear that the phobia is realistic. 3 Instructing the child as to why school attendance is necessary is not effective. 4 Allow the child to enter the classroom before other children will increase, not decrease, the child's fear.

Client Need: Psychosocial Integrity; **Cognitive Level:** Application; **Integrated Process:** Teaching/Learning; **Nursing Process:** Planning/Implementation

18. **1 School phobia is a disorder that cannot legally be ignored for long because children must attend school. It requires intervention to alleviate the separation anxiety and/or to promote the child's increasing independence.**

2 Fear of animals is a clinical manifestation and requires the parents to comfort, to reorient to reality, and to help the child regain self-control. Legally, there are no requirements mandating treatment for this common childhood problem. 3 Fear of monsters is a clinical manifestation requires the parents to comfort, to reorient to reality, and to help the child regain self-control. Legally, there are no requirements mandating treatment for this common childhood problem. 4 Sleep disturbances are clinical manifestations that require the parents to comfort, to reorient to reality, and to help the child regain self-control. Legally, there are no requirements mandating treatment for this common childhood problem.

Client Need: Management of Care; **Cognitive Level:** Knowledge; **Nursing Process:** Assessment/Analysis

19. **3 Neurologic aging causes forgetfulness and a slower response time; repetition increases learning.**

1 That knowledge reduces general anxiety is a principle applicable to all learning regardless of the client's age. 2 Learning occurs, but it may take longer. 4 That readiness of the learner needs to precede instruction is a principle applicable to all learning regardless of the client's age.

Client Need: Health Promotion and Maintenance; **Cognitive Level:** Knowledge; **Integrated Process:** Teaching/Learning; **Nursing Process:** Planning/Implementation

20. **4 Osteoporosis is not restricted to women; it is a potential major health problem of all older adults; estimates indicate that half of all women have at least one osteoporotic fracture, and the risk in men is estimated between 13% and 25%; a bone mineral density (BMD) measurement assesses the mass of bone per unit volume or how tightly the bone is packed.**

1 Osteoporosis also can occur in men. 2 Exercise may decrease the occurrence of osteoporosis, but will not prevent it; a regimen including weight-bearing exercises is advised. 3 A small frame is a risk factor for osteoporosis.

Client Need: Health Promotion and Maintenance; **Cognitive Level:** Application; **Integrated Process:** Teaching/Learning; **Nursing Process:** Planning/Implementation

21. **2 Bones become more fragile because of loss of bone density associated with the aging process; this often is associated with lower circulating levels of estrogens or testosterone.**

1 Carelessness is a characteristic applicable to certain individuals rather than to people within a developmental level. 3 Although prolonged lack of weight-bearing activity is associated with bone demineralization, hip fractures also occur in active older adults. 4 Rheumatoid diseases can affect the skeletal system but do not increase the incidence of hip fractures.

Client Need: Health Promotion and Maintenance; **Cognitive Level:** Knowledge; **Nursing Process:** Assessment/Analysis

22. **Answers: 3, 4.**

3 Changes in the ciliary muscles, decrease in pupil size, and a more rigid pupil sphincter contribute to an increased sensitivity to glare. 4 Diminished pain sensation may make an older individual unaware of a serious illness, thermal extremes, or excessive pressure.

1 There should be no interference with swallowing in older individuals. 2 Older individuals tend to feel the cold and rarely complain of the heat. 5 There is a decreased response to stimuli in the older individual.

Client Need: Health Promotion and Maintenance; **Cognitive Level:** Knowledge; **Nursing Process:** Planning/Implementation

23. **Answers: 1, 3.**

   1 Cerumen (ear wax) becomes drier and harder as a person ages. **3** Generally, female voices have a higher pitch than male voices; older adults with presbycusis (hearing loss caused by the aging process) have more difficulty hearing higher-pitched sounds.

   2 There is no greater incidence of tympanic tears caused by the aging process. **4** The hair in the auditory canal increases not decreases. **5** The epithelium of the lining of the ear becomes thinner and drier.

   Client Need: Health Promotion and Maintenance; **Cognitive Level:** Knowledge; **Nursing Process:** Assessment/ Analysis

24. **3 Aged clients may display psychomotor retardation and need more time to complete the tasks associated with the activities of daily living; mealtimes should be relaxing and social.**

   1 Supplemental drinks should augment meals and be offered between meals, not as a substitute for meals. **2** Clients should be encouraged to feed themselves to remain as independent as possible; spoon feeding may not mirror the pace of eating preferred by the client, and forcing the client to eat all of the food may precipitate anxiety, frustration, and agitation. **4** Placement of a gastrostomy tube is premature.

   Client Need: Health Promotion and Maintenance; **Cognitive Level:** Application; **Nursing Process:** Planning/ Implementation

25. **2 With aging there is a decreased vasomotor response and diminished elasticity of blood vessels that do not respond quickly to changes from horizontal to vertical; orthostatic hypotension may occur. Changing positions slowly allows the body to adjust, which prevents dizziness and loss of balance.**

   1 Usual fluid intake patterns can be maintained. **3** Furosemide should be taken with meals to prevent gastric irritation. It is best to take it in the morning rather than at night so that sleep is not interrupted with the need to void. **4** There is no link between furosemide and skin breakdown.

   Client Need: Health Promotion and Maintenance; **Cognitive Level:** Application; **Nursing Process:** Planning/ Implementation

Memory Aid: Fall Risk Assessment is important in the elderly for many reasons, including: furosemide's effects on fluid balance, retardation of reflexes, aging of joints.

Bibliography

American Psychiatric Association. (2003). Practice guidelines for the assessment and treatment of patients with suicidal behaviors. *American Journal of Psychiatry*, 160(Suppl. 11), 12.

American Psychiatric Association. (2015). *DSM-5 Fact Sheets*, www.psychiatry.org.

Anandarajah, G., & Hight, E. (2001). Spirituality and medical practice: Using the HOPE questions as a practical tool for spiritual assessment. *American Family Physician*, 63, 81.

Bailey, B. A. (2010). Partner violence during pregnancy: Prevalence, effects, screening, and management. *Int J Womens Health*, 2, 183–197.

Beck, A. T. (1967). *Depression: Clinical, experiential, and theoretical aspects*. New York: Hober.

Bureau of Justice Statistics & U.S. Department of Justice. (2017). *Crime Against Persons With Disabilities*. https://www.bjs.gov/index.cfm?ty=pbdetail&iid=5986.

Centers for Disease Control and Prevention, National Center for Health Statistics. (2015). https://www.cdc.gov/nchs.

Centers for Disease Control and Prevention, National Center for Injury Prevention and Control. (2015). *Suicide facts at a glance*. https://www.cdc.gov/violenceprevention/pdf/suicide-datasheet-a.pdf.

Centers for Disease Control and Prevention. (2013). *Mental Health Basics*. www.cdc.gov/mentalhealth/basics.htm.

Centers for Disease Control and Prevention. (2013). *Alcohol Related Disease Impact (ARDI) application*. https://www.cdc.gov/ARD.

Centers for Disease Control and Prevention. (2016). *Workplace Violence Prevention for Nurses Revolving Door Syndrome*. https://wwwn.cdc.gov/wpvhc/Course.aspx/Slide/Unit3_11.

Fitch, W. L. *Laws and programs for the special civil commitment of sex offenders*, presented at the NASMHPD Commissioners Summer 2007 Meeting, Denver, CO.

Fortinash, K., & Holoday-Worret, P. (2015). *Psychiatric Mental Health Nursing* (revised 5th ed.). St. Louis, MO: Mosby/Elsevier.

Halter, M. (2014). *Varcarolis' Foundations of Mental Health Nursing*. (7th ed.). St. Louis: Saunders.

Holmes, T. H., & Rahe, R. H. (1967). The social readjustment rating scale. *J Psychosom Res*, 11, 213–218.

Keltner, N. L., & Steele, D. (2015). *Psychiatric Nursing* (7th ed.). St. Louis, MO: Mosby/Elsevier.

Kurlansik, S. L., & Maffei, M. S. (2016). Somatic Symptom Disorder. *Am Fam Physician*, 93(1), 49–54A.

Levine, J. (2009). What's the matter with teen sexting? *The American Prospect* 1–2, www.prospect.org/cs/articles?articles=whats_the_matter_with_teen_sexting.

Lithwick, D. (2009). Teens, nude photos and the law: Ask yourself should the police be involved when a tipsy teen girl emails her boyfriend naughty Valentine's Day pictures? *Newsweek*, 153(8), http://proquest.umi.com.catalogue.fcsl.edu/pdqweb?index+18&sid=1&srchmode=1&inst.

Mattila, A. K., et al. (2008). Alexithymia and somatization in general population. *Psychosom Med*, 70(6), 716–722.

Mosby's Dictionary of Medicine. (2013). *Nursing & Health Professions* (9th ed.). St. Louis, MO: Mosby/Elsevier.

National Institute of Mental Health. (2016). *Post-Traumatic Stress Disorder*. https://www.nimh.nih.gov/health/topics/post-traumatic-stress-disorder-ptsd/index.shtml.

National Institute of Mental Health. (2013). *The numbers count: Mental disorders in America* (website). www.nimh.nih.gov/health/publications/the-numbers-count-mental-disorders-in-america/index.shtml.

National Institute on Alcohol Abuse and Alcoholism. (2012). A Family History of Alcoholism: Are you at risk? NIH Publication No. 03–5340. Reprinted June 2012 https://pubs.niaaa.nih.gov/publications/FamilyHistory/famhist.htm.

National Institute on Alcohol Abuse and Alcoholism. (2017). *Alcohol Facts and Statistics*. https://pubs.niaaa.nih.gov/publications/AlcoholFacts&Stats/AlcoholFacts&Stats.htm.

National Institute on Alcohol Abuse and Alcoholism. (2017). *Alcohol Use Disorder*. https://www.niaaa.nih.gov/alcohol-health/overview-alcohol-consumption/alcohol-use-disorders.

National Institute on Drug Abuse. (2015). *Hallucinogens and Dissociative Drugs*. https://www.drugabuse.gov/publications/research-reports/hallucinogens-dissociative-drugs/what-are-effects-common-dissociative-drugs-brain-body.

Nugent, P. M., Green, J. S., Hellmer, M. A., & Pelikan, P. K. (2012). *Mosby's Comprehensive Review of Nursing for the NCLEX-RN Examination* (20th ed.). St. Louis: Mosby/Elsevier.

Ortman, J. M., Velkoff, V. A., & Hogan, H. (2014). *An Aging Nation: The Older Population in the United States, U.S. Census Bureau.* https://www.census.gov/prod/2014pubs/p25-1140.pdf.

Poland, S. (2009). *Youth suicide prevention: Physicians can make the difference.* Retrieved from https://www.Medscape.com/viewarticle/588917.

Stuart, G. W. (2013). *Principles and Practice of Psychiatric Nursing* (10th ed.). St. Louis, MO: Mosby/Elsevier.

Substance Abuse and Mental Health Services Administration (SAMHSA). (2015). *National Survey on Drug Use and Health (NSDUH). Table 2.41B—Alcohol Use in Lifetime, Past Year, and Past Month among Persons Aged 12 or Older, by Demographic Characteristics: Percentages, 2014 and 2015.* Available at: https://www.samhsa.gov/data/sites/default/files/NSDUH-DetTabs-2015/NSDUH-DetTabs-2015/NSDUH-DetTabs-2015.htm#tab2-41b.

Substance Abuse and Mental Health Services Administration (SAMHSA). (2015). *National Survey on Drug Use and Health (NSDUH). Table 2.46B—Alcohol Use, Binge Alcohol Use, and Heavy Alcohol Use in Past Month among Persons Aged 12 or Older, by Demographic Characteristics: Percentages, 2014 and 2015.* Available at: https://www.samhsa.gov/data/sites/default/files/NSDUH-DetTabs-2015/NSDUH-DetTabs-2015/NSDUH-DetTabs-2015.htm#tab2-46b.

Substance Abuse and Mental Health Services Administration (SAMHSA). (2015). *National Survey on Drug Use and Health (NSDUH). Table 5.6A—Substance Use Disorder in Past Year among Persons Aged 18 or Older, by Demographic Characteristics: Numbers in Thousands, 2014 and 2015.* Available at: https://www.samhsa.gov/data/sites/default/files/NSDUH-DetTabs-2015/NSDUH-DetTabs-2015/NSDUH-DetTabs-2015.htm#tab5-6a.

Substance Abuse and Mental Health Services Administration (SAMHSA). (2015). *National Survey on Drug Use and Health (NSDUH). Table 5.6B—Substance Use Disorder in Past Year among Persons Aged 18 or Older, by Demographic Characteristics: Percentages, 2014 and 2015.* Available at: https://www.samhsa.gov/data/sites/default/files/NSDUH-DetTabs-2015/NSDUH-DetTabs-2015/NSDUH-DetTabs-2015.htm#tab5-6b.

Substance Abuse and Mental Health Services Administration (SAMHSA). (2015). *National Survey on Drug Use and Health (NSDUH). Table 5.56A—Need for and Receipt of Treatment at a Specialty Facility for an Alcohol Problem in the Past Year among Persons Aged 18 or Older, by Demographic Characteristics: Numbers in Thousands and Percentages, 2014 and 2015.* Available at: https://www.samhsa.gov/data/sites/default/files/NSDUH-DetTabs-2015/NSDUH-DetTabs-2015/NSDUH-DetTabs-2015.htm#tab5-56a.

Substance Abuse and Mental Health Services Administration (SAMHSA). (2015). *National Survey on Drug Use and Health (NSDUH). Table 5.5A—Substance Use Disorder in Past Year among Persons Aged 12 to 17, by Demographic Characteristics: Numbers in Thousands, 2014 and 2015.* Available at: https://www.samhsa.gov/data/sites/default/files/NSDUH-DetTabs-2015/NSDUH-DetTabs-2015/NSDUH-DetTabs-2015.htm#tab5-5a.

Substance Abuse and Mental Health Services Administration (SAMHSA). (2015). *National Survey on Drug Use and Health (NSDUH). Table 5.5B—Substance Use Disorder in Past Year among Persons Aged 12 to 17, by Demographic Characteristics: Percentages, 2014 and 2015.* Available at: https://www.samhsa.gov/data/sites/default/files/NSDUH-DetTabs-2015/NSDUH-DetTabs-2015/NSDUH-DetTabs-2015.htm#tab5-5b.

Substance Abuse and Mental Health Services Administration (SAMHSA). (2015). *National Survey on Drug Use and Health (NSDUH). Table 5.36A—Received Substance Use Treatment at a Specialty Facility in the Past Year among Persons Aged 12 to 17, by Demographic Characteristics: Numbers in Thousands, 2014 and 2015.* Available at: https://www.samhsa.gov/data/sites/default/files/NSDUH-DetTabs-2015/NSDUH-DetTabs-2015/NSDUH-DetTabs-2015.htm#tab5-36a.

U.S. Department of Health and Human Services (HHS), Substance Abuse and Mental Health Services Administration (SAMHSA). (2015). Behavioral Health Trends in the United States: Results from the 2014 National Survey on Drug Use and Health. https://www.samhsa.gov/data/sites/default/files/NSDUH-FRR1-2014/NSDUH-FRR1-2014.pdf

U.S. Department of Health and Human Services. (2017). *What is Long-Term Care?* LongTermCare.gov.

U.S. Department of Health and Human Services. (2016). *National Institutes of Mental Health, Bipolar Disorder.* https://www.nimh.nih.gov/health/topics/bipolar-disorder/index.shtml.

U.S. Department of Health and Human Services. (2017). *National Institutes of Health, National Institutes of Mental Health.* www.nimh.nih.gov/health/statistics.

U.S. Department of Health and Human Services. (2016). *National Institutes of Health, National Institutes of Mental Health, Autism Spectrum Disorder.* https://www.nimh.nih.gov/health/topics/autism-spectrum-disorders-asd/index.shtml

Varcarolis, E. (2017). *Essentials of Psychiatric Mental Health Nursing.* (3rd ed.). St. Louis: Saunders.

World Health Organization. (2017). http://www.who.int/features/factfiles/mental_health/en/.

World Health Organization. (2008). *The global burden of disease.* Geneva: World Health Organization.

A

D

DAR acronym, 43
Date rape, 298
  drugs for, 298
Death
  alcohol-related, 244
  with dignity, 52–53
Decision making, ethical, 47–48
  questions in, 47t
  steps in, 47, 47t
Defense mechanisms, for anxiety, 199, 199t
Delayed posttraumatic stress disorder, in sexual
    abuse of children, 312
Delirium, 143, 145
  alcohol withdrawal, 246
  assessment/analysis of, 146–147
  behavioral/clinical findings of, 145
  comparison of, 146, 146t
  definition of, 145
  etiologic and predisposing factors of, 145–146
  evaluation/outcomes of, 147
  nursing care of clients with, 146
  planning/implementation for, 147
  therapeutic interventions for, 146
Delusion, schizophrenia and, 160
Delusion of influence, 167
Delusion of reference, 167
Delusional disorder, 167–168
  assessment/analysis of, 168
  behavioral/clinical findings of, 167
  etiologic factors of, 167
  evaluation/outcomes of, 168
  nursing care of clients with, 168
  planning/implementation for, 168
  therapeutic interventions for, 168
  types of, 167
Dementia, 143
  assessment/analysis of, 149–150, 150t
  classification of, 143
  comparison of, 146, 146t
  evaluation/outcomes of, 151
  nursing care of clients with, 149–151
  planning/implementation for, 150
  types of, 143
Dendrite, 70
Denial, in anxiety, 200
Dependence, to substance, 240
Dependent personality disorder, 221, 223
Depersonalization/derealization disorder, 280,
    281
Depressants, 254–256
Depression, 367t
  in childhood and adolescence, 387

Depressive disorders, 115, 174, 179–180
  assessment/analysis of, 185
  bipolar disorder and, 185, 186t
  epidemiology of, 174–175
  etiology of, 175–179
    biologic theories, 176
    cognitive theory, 178
    genetic theories, 177
    life events and stress theory, 178–179
    neurochemical alteration in, 176
    neuroendocrine dysregulation in, 177
    psychoanalytic theory, 178
    psychologic theories, 177–178
  evaluation/outcomes of, 186
  major, 179–180
  nursing care of clients diagnosed with, 179
  persistent depressive disorder (dysthymia), 180
  planning/implementation for, 185–186
  prognosis of, 188–189
  terminology of, 174
Desensitization, 118
"Designer drugs," 259. *see also* Hallucinogens
Destructive aggression, 291
Developmental level, and therapeutic communication, 22
Developmental theories, 112
Dextroamphetamine, 258
Diagnoses, general purposes of, 115
Diagnostic and Statistical Manual of Mental Disorders, in
    mental health disorders, 114, 115
  format of, 115–116
Dialectical behavioral therapy, 225, 232
Diencephalon, 68
Disabled persons, assault of, 322
Disasters, 88
Disengagement theory, of aging, 392–393
Disorganized clients, with schizophrenia, 163–164b
Displacement, in anxiety, 200
Disruptive clients, with schizophrenia, 163–164b
Disruptive disorders, 116
Dissociation, in anxiety, 200
Dissociative amnesia, 280, 281
Dissociative disorders, 116, 279–280
  assessment/analysis of, 282, 283b
  etiology of, 271–272
  evaluation/outcomes of, 283–285
  general behavioral/clinical findings of, 280
  nursing care of clients with, 281–282
  planning/implementation for, 282–283, 284t
  therapeutic interventions for, 280
  types of, 280
    depersonalization/derealization disorder, 281
    dissociative amnesia, 281
    dissociative identity disorder, 280